The Patient's Brain
The neuroscience behind the doctor–patient relationship

D1555516

The Patient's Brain
The neuroscience behind the doctor–patient relationship

Fabrizio Benedetti, M.D.

Professor of Physiology and Neuroscience
Department of Neuroscience
University of Turin Medical School
and
National Institute of Neuroscience
Turin, Italy

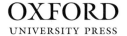
OXFORD
UNIVERSITY PRESS

OXFORD
UNIVERSITY PRESS

Great Clarendon Street, Oxford OX2 6DP

Oxford University Press is a department of the University of Oxford.
It furthers the University's objective of excellence in research, scholarship,
and education by publishing worldwide in

Oxford New York

Auckland Cape Town Dar es Salaam Hong Kong Karachi
Kuala Lumpur Madrid Melbourne Mexico City Nairobi
New Delhi Shanghai Taipei Toronto

With offices in

Argentina Austria Brazil Chile Czech Republic France Greece
Guatemala Hungary Italy Japan Poland Portugal Singapore
South Korea Switzerland Thailand Turkey Ukraine Vietnam

Oxford is a registered trade mark of Oxford University Press
in the UK and in certain other countries

Published in the United States
by Oxford University Press Inc., New York

British Library Cataloging in Publication Data
Data available

Library of Congress Cataloging in Publication Data
Data available

Typeset in Minion by Glyph International, Bangalore, India
Printed in Great Britain
on acid-free paper by
CPI Antony Rowe, Chippenham, Wiltshire

ISBN 978–0–19–957951–8

10 9 8 7 6 5 4 3 2 1

To the memory of my mother

Contents

Preface

There is a vast amount of literature on what has often been called 'doctor–patient relationship', 'patient–provider interaction', 'therapist–patient encounter', and such like. This special, and indeed intriguing, social interaction has been analysed from different perspectives, so that today the medical, psychological, social, philosophical, and even socioeconomical and health-policy literature is full of accounts and essays that deal with this topic. Needless to say, this literature has provided valuable information to physicians, health professionals, psychologists, philosophers, and policymakers. Basically, what has emerged in the course of the years is that not only should health professionals develop and take care of their own technical skills, but that they also should strengthen their social skills in order to better interact with their patients. This might seem quite obvious indeed, nonetheless a large amount of scientific investigation has provided compelling evidence that not only is a good doctor–patient relationship desirable because politeness is better than rudeness, but also because the former may have beneficial effects on health, whereas the latter may lead to negative outcomes.

With the recent advances of neuroscience, I believe we are today in a good position to also describe and discuss the biological mechanisms that underlie the doctor–patient relationship. No attempt of this kind has been made thus far and the task is not an easy one. Many neuroscientific facts must be put into the context of the clinical setting, routine medical practice, social issues, and psychological theories, in order to provide evidence that the doctor–patient relationship can indeed be approached in neurobiological terms.

Neuroscience is a very broad discipline, and actually many sub-disciplines do exist, like molecular and cellular neuroscience, as well as cognitive neuroscience. Social and cognitive neuroscience are in a good position to tackle the doctor–patient relationship from a biological perspective, for many neurobiological underpinnings of complex social interactions have been unravelled in recent years and many neuroscientific hypotheses have been put forward. For example, we now know that different physiological and biochemical mechanisms take part in complex functions, like trust, hope, empathy, and compassion, which are all key elements in the therapist–patient encounter. If on the one hand the patient must trust and hope, on the other hand the therapist must be empathic and compassionate.

Neuroscientific facts should also be put into an evolutionary context. Neuroscience investigates biological systems, and any simple or complex neurobiological system is a product of evolution which has emerged in animals and humans with a precise and specific purpose. For example, brain circuits subserving trust have emerged in the course of evolution in order to strengthen social interactions. Trustworthy behaviour is a prosocial behaviour, and if the patient who seeks relief does not trust therapists and therapies, the doctor–patient encounter has no meaning to exist at all. Therefore, an evolutionary understanding of why and how these social mechanisms have emerged and have evolved is of paramount importance. They give us insights into the evolutionary emergence of altruism and subsequent medical care.

In this book I propose to give scientific facts on the most recent discoveries and advances of neuroscience that can explain both the biological systems involved in the doctor–patient interaction and their evolutionary meaning. The basic concept is that from a neuroscientific perspective, I aver, the doctor–patient relationship can be subdivided into at least four steps. The first is 'feeling sick', a key starting point that triggers the subsequent behaviour. Neuroscience has a lot to say about feeling sick. It involves sensory systems and cortical areas that generate conscious awareness, and indeed the perception of a symptom, like pain, is the product of bottom-up processes and top-down modulation. The second step is 'seeking relief', a kind of motivated behaviour which is aimed at suppressing discomfort. This behavioural repertoire is not very different from the one aimed at suppressing hunger or thirst, and the brain reward circuits are of great importance in this regard. The third step is 'meeting the therapist', a special and unique social encounter whereby the therapist represents the means to suppress discomfort. Here many intricate mechanisms are at work, such as the patient's trust and hope and the therapist's empathy and compassion. Neuroscience is beginning to understand these complex functions and, interestingly, not only can we study the patient's brain but we can also have a look into the doctor's brain, in which many regions are responsible for empathic and compassionate behaviour. Finally, the fourth step is 'receiving the therapy', the final act of the doctor–patient interaction. The mere ritual of the therapeutic act may generate therapeutic responses (placebo responses) which sometimes may be as powerful as those generated by real medical treatments. In this regard, the present book wants to put the placebo effect into a broader context compared to my previous book *Placebo Effects: Understanding the Mechanisms in Health and Disease* (Oxford University Press 2008).

I believe these four steps, as described from a neurobiological point of view, represent a social-neural system which has evolved as a defence mechanism in all respects. In the same way as cellular immune responses evolved for protecting living organisms from external microinvaders, and the fight-or-flight response evolved for tackling environmental dangers, so the 'sick–healer interaction' emerged for providing psychological and social support to the weak, the sick, the elderly, and for guaranteeing suppression of discomfort by a mere social event, that is, meeting the healer. A person whose brain is capable of shutting down pain when the presence of medical help is detected may have an advantage over someone whose brain lacks this capacity. This system is always at work, regardless of effective or ineffective therapies. Even if the therapy is totally ineffective, expectation of benefit (the placebo response) may be sufficient to inhibit discomfort and eventually to influence the course of illness. What makes the difference between shamans and modern doctors is that, whereas shamanic procedures are likely to lack specific effects completely, at least in most circumstances, modern doctors rely on effective procedures and medications with specific mechanisms of action. But this social-neural system is always there, as an ancestral system which is ready to come out, both with shamans and with doctors.

The plan of the book can be summarized as follows. Chapter 1 is a brief evolutionary account of medical care, in which it will be described that simple self-defence mechanisms, such as withdrawal and scratch reflexes, evolved into more complex social events, like social grooming in nonhuman primates and altruism and shamanism in humans. Chapter 2 is about the more recent history of medicine, from the emergence of scientific medicine and the problem of animal experimentation, to the need to include a psychosocial component into modern medicine. Chapter 3, 4, 5, 6 are about 'feeling sick', 'seeking relief', 'meeting the therapist', and 'receiving the therapy', respectively (see above for an anticipated description). In Chapter 7, the brain of the non-communicative demented patient is described. The approach to the cognitively impaired patient is quite interesting for it gives us the flavour of what happens when the doctor–patient interaction is disrupted because of lack of communication. Chapter 8 tries to put the social-neural system 'patient+therapist' within the context of the body defence mechanisms, and emphasizes that this system can be conceptualized as a true social defence mechanism.

Is there any advantage to approach the doctor–patient relationship from a neuroscientific perspective? I believe so, for a number of reasons. The first is obvious. Neuroscience is interested in understanding how brains work, and this special social encounter may uncover the mechanisms of higher brain functions, such as trust and hope. The second reason is that physicians, psychologists, and health professionals can better understand the kind of changes they can induce in their patients' brains. With this neuroscientific knowledge in their hands, health professionals 'see' directly how their words, attitudes, and behaviours activate and inactivate molecules, cortical areas and sensory systems in the brains of their patients. I believe that this 'direct vision' of the patient's brain will hopefully boost health professionals' empathic and compassionate behaviour further. The third reason is related to the second one. I think doctors, nurses, and other medical personnel would benefit from the teaching of Neuroscience of the Doctor–Patient Relationship in Medical Schools and Schools of Nursing, as well as in Psychology courses. Including such teaching in the education of health professionals, as we are trying to do in our Medical School, would lead to a better awareness of the potential power that the doctor's behaviour may have on the patient's behaviour and capacity of recovery from illness. Last but not least, understanding the neurobiological underpinnings of the doctor–patient relationship may lead to better medical practice and clinical profession, as well as to better social/communication skills and health policy. The recent advances in placebo research are a good example of how neurobiological mechanisms may lead to important implications in the clinic (Chapter 6).

Acknowledgements

This book is based on research work and scientific discussions which are a continuation of my previous book *Placebo Effects: Understanding the Mechanisms in Health and Disease* (Oxford University Press 2008). Therefore, all the persons I want to thank here are the very same as those I acknowledged in my previous book. They helped and supported me in a number of ways, both directly and indirectly, both from my own Institution, such as Piergiorgio Strata, Piergiorgio Montarolo, Luana Colloca, Martina Amanzio, Antonella Pollo, Sergio Vighetti, Bruno Bergamasco, Leonardo Lopiano, Michele Lanotte, Elena Torre, Giovanni Asteggiano, Innocenzo Rainero, Giuliano Maggi, as well as from around the world, like Anne Harrington, Dan Moerman, Howard Fields, Nick Humphrey, Jamie Pennebaker, Ginger Hoffman, Stephen Strauss, Linda Engel, Manfred Schedlowski, Paul Enck, Damien Finniss, Don Price, Ron Kupers, Serge Marchand, Ted Kaptchuk, and Franklin Miller. Not to mention my family, both my wife Claudia and my daughter Federica. Without their continuous loving support and patience, this book could have never been written.

Chapter 1

A brief evolutionary account of medical care

Summary and relevance to the clinician

1) In this chapter, medical care is approached from an evolutionary perspective. It represents a complex form of social behaviour that is aimed at taking care of the weak, the sick, the elderly and, more in general, the individual who needs help.

2) This evolutionary account starts from unicellular organisms. These simple forms of life are capable of taking care of themselves through a variety of mechanisms, which are often aimed at tackling harsh environments. Mechanisms of self-care and self-protection then evolved in more complex forms, such as the withdrawal reflex, the wiping reflex, and the scratch reflex. All these simple behaviours allow a noxious stimulus to be removed from one's own body. The spinal cord neuronal circuits are sufficient to warrant the correct functioning of these reflexes.

3) Grooming is somehow more complex than these simple reflexes, and involves scratching, rubbing, licking, and the like. It is not triggered by peripheral stimuli on the skin, but rather it is generated in the central nervous system through a complex concertation of neural, hormonal, and genetic events, which take place mainly in subcortical areas. There is however a similarity between grooming and the simple scratch reflex: both are directed towards one's own body.

4) The big evolutionary step that is relevant to the mechanisms of the doctor–patient relationship occurred when animals started grooming others rather than themselves. Grooming others, the so-called social grooming or allogrooming, is one of the first examples of social interaction. It represents a very elementary form of medical care, whereby the groomer takes care of the groomee. The neocortex and some hormones, e.g. oxytocin, are involved in this social behaviour.

5) Social grooming in apes and early hominids was likely to pave the road to altruistic behaviour. In real altruism, the conscious intentions to help

other individuals are critical, the so-called psychological altruism. There are many examples of supposed altruistic behaviour in *Homo erectus* and in Neanderthal's men.

6) Whereas the very early forms of altruism and medical care in a social group relied on the involvement of many members of the group, in the course of evolution a single individual started taking care of the sick: the shaman. Shamanistic practices are common in prehistoric, historic, and modern medicine, and help us understand how medical care may have emerged among early hominids. Shamans have then been replaced with doctors, e.g. in Ancient Greece, but a real scientific medicine has emerged only very recently.

7) It is important to look at the doctor–patient relationship from an evolutionary perspective because it reminds us that it is a sort of social interaction aimed at taking care of the members of a social group, and thus at protecting both the single individual and the social group from possible dangers and damages. Medical care must also be considered within the context of self-care in unicellular organisms, invertebrates, and vertebrates, and within the context of social care in apes and humans. Therefore, the doctor–patient relationship is a product of the evolution of the nervous system and behaviour and can be studied with a neuroscientific and evolutionary approach.

1.1 Simple organisms can take care of themselves

1.1.1 Unicellular organisms use simple strategies to protect themselves

Living organisms take care of themselves and others for a better survival, and in so doing adopt different strategies, from the shape of intracellular organelles and the movement of the cilia in unicellular protists to the verbal communication between members of a social group. Of course, we should not think about a phylogenetic scale, from unicellular mechanisms of self-defence to human social interactions, whereby the amoeba is at the bottom and primates at the top. There is today compelling evidence for an extensive divergence of evolutionary lines, which involves both parallel evolutionary lines and extinction of intermediary lines (Simpson 1949). Therefore, some of the strategies adopted by simple organisms, e.g. unicellular, do not necessarily mean that these have then evolved into those strategies that are used by higher mammals. Nevertheless, it is crucial to understand that both simple and complex organisms can take care of themselves at different stages of evolution, and this occurs on the basis of different physiological mechanisms and behavioural repertoires.

Some relatively simple mechanisms and strategies are already present in unicellular organisms, such as the paramecium, also known as Lady Slipper, a freshwater protist especially found in scums. The paramecium takes care of itself in different ways. For example, it contains intracellular organelles, the contractile vacuoles, which are used to pump excess water out of the cell (Wichterman 1986). These intracellular structures are surrounded by several pores that absorb water from the cytoplasm by osmosis. If there is an overload of water in the cell, the contractile vacuole can expel it through a pore that can be opened and closed (Fig 1.1A). Without such a mechanism, the paramecium would explode when excess intracellular water is present.

The paramecium, like many other unicellular organisms, can also solve simple problems of locomotion when, for example, it hits an obstacle. It has a

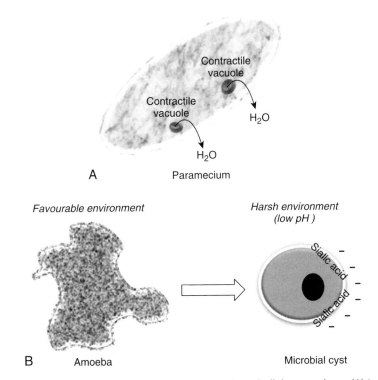

Fig 1.1 Two examples of self-defence mechanisms in unicellular organisms. (A) In the paramecium, excess water is pumped out by means of the so-called contractile vacuoles. (B) In harsh conditions, such as low pH, the amoeba turns into a microbial cyst. Its wall may become negatively charged, due to sialic acid, thus preventing its attachment to the intestinal wall and facilitating its passage to a more favourable environment.

series of cilia on the membrane surface that allow movement in water (Wichterman 1986). When the cilia beat backward simultaneously, the paramecium moves forward with a spiral trajectory. However, it may happen that it run into an obstacle. If so, the cilia change their direction and beat forward, causing the paramecium to go away from the obstacle. After a while, the cilia beat backward again, and the paramecium too moves forward. If it hits the obstacle again, this process will go on till the obstacle is overcome.

Other unicellular protists show similar mechanisms. The amoeba has vacuoles that can regulate intracellular osmosis by expelling excess water through exocytosis (Jeon 1973). In this case, the overloaded vacuole moves towards the surface of the cell in order to expel the water into the extracellular environment. The amoeba can also face harsh conditions, such as an acid environment. In this case, it turns into a dormant state, whereby the metabolic activities, feeding, and locomotion are slowed down, the so-called state of microbial cyst (Fig 1.1B). In a microbial cyst, a wall surrounding the cell membrane is built up, and this wall increases the resistance of the organism to the new harsh environment. For example, the wall of the Entamoeba histolytica contains sialic acid which confers a negative charge to the cyst. This negativity, in turn, prevents the attachment of the cyst to the intestinal wall, thus facilitating its elimination with the faeces and its passage to a more favourable environment.

These forms of self-protection are crucial to survival, of course. Both the paramecium and the amoeba use strategies that allow taking care of themselves, so as to tackle difficult conditions and environments. Therefore, at these very early stages of evolution, we already observe simple mechanisms of self-care, although they do not require a nervous system. It goes without saying that unicellular organisms do not have neurons, but only specialized intra- and extra-cellular structures which confer some self-defence properties to the cell. Without such specialized structures, these cells would have not survived throughout evolution.

1.1.2 The withdrawal reflex is present in both invertebrates and vertebrates

Withdrawal reflexes are common in those organisms with a nervous system. The withdrawal reflex is a somatic-motor reflex act which protects some parts of the body from threatening stimuli. In general, when a body part is touched by a potentially threatening stimulus, be it non-painful or painful, it is suddenly withdrawn so as to warrant protection from possible damage. This reflex is present in both invertebrates and vertebrates, including man. Without it, an organism would be exposed to a number of noxious environmental stimuli, with no possibility to retract from them.

In the marine snail Aplysia, the neuronal organization of the withdrawal reflex has been analysed in detail. In particular, Aplysia shows two interesting reflexes, the siphon-withdrawal reflex and the gill-withdrawal reflex (Kandel 1976). A tactile stimulus to the siphon or mantle causes the gill to contract and withdraw into the mantle cavity and the siphon to contract beyond the parapodia, thus preventing potential damage. A relatively simple circuit is needed for this reflex (Fig 1.2A). Basically, the reflex arc that has developed in Aplysia is represented by an afferent pathway, a centre in the nervous system, and an efferent pathway. The afferent pathway is made up of sensory neurons innervating both siphon and gill which, in turn, make synapses with several clusters of motor neurons in the abdominal ganglion of the snail. On the whole, there are about 24 identified sensory neurons innervating the siphon, while there are 13 identified motor cells (Kandel 1976). Although most of the connections between sensory and motor neurons involve one synapse only, it should be noted that some of these connections are not direct, as they occur via either excitatory or inhibitory interneurons.

The circuit depicted in Fig 1.2A is sufficient to guarantee the efficient withdrawal of both siphon and gill. It can be explained in terms of the features of its components. First, the afferent discharge is in fact proportional to the intensity of the stimulus. Second, there is a linear summation of the synaptic actions induced by the sensory afferents onto motor neurons. Third, the frequency of the action potentials is a linear function of the amplitude of the excitatory post-synaptic potential. Fourth, the motor response, i.e. the muscle contraction of siphon and gill, is linearly related to motor cell discharge (Kandel 1976).

Withdrawal reflexes are present in vertebrates as well. They are somehow more complex in mammals, including man, than in invertebrates, as they involve different muscles for the maintenance of posture (Sherrington 1947). The withdrawal reflex in mammals obeys to the law of reciprocal innervation, whereby the flexor muscles of the stimulated limb contract whereas the extensor muscles of the same limb are inhibited (Fig 1.2B). Along with these effects in the stimulated limb, this reflex yields opposite outcomes in the contralateral limb: extensor muscles are excited while flexor muscles are inhibited. These opposite effects in the two limbs, e.g. the legs, strengthen the postural adjustment during the withdrawal of the stimulated leg from the noxious stimulus. In fact, posture is maintained through the extension of the non-stimulated leg.

Due to the complex nature of the flexor-extensor reciprocal innervations for the withdrawal and the postural maintenance, the withdrawal reflex in man and other mammals is polysynaptic, as it involves a number of interneurons (Kandel et al. 2000) (Fig 1.2B). Nonetheless, the withdrawal reflex is a relatively simple

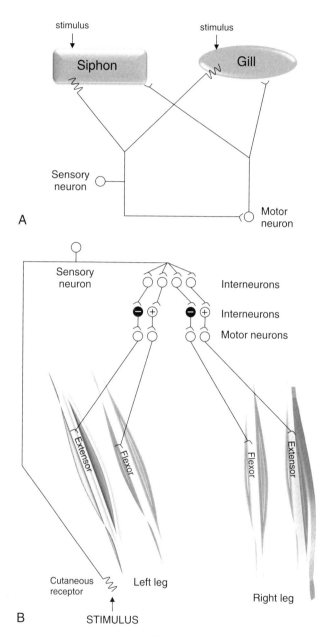

Fig 1.2 Organization of the withdrawal reflex in the snail Aplysia (A), and in mammals, including man (B). In the simple circuit in A, sensory neurons innervating both siphon and gill make synapses with motor neurons which innervate the muscles of siphon and gill. In the more complex circuit in B, the reflex is governed by the law of reciprocal innervation, which warrants postural adjustment while the stimulated leg is retracted. In fact, the reciprocal innervation of flexor and extensor muscles guarantees that, while a limb is withdrawn, the other is extended to maintain the posture.

neuronal circuit that warrants self-protection from environmental noxious stimuli. Without it, the organism would be exposed to possible damage of different parts of the body.

1.2 From the scratch reflex to grooming

1.2.1 The scratch reflex is a simple purposive behaviour

Like the withdrawal reflex, the scratch reflex has a purpose, for the movement is aimed at protecting against potential damage. However, from an evolutionary perspective, the scratch reflex is particularly interesting because the reflex movement is aimed at targeting the potential noxious stimulus and at removing it from the body. The wiping reflex in the frog is similar to the scratch reflex, with the notable difference being that in the former there is no rhythmic activity.

In the frog, the wiping reflex only requires the spinal cord, even for some complex features of this purposive behaviour (Fig 1.3). For example, if a weak acid solution is placed on the forelimb of a spinalized frog, the hindlimb is moved towards the irritated skin so as to wipe the acid solution away. However, if the position of the forelimb is changed, but the irritated skin is always the same, the direction of the movement of the hindlimb changes so as to reach the new spatial position of the irritated skin. Therefore, the spatial characteristics of the wiping reflex depend on the joint position at the moment of the application of the acid solution, and these spatial coordinates and relative adjustments are specified in the spinal cord (Fukson et al. 1980).

The scratch reflex differs from the wiping reflex as in the former the spinal cord is capable of generating rhythmic movements. This reflex is typical of those animals with fur, and is clearly aimed at removing the bothering stimulus produced, for instance, by a flea's bite. It starts with a movement of the hindlimb which is positioned in proximity of the stimulus. Then the rhythmic movements take place. It is crucial that the upright position of the body be maintained, thus the contralateral extensor muscles are excited (Sherrington 1947). In this case also, the spinal cord is sufficient in evoking this reflex. If a stimulus, such as a mild electrical shock is applied to a side of the body of a spinalized animal, the features of the reflex response depend on both intensity and duration of the stimulus. By increasing the intensity of stimulation, the latency of the reflex decreases and the strength of the muscle contractions as well as the number of alternated movements increase. Interestingly, the rhythm of these movements is independent of the stimulus. Thus the frequency of the rhythmic movements stays the same when stimulus duration and intensity change. The neuronal circuits that are responsible for the alternated flexor and extensor movements during scratching are located in the spinal cord, and they

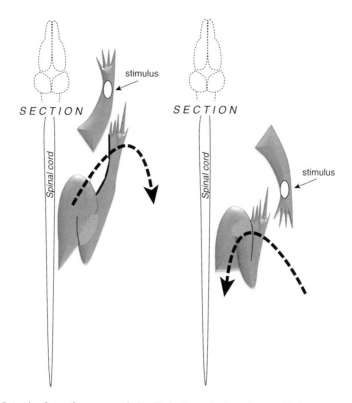

Fig 1.3 In the frog, the neuronal circuits in the spinal cord are sufficient to guarantee even complex motor reflexes. In the wiping reflex of the spinalized frog, whereby the hindlimb movement is aimed at removing a noxious stimulus from the forelimb (left), the spatial position of the forelimb is critical. In fact, if it changes its position (right), the hindlimb movement is adjusted so as to reach the new spatial location of the noxious stimulus.

require neither descending influences from supraspinal centres nor ascending influences from the periphery, such as muscles and joints (Sherrington 1947).

The scratching reflex is present not only in animals with fur, such as mammals, but in other species as well. For example, the semi-aquatic turtle *Trachemys scripta elegans* shows a typical scratch reflex, whose spinal circuits are partially understood. First of all, it is interesting to note that those neurons involved in scratching are also involved in other motor behaviours, like swimming. Therefore, a given cluster of spinal neurons, both interneurons and motor neurons, has not developed to give rise to a single and unique behavioural repertoire, but rather different motor patterns (scratching and swimming) share common neuronal circuits (Stein 2005). In addition, there is experimental evidence for a modular organization of turtle spinal networks.

For example, during scratching, hip-extensor motor neurons are active when hip-flexor motor neurons are silent. The same holds true for interneurons, which suggests a population of hip-extensor motor neurons and interneurons, the hip-extensor module, during scratching. This holds true for knee-extensor and knee-flexor modules as well (Stein 2005).

Therefore, both the occurrence of the wiping and scratch reflexes and the adaptability of the wiping reflex are warranted by circuits in the spinal cord. A purposive behaviour of this kind does not require a complex nervous system. During evolution, simple networks in the spinal cord have acquired the capability of generating a behavioural repertoire that is aimed at preventing damage of a body part. In so doing, relatively elementary circuits subserve a very elementary form of self-care which involves the removal of the potentially noxious stimulus from the body.

1.2.2 Grooming involves a complex behavioural repertoire

Whereas scratch and wiping reflexes are triggered by cutaneous stimuli, such as a bug's bite, a quite different motor behaviour emerged during evolution in order to take care of one's own body. Grooming is a self-directed behaviour which represents a biological function aimed at caring for the body surface (Spruijt et al. 1992). It has an important role in the control of ticks and ectoparasites across many animal species, and is characterized by a complex behavioural repertoire involving scratching, preening, rubbing, nibbling, wallowing, as well as dust, sand and mud bathing. Insects too show some forms of simple grooming, such as rubbing of the wings. Interestingly, ants spread antibiotic secretions over their body, thus self-protecting against bacteria and fungi (Spruijt et al. 1992).

Although grooming behaviour is concerned with care of the body surface, there is compelling experimental evidence that, in contrast to scratch and wiping reflexes, it is not triggered by cutaneous stimuli, but it is generated centrally in the brain. In fact, grooming is usually not associated with a particular stimulation of the skin but rather with a given state of the animal. Therefore, the structure and initiation of grooming bouts seem to be independent of any particular stimulus (Spruijt et al. 1992). In addition, peripheral deafferentation, such as sectioning of the trigeminal nerve in mice, does not abolish grooming behaviour, which suggests centrally generated grooming acts (Berridge and Fentress 1987).

The big evolutionary step from the peripherally driven scratch reflex to the centrally driven grooming behaviour helps us understand how the nervous system developed from a simple form of reflex act aimed at preventing potential damage of the skin to a more complex motor pattern aimed at taking care

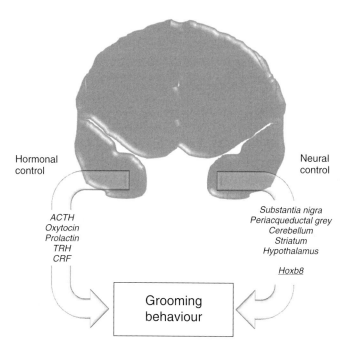

Fig 1.4 Grooming behaviour is under hormonal and neural control. It is induced by several hormones as well as by the activation of a variety of brain areas. *Hoxb8* genes may take part in the genetic programme of grooming. ACTH: adrenocorticotropic hormone. TRH: thyrotropin-releasing hormone. CRF: corticotrophin-releasing factor.

of the whole body surface. Grooming motor pattern is controlled by at least two mechanisms: on the one hand, it is modulated by several hormones, on the other hand, it is generated by some specific regions of the brain (Fig 1.4).

The most effective hormone that induces grooming behaviour is the adreno-corticotropic hormone (ACTH). Intracerebral administration of ACTH induces excessive grooming in the rat (Ferrari 1958; Ferrari et al. 1963; Gispen et al. 1975), an observation that has been confirmed by many subsequent studies. However, it should be noted that other peptides have been found to produce grooming, like vasopressin, oxytocin, prolactin, substance P, bombesin, somatostatin, thyrotropin-releasing hormone, corticotrophin-releasing factor (Spruijt et al. 1992). ACTH-induced grooming is mediated by endogenous opioids, as it can be prevented by the opioid antagonist naloxone (Gispen and Wiegant 1976). In addition, dopamine, gamma-aminobutyric acid (GABA), and serotonin have been found to take part to ACTH-induced grooming, which indicates the high complexity of the endocrine control of grooming behaviour (Spruijt et al. 1992).

As far as specific brain regions are concerned, it is now clear that grooming behaviour is still present in the decerebrated animal, thus showing that it is a subcortical function. There is not a single area involved in the motor pattern but many. Lesions of the substantia nigra and of the dorsal periaqueductal grey in the rat are crucial in suppressing ACTH-induced grooming (Gispen and Isaacson 1986; Spruijt et al. 1986), and stimulation of the cerebellum in the cat induces grooming bouts (Berntson et al. 1988). The striatum and hypothalamus are also involved. For example, the stimulation of some hypothalamic areas induces grooming in the cephalo-caudal direction which is characterized by licking paws and fur, and washing movement over the head (Kruk et al. 1998).

Knock-out mice with disruptions of *Hoxb8* show excessive grooming, without any sign of abnormality in the skin or peripheral nerve fibres (Greer and Capecchi 2002). *Hoxb8* is a member of the mammalian *Hox* complex, a group of 39 transcription factors known for their role during development. Interestingly, *Hox* genes are expressed in the adult brain and, in particular, *Hoxb8* is expressed in those regions that are implicated in the control of grooming behaviour in rodents. This suggests that the innate pre-programmed grooming behaviour involves neuronal networks that are specified using a genetic program, in which *Hoxb8* may take part.

1.3 Scratching somebody else: a big evolutionary jump to social behaviour

1.3.1 Primates spend plenty of time in social grooming

Not only do animals scratch, rub, and lick themselves, but they scratch and rub their companions as well, devoting as much as 20% of their total daytime to this one activity, depending on the animal species. This social grooming, or allogrooming, represents an important step in the evolution of social behaviour, and is a characteristic in many mammals, such as kangaroos, antelopes, horses, dogs, cats, and rodents; however it is typical, above all, of primates (Spruijt et al. 1992). It is important to realize that allogrooming is not only involved in the care of body surface, but has also a function in the regulation of social relationships. One of major forms of social grooming is maternal grooming, whereby the relation between mother and pups is cemented as well as the body surface of the offspring is maintained.

Although social grooming may have a function in the care of the skin of the companions and may help groom areas that cannot be easily reached by the animal itself, in primates it should be noted that individuals who are virtually free of parasites, still solicit for and submit themselves to being groomed. Therefore, the social functions of allogrooming appears to be as important as, or even more important than the cleaning function of the skin. For example, if grooming were purely hygienic in function, then one should expect a correlation with surface area, but it does not. Moreover, social grooming time correlates with social group size, which suggests that allogrooming has to do with intense social relationships (Dunbar 2010).

There is thus compelling evidence that social grooming serves to establish, renew, maintain, and strengthen social bonds. It may also regulate social tension and reconciliation among the members of a group, and may also play a role in consolation behaviour. For example, there is some evidence in chimpanzees that relatives or allies of a victim are capable of restoring his emotional balance by soothing him (de Waal and van Roosmalen 1979). It is also worth noting that relationships established by social grooming may have lifelong consequences. In fact, among wild gelada baboons, the likelihood of a female going to the aid of another female when the latter is under attack is significantly correlated with the amount of time the two of them spend grooming with each other, and the reproductive success of wild female savannah baboons is correlated with the number and intensity of their grooming-associated relationships (Dunbar 2010).

In contrast to scratch reflexes and self-grooming, which require neuronal circuits in the spinal cord and in the brainstem, respectively, allogrooming is tightly linked to social interactions, a complex function that requires a complex integration in the cerebral cortex (Fig 1.5). The relative neocortex volume in primates in fact correlates with several behavioural indices of social complexity (Dunbar 1998; Dunbar and Shultz 2007). In the social brain hypothesis, brain size is correlated to social group size and social relationships (Dunbar 2010). Bonded relationships are cognitively very demanding and a large increase in the development of the neocortex should be expected in these cognitive/social activities.

Being groomed is physiologically relaxing, as shown by the decrease of heart rate, the reduction of some indices of stress, and sometimes falling asleep (Dunbar 2010). A role for endogenous opioids has been suggested in these effects. For example, the opioid-blocker naltrexone has been found to increase the frequency with which monkeys solicit grooming from others (Keverne et al. 1989). Similarly, oxytocin and vasopressin, two neuropeptides widely distributed in the brain, have been found to have prosocial effects (see also section 5.1.3). In particular, oxytocin receptors can be found in the nucleus accumbens, a region involved in reward mechanisms, thus suggesting that oxytocin may be involved in reward. Massage-like stroking in rats raises plasma oxytocin, and increases pain tolerance, which indicates that the mechanical stimulation of the skin affects oxytocin secretion (Agren et al. 1995). More interestingly,

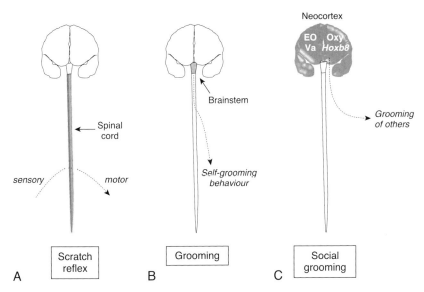

Fig 1.5 The evolutionary steps from the care of oneself to the care of others. (A) The neuronal circuits in the spinal cord warrant the simple sensory-motor integration of the scratch reflex. (B) Centrally (subcortical) generated grooming behaviour is aimed at the care of one's own body. (C) The neocortex, together with some hormones, like oxytocin (Oxy) and vasopressin (Va), endogenous opioids (EO), and *Hoxb8* genes, are crucial to generate social grooming, whereby the grooming behaviour is directed towards other members of the social group.

vasopressin has been found to affect social memory in male mice: vasopressin V1a receptor knockout males show a marked impairment of social, but not spatial, memory (Bielsky et al. 2004).

An important aspect of *Hoxb8* mutant mice (see the previous section 1.2.2) is that they show both excessive self-grooming and excessive allogrooming. Therefore, *Hoxb8* excessive grooming includes a social component. In fact, when *Hoxb8* mutants are caged with control littermates, the control animals show bald patches over the body and the head (Greer and Capecchi 2002). These findings suggest that genetic programmes specify the neuronal networks for both self- and allogrooming (Fig 1.5).

1.3.2 **From social grooming to altruistic behaviour**

In social grooming, there are at least two actors: the one being groomed and the groomer. Whereas the former benefits from it in a number of ways, such as touch-induced pleasure, relaxation and hygiene, it is less clear what the benefits are for the latter. Indeed, there are no immediate benefits to the groomer, for he spends energies and time to the advantage of others. The act of grooming can thus be considered an altruistic behaviour.

In the strict biological sense, altruistic behaviour benefits other organisms at a cost to itself. What counts in biological altruism is not so much the intention to be altruistic but rather the consequences of an action. Indeed, altruism is common in many animals but most of them, if any, are not capable of conscious intentions at all. For example, in social insects, such as ants, bees, and termites, sterile individuals devote their lives to caring for the queen, and vampire bats regurgitate blood and give it to other members of the group who have failed to feed that night. It is hard to believe that insects or bats have conscious altruistic intentions. Therefore, the biological notion of altruism has to do with the action itself, not with what causes that action. Through the altruistic act, the altruist reduces the number of offspring it is likely to produce itself, but boosts the number that other organisms are likely to produce. Self-sacrificial behaviour, though disadvantageous for the individual altruist, might be beneficial at the group level (Darwin 1871).

The role of the groomer and the gromee are related, of course. Any individual can be either a groomer or a groomee, depending on the circumstances. Thus altruism is reciprocal and, if there is no immediate advantage to the groomer, the service can be returned by the one who is being groomed. This idea of reciprocal altruism was introduced to explain cases of altruism among unrelated organisms (Trivers 1971). If the groomer scratches the back of the gromee, the groomee will eventually return the same service to the groomer in the near future. In other words, it may pay an organism to help another, if there is an expectation of the favour being returned in the future.

The main objective of the theory of reciprocal altruism is to explain why some altruistic acts are performed towards non-kin. Indeed, kin selection theory explains altruism when the altruistic action is towards kin. It predicts that animals are more likely to behave altruistically towards their kin than towards unrelated members of their species, and that the closer the relationship, the greater the degree of altruism (Hamilton 1964). Indeed, grooming behaviour often takes place among relatives, like in chimpanzees, macaques, and baboons. However, this is not a general rule, and in many species of primates grooming occurs between both kin and non-kin (Spruijt et al. 1992). Thus kin selection alone cannot explain grooming among non-kin.

In primates, complex patterns of grooming behaviour have been described. In a study in chimpanzees (Nakamura 2003), these included 27 types of grooming cliques and the largest one consisted of 7 individuals. The proportion of multi-interaction-grooming cliques was more than 25% compared to less than 10% in other primate species. Overlap of grooming interactions, such as grooming and being groomed simultaneously or being groomed by multiple individuals, accounted for about 20% of individual grooming, and the maximum number of interactions for one individual at one time was 4. Grooming clusters of 2–23 individuals were observed, and clusters of 3 or more members accounted for about 70% of total duration.

By taking this study as an example, it is clear that the roles of the groomer and the gromee overlap, and any member of the group can be both a groomer and a gromee. Thus, any individual experiences the pleasure and relaxation of being groomed and eventually adopt the altruistic act of grooming the companions. These continuous exchanges of roles boost social interactions and promote reciprocal social behaviour. In the course of evolution, these social interactions are accompanied by a dramatic increase of the neocortex, thus warranting a social brain specifically aimed at boosting sociality (Dunbar 1998, 2010).

Altruistic behaviour and sociality are far from being understood in humans. For example, reciprocal altruism is clearly the antithesis of real altruism, as behaving nicely to someone in order to procure return benefits from them in the future is just delayed self-interest. Adoption is a special case whereby reciprocal altruism does not seem to apply to *Homo Sapiens*. Biological fitness is reduced in parents who adopt children, for these children are usually unrelated to their adoptive parents. Adoption as well as other human altruistic acts seem to obey neither to kin selection nor to reciprocal altruism, so they probably need to be treated as real altruistic actions.

All those human altruistic acts that seem to be at odds with the evolutionary theory, are clearly related to conscious intentions. In contraposition to biological altruism (i.e. kin selection and reciprocal altruism), psychological altruism is used to mean the conscious intention of helping somebody else. Psychological altruism may represent a form of genuine altruism whereby individuals may indeed care about helping others. Many directed altruistic behaviours in humans are based on empathy, that is, the capacity to share the emotional state of another and to adopt his perspective. In this sense, the altruistic act may represent a self-reward, for it is aimed at placating the altruist's internal state.

A possible origin of empathy may be represented by the evolution from emotional contagion, whereby the emotional state of a subject is matched with an object, to sympathetic concern, whereby both concern about another's state and the attempts to ameliorate it are present (de Waal 2008) (see also section 5.4). In the latter, sympathy consists of feelings of sorrow for a distressed other. The best example of sympathetic concern is consolation, which is widely present in apes and humans but not in monkeys, and which may consist of putting an arm around a companion who has been defeated in a fight (de Waal 2008). The next evolutionary step occurs when the capacity to take another's perspective has emerged, the so-called empathic perspective-taking (de Waal 2008) (see also section 5.4). In *Homo*, and particularly in *Homo Sapiens*, the groomer and the groomee, with their sympathetic concern and empathic repertoire, evolved into those who helped each other in a number of circumstances, including the care of the sick.

1.4 **Taking care of the sick**

1.4.1 **From early forms of altruism to the emergence of the shaman**

The evolution of prosocial behaviour in early hominids went on in a number of ways. One of these is certainly the care to the weak, the sick, the elderly and, more in general, the individual who needs help. For example, in order to survive in harsh conditions, it was crucial for our ancestors to obtain a daily nutritious diet of meat and other food. However, this daily provision was not guaranteed, because of the high variability of hunting success. Therefore, there were days with a food excess and days with a food shortage. Although the first altruistic exchanges were likely to occur among relatives, thus favouring kin selection, in the course of evolution further food exchanges occurred with non-kin that were less lucky on that particular hunting day. These non-kin recipients eventually returned this favour, according to the reciprocal altruism theory (Van Vugt and Van Lange 2006).

Living in social groups is advantageous to individuals and sharing food and other goods may be critical for survival. This is nicely shown by some social decision dilemmas, such as the *ultimatum game* or the *prisoner's dilemma*, whereby the individual has to choose among different possibilities that can be either advantageous or disadvantageous to him. In such social dilemmas, cooperation turns out to be the best choice. In the example by Van Vugt and Van Lange (2006), two subjects, A and B, share a house together. Each of them would be better off if they relied upon the other to clean the house (assuming that for most cleaning is time-consuming, energy-consuming, and tiring). However, if neither of them makes an effort to clean the house, the house becomes a mess and they will both be worse off. The altruistic or cooperative choice (C-choice) in this example stands for cleaning the house, whereas the defecting choice (D-choice) stands for not cleaning the house. If A cleans the house by himself, but B does nothing, the outcomes for B are very good (e.g. 10 on a personal satisfaction-scale), but they are poor for A (e.g. 0). Conversely, if B cleans by himself, but A does nothing then the outcomes for A are good (10), but for B they are bad (0). If A and B share the cleaning, the outcomes for both of them are moderately good (e.g. 5 each), which is not as good as when the other subject does all the cleaning. The gist of the social dilemma is that, if neither A nor B cleans the house, their outcomes will be relatively poor (e.g. 2 each), which is worse than their outcomes had they both shared the cleaning (5 each). Altruism and cooperation is thus advantageous in a society. Once the members of a social group understand that their interests are at least partly over-lapping, and that they have some sense of a shared future, they will tend to act benevolently towards each other.

By taking kin selection, reciprocal altruism, psychological altruism, and social dilemmas into account, in a social group it is very important to help and support the weak, the sick, and the elderly. Individuals who cannot hunt and feed themselves are not abandoned, but rather they are looked after and fed. Maybe the first example of human compassion is represented by a toothless skull that was found in the site of Dmanisi in the Eurasian republic of Georgia (Lordkipanidze et al. 2005). It belongs to a *Homo erectus* dating back 1.7 million years, who had lost all but one tooth several years before death. This specimen represents the earliest case of severe masticatory impairment which raises questions about subsistence strategies in early *Homo*. In fact, it may attest to evolution's oldest known example of some kind of altruism and compassion for the elderly and handicapped in the social group. As all his teeth, except the left canine, were missing at least two years before he died, it would have been difficult for him to survive that long, unable to chew the food of a mainly meat-eating society. Companions might have helped him in finding soft plant food and hammering raw meat with stone tools.

There are other examples of this kind in *Homo erectus*, such as the one who presented severe bone lesions that were attributable to hypervitaminosis A (Walker et al. 1982). These lesions were likely to be due to the high dietary intake of animal liver and were painful and disabling. In this case also, surviving for weeks or months in these conditions requires help from the group the individual belongs to.

Neanderthal's men have been found to show signs of compassion towards their companions as well, dating back to about 60 000 years ago. For example, due to the many lesions to the bones, the La Chapelle-aux-Saints and Shanidar individuals must have been severely incapacitated and would have died even earlier without substantial help and care from the group they belonged to (Klein 1989). The analysis of undeveloped bone structure indicates that a man at Shanidar caves was a severe cripple from birth. His right upper limb was entirely useless and may have been amputated just above the elbow. Extensive bone scar tissue indicates that he was blind in his left eye. He was apparently cared for by his companions until his death at age forty, which represents a very old age by Neanderthal standards (Wiester 1983).

Although at the very beginning of human evolution these altruistic acts were probably adopted by different members of the groups, in the course of evolution a single member of the group assumed the role of the one who takes care of the sick. This member is usually named shaman, and represents a very important component of any social group, both in prehistoric, historic, and modern times. Although there are plenty of variations of shamanisms throughout the world, there are some common factors that are present in virtually all kinds of shamanism (Eliade 1964). For example, the shaman can communicate with the spirit world, in which spirits can be good or evil, and ecstasy, trance, and altered states of consciousness are central to shamanistic practices. A typical feature in all forms of shamanism is that the shaman can treat sickness caused by evil spirits and to do this he adopt a number of procedures that vary from culture to culture, such as the evocation of animal images as spirit guides or the use of different symbolic objects and rituals.

Shamanistic practices are likely to date back to the Paleolithic, and certainly to the Mesolithic and Neolithic. For example, a shamanic figure was found in *Les Trois Freres* cave in France, dating back to approximately 13 000 BC. This is a therianthropic figure, i.e. part man and part beast, which is likely to represent a sorcerer, or magician, wearing a horned mask and costume and in the process of transforming into an animal, as drawn by Henri Breuil (Boyle 1952). Prehistoric shamanism represents the first example of real medical care. This is a form of good relationship between the sick and the shaman. The sick trusts the shaman and has strong beliefs in his therapeutic capabilities, thus he refers to him for any kind of psychological, spiritual, or physical discomfort. In this way, the shaman became a central figure in any social group and acquired more and more prestige and a higher social status over the centuries and across different cultures.

1.4.2 More rational treatments emerge slowly from prehistoric to historic medicine

The term prehistoric medicine refers to medicine that predates written records. Its study is mainly dependent on sources such as skeletons and cave paintings as well as anthropological studies of indigenous cultures in Asia, Australia, Africa, and the Americas. Despite the central figure of prehistoric medicine being the shaman, with his shamanistic procedures, it should be noted that several rational treatments emerged over the centuries. For example, besides the many spiritual and irrational healing practices, some rational treatments were also adopted, like those aimed at treating a broken bone resulting from an accident. In order to protect the bone during healing, a broken arm or leg was covered in river clay or mud and the cast allowed to dry hard in the sun. Herbal concoctions were administered or applied to wounds, and animal skin was used for bandages. Surgical procedures, such as skull trepanning, were also used, although these were likely to be carried out with a spiritual meaning, that is, to free the soul from the body.

Although these procedures refer to prehistoric medicine before the emergence of writing, little progress has been made over the centuries, as documented by writing records. In fact, plenty of bizarre treatments were developed over the centuries and across different cultures. These were mainly based on spiritual beliefs and social influences and consisted, for instance, of different types of concoctions that were made of a variety of ingredients, like moss from the skull of victims of violent death, viper's flesh, frogs, worms, crabs' eyes, bee glue, fox lung, feathers, hair, horns, hoofs, ants, scorpions, spider webs, teeth, sexual organs, as well as several procedures, such as purging, puking, cutting, blistering, bleeding, freezing, heating, sweating, and leeching. Most, if not all, of these drugs and procedures were ineffective, with only a few possible but unlikely speculative exceptions. For example, if opium was added to the concoction, it was likely to produce specific analgesic effects. Likewise, bleeding was likely to have specific effects in some circulatory diseases (Shapiro and Shapiro 1997; Benedetti 2008).

Therefore, a clear-cut distinction between shamans and ancient doctors is somehow difficult to be made, and this is true until a few centuries ago, when modern scientific medicine emerged (see Chapter 2). For example, in ancient Egypt, doctors were magicians and priests and most, if not all, of their procedures where shamanic in nature, with the possible exception of external and visible disorders, like trauma. However, it should be noted that during the course of the history there was a slow tendency to rely on naturalistic observations while abandoning the spiritual and religious nature of diseases. For example, Greeks used a more empirical and rational approach, whereby several anatomical observations started to take place. The transition from shamans to modern doctors is thus very recent and mostly depended on the emergence of modern scientific medicine. In spite of this transition, it should be pointed out that today plenty of shamanistic practices still persist throughout the world.

References

Agren G, Lundeberg T, Uvnas-Moberg, K and Sato A (1995). The oxytocin antagonist 1-deamino-2-D-Tyr(Oet)-4-Thr-8-Orn oxytocin reverses the increase in the withdrawal response latency to thermal, but not mechanical stimuli following oxytocin administration or massage-like stroking in rats. *Neuroscience Letters*, **187**, 49–52.

Benedetti F (2008). *Placebo effects: understanding the mechanisms in health and disease.* Oxford University Press, Oxford.

Berntson GG, Jang JF and Ronca AE (1988). Brainstem systems and grooming behavior. *Annals of New York Academy of Science*, **525**, 350–62.

Berridge KC and Fentress JC (1987). Deafferentation does not disrupt natural rules of action syntax. *Behavioral Brain Research*, **23**, 69–76.

Bielsky IF, Hu S-B, Szegda KL, Westphal H and Young LJ (2004). Profound impairment in social recognition and reduction in anxiety-like behavior in vasopressin V1a receptor knockout mice. *Psychoneuroendocrinology*, **29**, 483–93.

Boyle ME (1952). *Four Hundred centuries of Cave Art*. Zwemmer, London.

Darwin C (1871). *The descent of man*. Appleton, New York, NY.

De Waal FBM (2008). Putting the altruism back into altruism: the evolution of empathy. *Annual Review of Psychology*, **59**, 279–300.

de Waal FBM and van Roosmalen A (1979). Reconciliation and consolation among chimpanzees. *Behavioral Ecology and Sociobiology*, **5**, 55–66.

Dunbar RIM (1998). The social brain hypothesis. *Evolutionary Anthropology*, **6**, 178–90.

—— (2010). The social role of touch in humans and primates: behavioural function and neurobiological mechanisms. *Neuroscience and Biobehavioral Reviews*, **34**, 260–8.

Dunbar RIM and Shultz S (2007). Understanding primate brain evolution. *Philosophical Transactions of the Royal Society of London B*, **362**, 649–58.

Eliade M (1964). *Shamanism*. Princeton University, Princeton, NJ.

Ferrari W (1958). Behavioural changes in animals after intracisternal injection with adrenocorticotrophic hormone and melanocyte stimulating hormone. *Nature*, **181**, 925–6.

Ferrari W, Gessa GL and Vargiu L (1963). Behavioral effects induced by intracisternally injected ACTH and MSH. *Annals of New York Academy of Science*, **104**, 330–45.

Fukson OI, Berkinblit MB and Feldman AG (1980). The spinal frog takes into account the scheme of its body during the wiping reflex. *Science*, **209**, 1261–3.

Gispen WH and Isaacson RL (1986). ACTH-induced excessive grooming in the rat. *Pharmacology and Therapeutics*, **12**, 209–46.

Gispen WH and Wiegant VM (1976). Opiate antagonists suppress ACTH1–24-induced excessive grooming in the rat. *Neuroscience Letters*, **2**, 159–64.

Gispen WH, Wiegant VM, Greven HM and deWied D (1975). The induction of excessive grooming in the rat by intraventicular application of peptides derived from ACTH: structure-activity studies. *Life Sciences*, **17**, 645–52.

Greer JM and Capecchi MR (2002). *Hoxb8* is required for normal grooming behaviour in mice. *Neuron*, **33**, 23–34.

Hamilton WD (1964). The genetical evolution of social behaviour I and II. *Journal of Theoretical Biology*, **7**, 1–32.

Jeon KW, ed. (1973). *The biology of amoeba*. Academic Press, New York, NY.

Kandel ER (1976) *Cellular basis of behavior*. WH Freeman and Company, San Francisco, CA.

Kandel ER, Schwartz JH and Jessell TM (2000) *Principles of neural sciences*. 4th Edition. McGraw-Hill, New York.

Keverne EB, Martensz N and Tuite B (1989). Beta-endorphin concentrations in cerebrospinal fluid of monkeys are influenced by grooming relationships. *Psychoneuroendocrinology*, **14**, 155–61.

Klein RG (1989). *The human career*. The University of Chicago Press, Chicago, IL.

Kruk MR, Westphal KGC, Van Erp AMM et al. (1998). The hypothalamus: cross-roads of endocrine and behavioural regulation in grooming and aggression. *Neuroscience and Biobehavioral Reviews*, **23**, 163–77.

Lordkipanidze D, Vekua A, Ferring R, Rightmire GP, Agusti J, Kiladze G et al. (2005). Anthropology: the earliest toothless hominin skull. *Nature*, **434**, 717–8.

Nakamura M (2003). 'Gatherings' of social grooming among wild chimpanzees: implications for evolution of sociality. *Journal of Human Evolution*, **44**, 59–71.

Shapiro AK and Shapiro E (1997). *The powerful placebo: from ancient priest to modern physician*. Johns Hopkins University Press, Baltimore, MD.

Sherrington C (1947) *The integrative action of the nervous system*. 2nd Edition. Yale University Press, New Haven, CT.

Simpson GG (1949). *The meaning of evolution*. Yale University Press, New Haven, CT.

Spruijt B, Cools AR and Gispen WH (1986). The periaqueductal gray: a prerequisite for ACTH-induced excessive grooming. *Behavioral Brain Research*, **20**, 19–25.

Spruijt BM, Van Hoof JARAM and Gispen WH (1992). Ethology and neurobiology of grooming behavior. *Physiological Reviews*, **72**, 825–52.

Stein PSG (2005). Neuronal control of turtle hindlimb motor rhythms. *Journal of Comparative Physiology A*, **191**, 213–29.

Trivers RL (1971). The evolution of reciprocal altruism. *Quarterly Review of Biology*, **46**, 35–57.

Van Vugt M and Van Lange PAM (2006). The altruism puzzle: psychological adaptations for prosocial behaviour. In: M Schaller, JA Simpson and DT Kenrick, eds. *Evolution and social psychology*, pp. 237–62. Psychology Press, New York, NY.

Walker A, Zimmerman MR and Leakey RE (1982). A possible case of hypervitaminosis A in Homo erectus. *Nature*, **296**, 248–50.

Wichterman R (1986) *The biology of paramecium*. Plenum Press, New York, NY.

Wiester J (1983). *The genesis connection*. Thomas Nelson Publishers, Nashville, TN.

Chapter 2

Emergence and development of scientific medicine

Summary and relevance to the clinician

1) This chapter describes how scientific medicine has developed over the centuries, with particular emphasis on the scientific acquisitions in the fields of anatomy, physiology, as well as of specific medical branches. Besides these anatomical and physiological advances, scientific medicine also includes a biopsychosocial approach, whereby biological factors merge with psychological and social factors in both the pathophysiology and the management of diseases.

2) The transition from the shaman to the modern physician, and from shamanism (i.e. a spiritual-based notion of disease) to scientific medicine (i.e. an anatomophysiological-based concept of disease), was a slow process that took many centuries to develop. Today there are plenty of medical sub-disciplines that have increased their own knowledge and skills over time. The over-specialized physician has often great difficulty to understand and to practice medical specialties other than his own. Therefore, medical care has evolved from the shaman who takes care of the whole body and soul to the modern doctor who takes care of single organs and apparatuses.

3) Animal experimentation has been, and is today, a major ethical problem, both for the lay person and for the scientist/clinician. In particular, the clinician must understand, although he may refuse morally, that what he uses in his routine medical practice comes from experiments and observations that have been made in different animal species. It is also important to recognize that the opponents to animal research are motivated by particularly cruel experiments that have been performed in the past, such as the use of curare without anaesthesia.

4) Many therapies that are used in routine clinical practice are not the consequence of anatomical and physiological advances. For example, treatments such as deep brain stimulation are highly effective, yet their mechanisms are completely or partially unknown. This does not detract from the

significance and rigour of modern medicine, for it uses sophisticated methods to validate therapeutic efficacy. For example, pragmatic clinical trials are aimed at assessing efficacy, regardless of the understanding of the underlying mechanisms.

5) With the advent of psychoimmunology and the discovery that immune responses can be conditioned, modern medicine recognizes that the brain may play an important role in the pathophysiology of diseases. In addition, with the recent explosion of placebo research, particularly its biological underpinnings, modern medicine recognizes that the brain may also have an active role in the therapeutic outcome.

6) It is important to underscore that although medical approaches vary across different cultures, the interaction between the doctor and his patient does not change very much. For example, Western medicine explains the mechanisms of acupuncture differently from traditional Chinese medicine, nonetheless in both the psychosocial component, whereby the patient expects a therapeutic benefit, is crucial.

7) From these many aspects of modern scientific medicine, this chapter argues that the doctor–patient relationship can be made even more scientific by examining the patient's brain from a neuroscientific perspective. In so doing, four behavioural and biological steps can be identified that take place in the patient's brain. First, the subject starts feeling sick through both bottom-up and top-down processes. Second, he starts seeking relief from his discomfort by activating motivational and reward neural mechanisms. Third, trust and hope mechanisms are at work while the patient interacts with a doctor. At the same time, it is interesting to consider empathy and compassion mechanisms in the doctor's brain. Fourth, the very therapeutic act triggers expectation and placebo mechanisms in the patient's brain that only today begin to be understood. These four steps in the doctor–patient relationship will be treated throughout this volume, i.e. feeling sick in Chapter 3, seeking relief in Chapter 4, meeting the therapist in Chapter 5, and receiving a therapy in Chapter 6.

2.1 Emerging knowledge and the problem of animal experimentation

2.1.1 Scientific medicine requires basic anatomical and physiological knowledge

Whereas prehistoric medicine was likely to be based only on shamanic procedures and on a spirits-related concept of illness, writing records started documenting the first anatomical and physiological observations both in humans and in animals. In particular, the dissection of animals was common practice in different cultures and represented the first instance of animal experimentation. For example, Galen, who was born in Greece in the second century after Christ, moved to Rome when he was 30 and performed plenty of experiments in Italy on pigs and monkeys, cutting, removing different organs, tying up arteries and veins without using any sort of anaesthesia. In one of his most famous experiments, he first tied up the artery of an awake animal in two different loci, then he cut it in between, thus showing that there was blood inside (Fig 2.1). If the animal had not been alive, such discovery could not have been performed, as the arteries get empty after death (Paton 1994).

Vivisection was common practice over the following centuries, and many important scientists, such as Graaf, Harvey, Aselli, Pecquet, and Haller, used to work on animals without adopting any kind of anaesthesia. For example, in

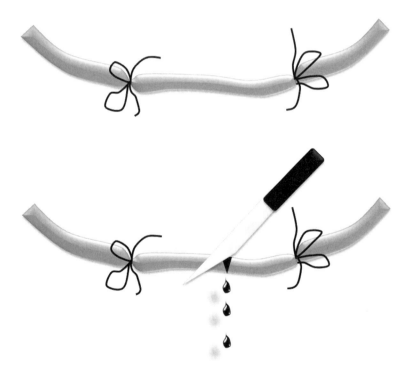

Fig 2.1 One of the most famous (and ethically questionable) experiments by Galen, performed in the second century after Christ. After tying up a blood vessel in a live animal in two loci, he cut it in between, causing bleeding and thus showing that there is blood inside the arteries. Such discovery could not have been performed in a dead animal, as the arteries get empty after death.

1600 William Harvey described blood circulation in great detail by using awake amphibians, reptiles, and mammals. Before 1800, there was no great concern about vivisection, and indeed many influential figures, like Descartes and Francis Bacon, justified vivisection. For example, Descartes asserted that animals are nothing but machines, while Bacon said that they were useful to understand human functioning.

In Victorian England, the *Royal Society for the Prevention of Cruelty to Animals* was founded in 1824, which led to *The Cruelty to Animals Act* in 1876, whose main points were the following: (i) a licence for animal experimentation was introduced; (ii) animal experiments were aimed at reducing suffering in humans and not at performing demonstrations; (iii) a special licence was needed for experiments on dogs, cats, horses, mules, and donkeys; (iv) curare should not be considered an anaesthetic, thus its use was forbidden (French 1975).

The Cruelty to Animals Act is important because people started recognizing that, although medical knowledge must advance, animal experimentation cannot be used loosely and without rules. In contrast to the previous centuries, when anatomy and physiology were learnt through the uncontrolled use of animals, in Victorian society, scientific medicine posed limits to its methods. An important concern that led to The Cruelty to Animals Act was due to the use of curare, a poison used in animal research. In 1844, the French physiologist Claude Bernard curare started studying curare – used by the natives of South America to put on their arrows for hunting. The main characteristic of curare is that it induces an apparently calm and sweet death, both in humans and in animals, with the progressive and quick disappearance of all movements, including respiration. As a matter of fact, this seemingly pacific death conceals profound suffering, as curare blocks nerve-muscle transmission leaving sensory input and consciousness unchanged. No pain reaction occurs because the animal cannot move, however pain perception is unchanged. After a while, the animal dies because of the paralysis of the respiratory muscles.

At the beginning of his experiments, Claude Bernard did not understand completely the suffering of the animal under the effects of curare. He then soon realized that sectioning a curarized animal produced terrible suffering. He asserted that our imagination cannot conceive anything more horrible than feeling pain and having no possibility to escape from it (Olmstead and Olmstead 1952). Nonetheless, he went on with his experiments by saying that scientists have the right to perform experiments on animals and that life sciences need animal experimentation because in this way many human beings can be saved, and this can be done only after the sacrifice of animals. He also asserted that the scientist hears neither the cry nor the suffering of the animal, nor does he see the flowing blood, but he only hears and sees his own idea (Bernard 1865).

It should be noted that, in contrast to *The Cruelty to Animals Act* in 1876 in England, many other countries, such as France, Germany, Italy, and Spain remained virtually insensitive to vivisection. Many English experimenters moved to France in order to do their experiments, like Joseph Lister who developed new surgical seams on animals. The difference among European countries was particularly evident in England and France. Whereas in the former the deductive approach, i.e. understanding from anatomical observation, was more common, in the latter the vivisectionist approach was more used. Interestingly, English science remained behind French science in this period. In this regard, the Bell-Magendie dispute represents a straightforward example (Phillips and Sechzer 1989). In 1822, the French scientist Francois Magendie conducted certain experiments on the spinal cord of live and awake animals. By sectioning the posterior nerves, he found that different body sensations disappeared whereas, by cutting the anterior nerves he observed the disappearance of movements. This represented one of the most important discoveries in 1800, as it gave a fundamental physiological principle to the anatomical organization of the spinal cord, that is, the posterior nerves have to do with the sensory input while the anterior nerves deal with motor output. In the same period, the conclusions by Sir Charles Bell in England were only partially correct, that is, he concluded that the anterior nerves were correlated both with movements and with sensations. In fact, Sir Charles Bell, who did not like vivisection, stunned the animal with a blow on the head, cut the posterior nerves and, not surprisingly, did not see anything. If he had cut the posterior nerves in the awake animal, he would have noticed the loss of sensation from the body, and would have reached the correct conclusions, as Magendie did. Bell himself said that he had to give up, for some experiments were too cruel to be done, and he criticized Magendie, thus boosting the anti-vivisectionist debate further (Gordon-Taylor 1958).

The curare experiments by Claude Bernard and the Bell-Magendie controversy represent good examples of the ethical problem of animal experimentation to reach the solution of physiological issues (French 1975). In other words, in contrast to prehistoric medicine, modern scientific medicine has acquired slow but progressive knowledge through the systematic observation of animal anatomy and physiology. As shown in the following sections, this approach went on over the centuries in more specific medical conditions and surgical interventions, and in all these situations the scientific and the ethical issue have always proceeded one against the other. The ethical concerns about scientific progress at the cost of cruelty to animals is also shown by Charles Darwin's ideas (Rupke 1987). Although he overtly favoured vivisection in a letter to *The Times* in 1881, he also condemned painful and unnecessary experiments without anaesthesia, thus boosting the ethical discussion further.

2.1.2 Acquiring new medical and surgical skills

If we consider the long history of medicine over the centuries, the acquisition of sophisticated medical and surgical skills is really very recent. Dying for a simple infection was the rule only two centuries ago. On 13 December 1799, at the end of a working day in his farm at Mount Vernon, the late president of the United States of America, George Washington, started developing speaking and respiratory problems due to a throat infection. Three physicians suggested gargling with water and vinegar, and bled him three times. Nonetheless, George Washington died after less than 48 hours, probably due to an acute infection. As quinsy was unlikely, considering old age and the quick evolution, he probably died of a common throat infection (Scheidemandel 1976).

The identification of infectious diseases, along with their pathogen agents, such as bacteria and viruses, dates back only some decades. Some preventive treatments, like vaccines, have been developed only very recently, such as anti-rabies in 1885, anti-tuberculosis between 1906 and 1921, anti-diphtheria in 1923, anti-tetanus in 1927, anti-polio between 1955 and 1960, and some very recent vaccines, like anti-measles in 1958 and anti-hepatitis B in 1986. Animal experimentation has been crucial in all these cases. For example, in 1869 Friedrich Trendelenburg took some diphtheria tissue from some patients and transplanted it into the trachea of several animals, showing that it is contagious and is mediated by a specific pathogen agent. Likewise, in 1889 Shibasaburo Kitasato injected the tetanus bacillus in several animals and found that the bacillus remained still in the locus of injection, without spreading throughout the organism. This observation allowed him to conclude that tetanus was due to a toxin produced by the tetanus bacillus. Louis Pasteur himself injected several pathogens in different animals in order to test the transmission of different infectious diseases (Bulloch 1938).

The history of antibiotics is also very recent. In 1928, Alexander Fleming noted that the zone around the muffle *Penicillum notatum* was free of bacteria, and in 1940 Howard Walter Florey and Ernst Boris Chain extracted a sufficient amount of penicillin to be tested in animals. The first experiment was done in mice – they were injected with highly infective pathogens. One group received a simultaneous injection of penicillin whereas a second group did not. Whereas the former survived, the latter died in 17 hours (Dowling 1977; Selwyn 1986). Following penicillin, other pharmacological agents were developed, such as the cephalosporins by Giuseppe Brotzu in 1945 and the sulfamides by Gerhardt Domagk in 1932–35 (Dowling 1977; Selwyn 1986).

Whereas the prevention and control of infectious diseases represent good examples of the recent development of medical skills, both for diagnosis and therapy, all fields of medicine have seen the development of specific skills only in very recent times. For example, diabetes had long been known as a disease whereby hyperglycaemia could be recognized but no treatment was available. Only in 1921 Frederic Banting and Charles Best discovered insulin as the hormone responsible for the control of glycaemia. Insulin was discovered in the dog through harsh experiments, in which the pancreas was removed and then pancreas extract administered. The course of diabetes changed radically from the discovery of insulin (Bliss 1982).

Similarly, although the history of the salicylic acid as a painkiller is very old, the discovery of the peripheral effects of aspirin (i.e. acetylsalicylic acid) is very recent. In 1964, Robert Lim showed that the analgesic effects of aspirin are not attributable to an action on the central nervous system, but rather to a peripheral effect (Collier 1984). To show this, Lim performed harsh experiments in awake dogs. The spleen of dog B was surgically connected to dog A, so that the blood of dog A supplied the spleen of dog B (Fig 2.2). Then the spleen of dog B was injected with a pain-inducing substance so as to induce a painful sensation in animal B. Lim showed that, by injecting aspirin in dog A, an analgesic effect was induced in dog B, which unequivocally indicates that aspirin does not

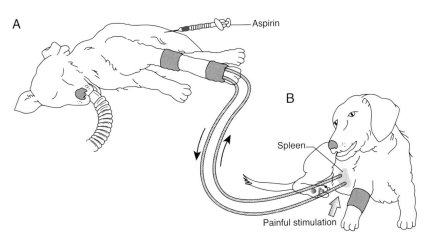

Fig 2.2 The experiment that allowed the identification of the peripheral effects of aspirin in the 1960s. The spleen of dog B was surgically connected to the circulation of dog A, so that it was supplied by the blood of dog A. By injecting aspirin in dog A, an analgesic effect was produced in dog B, which indicates that aspirin does not act on the brain, but on the spleen itself.

act on the brain but rather on the spleen itself. Following this experiment, John Vane showed that aspirin inhibits prostaglandins in rodents (Collier 1984).

In the history of medicine, the acquisition of sophisticated surgical skills is also very recent. For example, sophisticated heart surgery dates back a few decades only. In the 1940s, Blalock and Taussig performed the first operation on *blue babies*, i.e. children made cyanotic by a heart malformation. Both the anatomical knowledge of the animal and human heart and the acquisition of surgical skills on the heart of different animals, like dogs, pigs, sheep, goats, and monkeys, were crucial in the development of heart surgery (DeBakey 1985). This kind of surgery on the heart requires extra-body circulation, a procedure that was applied for the first time in man by John Gibbon in 1953. Like many other stories, the story of heart surgery is interesting because it shows the gradual progression and the gradual acquisition of new physiological, medical, and surgical skills. For example, it is worth pointing out that John Gibbon could use an extra-body circulation procedure in man because in 1929 Werner Forssmann introduced in his own heart a catheter and measured intracardiac pressure. Forssmann would have never introduced a catheter into his own heart if in mid-1800 Claude Bernard had not measured intracardiac pressure in many animals, such as horses, dogs, and sheep. Bernard could not have planned these experiments if in 1733 Stephen Hales had not introduced a catheter into the neck vessels of a horse up to the heart, and performed a gross measurement of blood pressure. Hales, in turn, based his experiment on some basic notions of heart and blood circulation that were developed starting from William Harvey in 1628 with experiments in amphibians, reptiles, and mammals.

Needless to say, many medical disciplines are tightly related to surgery. For example, in organ transplantation, immunology plays a key role, and the discovery of cyclosporine in 1976 was crucial to prevent rejection of different organs (Brent 1997). Another example is blood transfusion, which is also quite recent. In fact, although the first transfusion was performed by Richard Lower in 1667 from one dog to another, only in 1900 Karl Landsteiner identified the human blood groups. Between 1667 and 1900, different attempts had been made. For example, in 1842 Francois Magendie injected frog blood, which has oval-shaped red blood cells, into a mammal, which has round-shaped red blood cells, and observed that the oval red cells were destroyed.

Not to mention anaesthesia, which represents today the basis for a surgical operation. Without anaesthesia, no surgery would be possible, particularly long-lasting operations. Many sophisticated surgical procedures were developed because of the possibility to anaesthetize the patient, thus allowing the surgeon to carry out complex procedures. Interestingly, one of the main causes of the slow development of surgery in the past was the lack of anaesthesia.

When anaesthesia was developed, surgery procedures and techniques developed very quickly. Before the advent of modern anaesthesiology, surgery was performed by anesthetizing the patient with different substances, such as mandrake (*Mandragora officinalis*), Indian cannabis (*Cannabis sativa*), opium (*Papaver somniferum*), and alcohol. Some of these substances were used both 2000 and more years ago and in 1800, with no scientific progress over the centuries. Besides these drugs, many bizarre and dangerous methods were also adopted. For example, both Assires and Egyptians were used to occlude the carotids so as to block blood supply to the brain. In this way, there was a loss of consciousness that allowed surgery to be performed. Interestingly, 'carotid' means somnolence in Greek language, thus carotid artery means sleep artery. The complete lack of scientific progress over the centuries is shown by the fact that carotid compression was performed even in 1600. A similar procedure was developed in 1700 by Hunter and Moore, however the compression was performed on nerves. This compression, that was carried out with a bandage about one hour before surgery, made the limbs insensitive, thereby allowing amputation. It appears clear that in these conditions the real ability of the surgeon was his speed (Holzer and Lembeck 1983). In 1809, a 40-year-old woman, Jane Crawford, underwent the removal of an ovarian cancer, whose weight was 10 kg, without any anaesthesia. The operation, that was performed by Ephraim McDowell, lasted 25 minutes from the opening of the abdomen to the removal of the tumour (Livingston 1983).

In 1800, Humphrey Davy tested for the first time the anaesthetic properties of a gas, nitrous oxide, both in animals and on himself, and showed that it was possible to make the organism insensitive to pain. In 1824, Henry Hickman performed similar experiments with carbon dioxide, and in 1850, John Snow was the first to promote the development of anaesthetic techniques with a rigorous scientific approach. On the basis of the use of ether by William Morton and of chloroform by James Simpson, he improved the inhalation procedures by developing and building new devices and instruments (Atkinson and Boulton 1989). Besides these procedures of general anaesthesia, there are plenty of techniques that allow local anaesthesia to be performed (Holzer and Lembeck 1983). The first local anaesthetic was cocaine. Its effects were identified in 1884 by Carl Koller, who was looking for something that would make the eye insensitive to pain. Following the discovery of the anaesthetic properties of cocaine, in 1885 Corning injected cocaine in the spinal cord of the dog, and noted that it induced anaesthesia in the hind paws, thus setting the stage for epidural anaesthesia.

Interestingly, surgery has not been considered a medical discipline until recent times. In 1700, surgeons were not considered physicians, and operations were carried out by the so-called barber surgeons after consultation with a physician. For example, the barber surgeon Vylhoorn developed a sort of huge scissors that could cut the breast of a woman with a single cut. Horne used these scissors by pulling out the breast with some threads and then cutting it in a few seconds (Gabka and Vaubel 1983).

The acquisition of medical skills over the centuries does not involve only therapy, but diagnosis as well. Before the advent of modern and refined radiological techniques, the medical error was the rule, and many patients were surgically opened on the basis of gross and imprecise diagnoses. In 1895, the discovery of X-rays by Wilhelm Conrad Roentgen led to a diagnostic revolution. He performed the first radiography on his wife's hand, and then on other parts of the body, both in humans and animals. As soon as people realized that excessive exposition to X-rays was dangerous, plenty of experiments were carried out in animals in order to assess doses and tolerances, as well as to test new contrast agents such as barium sulphate, which are today routinely used in radiology (Rosenbusch et al. 1995).

This is not a volume on the history of medicine, thus other examples would be superfluous and redundant. It appears clear, however, that knowledge of the anatomy and physiology of animals and humans parallels the development of new therapeutic and diagnostic tools. In more recent times, new disciplines, such as genomics, proteomics, and molecular biology have emerged, and these represent a further advance in animal and human physiology. The transition from the shaman to the modern physician, and from shamanism (i.e. a spiritual-based notion of disease) to scientific medicine (i.e. an anatomophysiological-based concept of disease), was a slow process that took many centuries to develop. Today there are plenty of medical sub-disciplines that have increased their own knowledge and skills over time. The over-specialized physician has often great difficulty to understand and to practice medical specialties other than his own. Therefore, medical care has evolved from the shaman who takes care of the whole body and soul to the modern doctor who takes care of single organs and apparatuses.

2.1.3 Effective treatments need not be understood, but they do need validation

There is no doubt that many treatments, diagnostic methods, and procedures derive from a detailed knowledge of the anatomy, physiology, and biochemistry of the whole body. It is clear, for instance, that most surgical techniques have their origin in the knowledge of both the anatomy and the pathophysiology of the disease. Once the damaged organ has been identified, it can be removed, and once the malfunction of an anatomical part, like a heart valve, has been diagnosed, it can be replaced. Likewise, hormonal therapy originates from a detailed knowledge of the anatomy, physiology, and biochemistry of the endocrine system. Whenever a hyposecretion or hypersecretion of a given hormone has been identified, it can be either replaced or antagonized, respectively. For example, modern therapy of some forms of diabetes comes from the crucial discovery of insulin by Frederic Banting and Charles Best in 1921. This holds true for many drugs as well, whose development was based on anatomical, physiological, and biochemical findings. For example, the understanding of the physiology of the hydrogen/potassium adenosine triphosphatase enzyme system (the H^+/K^+ ATPase), or more commonly just gastric proton pump, of the gastric parietal cell, led to the development of omeprazole, one of most prescribed antiacid drugs in the world. These are only a few examples, but the list is long in many fields of medicine (see section 2.1.2).

Despite the causal connection between anatomical–physiological–biochemical advances and the development of many new therapies, there are also many examples whereby medical knowledge went in the opposite direction. In many cases, effective therapies led to the search of the underlying mechanisms. Thus, it is not necessary to know the underlying mechanisms for a therapy to be effective. Opium (*Papaverum somniferum*) and morphine are good examples of drugs with powerful analgesic properties but whose mechanisms have been unknown for many years. Even today, we do not know where morphine exerts its major effects, at the spinal and/or supraspinal level. Likewise, salicylates have been used over the centuries as analgesics, but the underlying mechanisms were completely unknown. Only in 1964 did Robert Lim show that the analgesic effects of aspirin are not attributable to an action on the central nervous system, but rather to a peripheral effect (see section 2.1.2). Figure 2.2 shows the experiment performed by Lim, whereby the spleen of dog B was supplied with the blood of dog A, and when the spleen of dog B was made painful, an aspirin injection in dog A induced an analgesic effect, thereby showing that aspirin does not act on the brain but rather has a peripheral action on the spleen itself. In 1971, John Vane showed that aspirin inhibits the prostaglandins (Collier 1984). Both morphine and aspirin are examples of highly effective drugs whose mechanisms have been unknown for centuries, thus emphasizing that efficacious treatments sometimes do not need to be understood.

Even modern effective therapeutic approaches are often used without knowing the underlying mechanism. Interestingly, sometimes the search of the mechanisms leads to a better knowledge of the physiology of a system. A good and timely example is deep brain stimulation for the treatment of several brain pathologies, such as motor disorders. Parkinson's disease is today treated surgically through the implantation of electrodes in the brain for the chronic stimulation of different regions. It was tested for the first time in the monkey that was made Parkinsonian by means of 1-methyl-4-phenyl-1,2,3,6-tetrahydropyridine (MPTP). Although the stimulation of the subthalamic nucleus was found to block the Parkinsonian symptoms, the underlying mechanism was completely unknown, and even today is only partially understood. It is interesting to note that the physiology of the basal ganglia is today better understood, thanks to the search of the mechanisms of deep brain stimulation. For example, today we know that the firing rate of subthalamic nucleus neurons is sustained in Parkinson patients, thereby inducing hyperactivity in the substantia nigra pars reticulata, a region which receives excitatory inputs from the subthalamic nucleus. The substantia nigra pars reticulata increases its inhibition upon the thalamus which, in turn, reduces its control upon the motor cortex. This decrease of the thalamic output to the motor cortex is believed to affect motor performance in Parkinson patients (Bergman et al. 1994; Benazzouz et al. 2000; Blandini et al. 2000; Maurice et al. 2003; Tai et al. 2003; Shi et al. 2006; Maltete et al. 2007).

The current idea is that the relief of Parkinsonian rigidity is associated with a decrease in neuronal firing rate in the subthalamic nucleus and substantia nigra pars reticulata. According to this model, an anti-Parkinson treatment, such as deep brain stimulation, would restore a normal activity in the subthalamic nucleus (Limousin et al. 1998; Benazzouz and Hallett 2000), and thus in the substantia nigra pars reticulata, with a decreased inhibition over the thalamus. The increased thalamic output would facilitate the control of movement by the motor cortex. Why high frequency deep brain stimulation, which is delivered at a frequency of about 130 Hz, inhibits the subthalamic nucleus is still a puzzle. At least three mechanisms might be involved (Fig 2.3). First, the electrode might stimulate afferent inhibitory GABAergic fibres to the subthalamic nucleus, thus exerting a powerful inhibitory effect upon its neurons. Second, high-frequency stimulation might induce changes in membrane excitability of the subthalamic nucleus neurons. A third mechanism might have to do with oscillatory activities. In fact, although the firing rate model of basal ganglia neurons seems to play a role in the motor Parkinsonian symptoms, recent findings suggest that synchronized activity between different regions may be impaired in Parkinson's disease (Brown 2003). For example, oscillations below 30 Hz have been described in experimental models of parkinsonism, such as in monkeys treated with MPTP (Nini et al. 1995). Likewise, intraoperative studies in Parkinson patients have shown synchronization of single neurons in both the subthalamic nucleus and the internal globus pallidus at 11–30 Hz (Levy et al. 2000, 2001, 2002). Oscillations greater than 60 Hz have also been

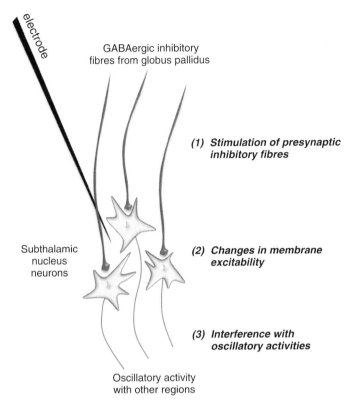

GABAergic inhibitory
fibres from globus pallidus

**(1) Stimulation of presynaptic
inhibitory fibres**

Subthalamic
nucleus
neurons

**(2) Changes in membrane
excitability**

**(3) Interference with
oscillatory activities**

Oscillatory activity
with other regions

Fig 2.3 High-frequency stimulation of the subthalamic nucleus by an electrode is highly effective in reducing motor symptoms in Parkinson's disease. However, the underlying mechanisms are virtually unknown. Three hypotheses are shown, but the debate is still open.

described between the subthalamic nucleus, the internal globus pallidus, and the cortex in Parkinson patients under treatment with levodopa (Brown et al. 2001; Williams et al. 2002). Overall, these data suggest that basal ganglia functioning is not mediated by neuronal firing rate only, but by different oscillatory activities as well (Brown 2003). According to this view, deep brain stimulation would interfere with these oscillations.

As can be seen from this example of a modern and timely neurological treatment for motor disorders, although deep brain stimulation is highly effective in relieving the motor symptoms, its mechanisms are virtually unknown. Figure 2.3 shows three hypotheses for the functioning of deep brain stimulation, but the debate is still open, and whether one mechanism is more important than the others is still an unanswered question.

Although many treatments are delivered without knowing anything about the possible underlying mechanisms, modern scientific medicine maintains its value compared to most of the medical procedures that were used in the past. In fact, although in both situations the mechanisms are virtually unknown, modern scientific medicine has learned to assess real effectiveness. The modern pragmatic clinical trials do not need to investigate the mechanisms, but merely whether or not a therapy works better than a placebo, i.e. an inert treatment. Therefore, the main focus of most trials is the effectiveness and not the mechanism. In this sense, scientific medicine is aimed at applying a rigorous methodology to assess efficacy, regardless of the anatomical–physiological–biochemical knowledge. For example, clinical trials are rigorously conducted in phases. With pharmacological agents, Phase 1 trials try to determine dosing, document how a drug is metabolized and excreted, and identify acute side effects. In this phase, usually a small number of healthy volunteers (between 20 and 80) are used. Phase 2 trials include more participants (about 100–300) who have the disease or condition that the medication potentially could treat. In Phase 2, researchers seek to gather further safety data and preliminary evidence of the drug's beneficial effects (efficacy). If the Phase 2 trials indicate that the pharmacological agent may be effective, and the risks are considered acceptable, given the observed efficacy and the severity of the disease, the drug moves on to Phase 3. In Phase 3 trials, the drug is studied in a much larger number of people with the disease (about 1000–3000). This phase further tests the medication's effectiveness, monitors side effects, and, in some cases, compares the medication's effects to a standard treatment, if one is already available. As more and more participants are tested over longer periods of time, even rare side effects can be revealed. Sometimes, Phase 4 trials are conducted after a drug is already approved and in the market, in order to better understand the treatment's long-term risks, benefits, and optimal use, as well as to test the medication in special populations, such as children.

This validation procedure does not take into account any mechanism. It is only based on the notion of efficacy. Plenty of drugs are assessed in this way, without understanding what they do, where they bind, and how they work. For example, gabapentin, which is used as both antiepileptic and antinociceptive drug, was developed by adding a cyclohexyl group to gamma-aminobutyric acid (GABA), which allowed this form of GABA to cross the blood–brain barrier. Therefore, it was originally designed as a GABAmimetic that could freely cross the blood–brain barrier. However, despite its structural similarity to GABA, gabapentin does not bind to GABA receptors in the central nervous system. The most likely mechanism seems to be the binding to the $\alpha_2\delta$ subunit of a voltage-dependent calcium channel, thereby exerting calcium channel-blocking effects

(Fink et al. 2000), but its exact mechanism is still a source of discussion. Of course, from a strict pragmatic point of view, the action of gabapentin on GABA receptors or on calcium channels does not make any difference. Being ignorant about the mechanism of action does not affect efficacy.

A further point to be considered is the placebo component of any medical and surgical treatment (Benedetti 2008b). Although this can be identified by using the appropriate paradigms and control groups, it is not always clear how much the specific effect of a treatment and its placebo component contribute to the therapeutic outcome. For example, the response rate in the placebo groups in antidepressant clinical trials is very high. In 1998, Kirsch and Sapirstein (1998) conducted a meta-analysis in 19 double-blind clinical trials which included 2 318 patients. It was found that 75% of the response to the active drug is attributable to a placebo effect, thus the specific pharmacodynamic effect of the drug would account for only the 25%. In addition, a high correlation was found between placebo effect and drug effect, which indicates that virtually all the variation in drug effect size was due to the placebo component. Kirsch and Sapirstein (1998) also assessed natural history effects, in order to evaluate how much of the 75% was attributable to the real placebo responses and how much to other factors. To do this another 19 trials of psychotherapy, whereby the use of no-treatment groups is more common, were analysed. Natural history accounted for the 23.87%, drug effect for 25.16%, and placebo effect for 50.97%. Therefore it was concluded that, in clinical trials for major depression, one quarter is due to the specific action of the active medication, one quarter to other factors, like spontaneous remission, and one half is a placebo effect. Despite the many controlled clinical trials that have been performed in the past, the real effectiveness of many antidepressant treatments still remains an open question, and certainly the underlying mechanisms are still virtually unknown.

2.1.4 Animal research impacts negatively on most people and raises many ethical concerns

The advances in our knowledge of anatomy and physiology mostly rely on experiments that have been performed in animals. There is no doubt that what we know today and what we use in clinical practice comes from a continuum of knowledge that has involved a very large number of animals. The experiments on live animals by Galen, the use of curare in awake dogs by Claude Bernard, the nerve section in conscious animals by Francois Magendie, as well as those experiments that have been performed without anaesthesia, are certainly harsh and brutal, and raise many ethical concerns. It is not surprising, therefore, that many people are against animal experimentation and certainly we cannot blame them for this. An emotional reaction to the use of curare in conscious animals and to those experiments with no anaesthesia is unavoidable and uncovers a sensibility towards non-human species and nature in general. Nevertheless, those who have this emotional reaction and are strong opponents of animal experimentation, do not realize that they too are users of animal research in everyday life.

This is not a volume on the ethics of animal experimentation, thus no details will be provided. However, it is worth noting that the vehement protest against conducting experiments on animals is not only voiced by lay persons, but also among scientists and physicians. There are many reasons to believe that the emotional impact of biomedical animal research is much stronger than the exploitation of animals in other situations. For example, an analysis of pro-animal movements showed that 63% of people were against animal research, 30% against slaughter for food, 2% against dog pounds, 2% against hunting, 0.8% against furs, and 0.6% against animal games, e.g. bull fighting (Nicoll and Russell 1990). This is quite surprising, considering the number of animals used in the United States for different purposes: 96% for food, 2.5% for hunting, 0.4% killed in dog pounds, 0.3% for biomedical research, and 0.2% for furs. Therefore, although only 0.3% of animals are used for biomedical research, up to 63% of the literature criticizes animal research. In Germany, 9 animals per citizen are killed yearly for food, whereas 0.03 animals per citizen are killed for scientific purposes. Nevertheless, 80% of the time devoted to animals by the mass media deals with biomedical research (Singer 1993).

The following example is quite interesting and instructive, and shows the greater emotional impact of biomedical animal research compared with other situations. Ehinger (1986) describes a case of rod and bait fishing. A sports fisherman caught a 16-kg river salmon and this took him a full hour to land the fish. A local newspaper depicted him proudly showing his catch. Most interesting, the article approvingly noted that the fisherman was exhausted by the long fight and that he is certainly going to return for more fishing at the same river in coming years. Ehinger (1986) points out how this appealing little piece of local news can very easily be changed into a quite appalling headline without changing anything in the actual event. What is needed is to assume that the fisherman was not fishing for sport but because of his profession. The headline would read 'Scientist struggled full hour to catch and kill his experimental animal'. The public reaction to such a title would certainly be strong. In fact, whereas hunting and catching animals for pleasure are activities which are acceptable to society even if they involve prolonged pain and agony to the prey, animal use in biomedical research is not regarded this way and is readily condemned. What is important in this example is that most people are not so much concerned with the real pain and agony of the animal, for the two situations are exactly the same from the animal perspective, but rather with human activities.

Today many animal experiments have been replaced with other approaches, such as cell cultures. However, the use of animals to answer certain biological questions is still widespread. Nonetheless, ethical rules must be followed, like the use of anaesthesia in most experiments, and in particular the use of adequate anaesthetic agents when curarization is necessary. Even by adopting the strictest rules to avoid suffering, many people still react against any kind of animal experiments, and this leads to a negative reaction to medical practice for many of them. For example, some suggest opposing animal research by stopping to take medications for different medical problems, such as pain, liver and kidney disorders, and insomnia (Ruesch 1978). Although this would be coherent indeed, like a vegetarian who has stopped eating meat, it would be also more difficult, as giving up to painkillers and anaesthetics would require a sacrifice which a few people would be ready to make.

2.2 Biological, psychological, and social factors all contribute to illness and healing

2.2.1 Modern scientific medicine includes a psychosocial component

Physicians have long known that many factors other than the disease itself may impact negatively on both the symptoms and the course of the illness. In other words, although the anatomy, physiology, and biochemistry of different organs, systems, and apparatuses, as understood from animal experimentation and human studies, take an important part in the emergence and course of illness, they are not enough, and additional factors must be included in a global model of illness. Although many psychological and social aspects have been recognized over the centuries by physicians and psychologists as contributing factors to the emergence of certain diseases, the scientific formulation of such a contribution is relatively recent. Engel (1977) challenged the medical and scientific community by putting forward a new medical model that takes into account biological, psychological, and social factors as important determinants of illness (Fig 2.4). Engel's biopsychosocial model has had a great impact upon the scientific community, and its scientific foundations have been partly supported by the emergence of modern concepts in psychosomatics, psychoneuroimmunology, and psychoneuroendocrinology.

The basic idea of the biopsychosocial model is not so much to deny biomedical research but rather to criticize its narrow focus on the anatomical, physiological, and molecular mechanisms. There is no doubt that the new acquisitions of anatomy, physiology and, more recently, molecular biology, have been crucial to the advancement of biomedical research. The detailed knowledge of the origin and possibly the management of a disease have mainly relied on these biological acquisitions and, accordingly, have positively impacted on the medical profession. However, emerging experimental evidence in modern medicine indicates powerful influences of the mind over the body, whereby the patient's psychological state and the social factors impinging onto him are all involved in both the pathophysiology and the treatment outcomes of a given disease.

At least two milestones should be highlighted. In 1964, Solomon and Moos (1964) coined the term psychoimmunology, and in 1975 Ader and Cohen (1975) demonstrated classical conditioning of immune function, which triggered the explosive growth in both animal and human research. Many models of positive and negative psychosocial influences on the body were created over the years, and many social–psychological–immune–hormonal links were identified. For example, the hypothalamic-pituitary-adrenal axis, whereby the hypothalamic corticotrophin releasing hormone (CRH) stimulates pituitary secretion of adrenocorticotropic hormone (ACTH) which, in turn, stimulates cortisol secretion at the level of the adrenal glands, is typically activated in stressful situations, and cortisol, one of the main glucocorticoids of the adrenal glands, is intimately related to immune functions. In fact, at physiological concentrations it causes a shift in immune responses from a type-1 pro-inflammatory cytokine pattern (e.g. tumour necrosis factor alpha) to a type-2 anti-inflammatory cytokine patterns (e.g. interleukin-10) (Elenkov and Chrousos 1999). At higher concentrations, cortisol is immunosuppressive, thus the hyperactivity of the hypothalamic-pituitary-adrenal axis tends to suppress immune responses and predisposes to infections (Sternberg 1997a, b). Other pathways connecting the brain to the immune system involve the autonomic nervous system. For example, the ventromedial hypothalamus controls the sympathetic innervation of the spleen and the splenic nerve in turn controls, at least in part, natural killer cell activity (Katafuchi et al. 1993, 1994; Okamoto et al. 1996). Besides the sympathetic system (Elenkov et al. 2000), the vagus/parasympathetic cholinergic system has been found to affect immune functions as well (Tracey 2002; Pavlov and Tracey 2005). Therefore, the opposite activation of the sympathetic and parasympathetic system has profound effects on immune responses.

These are only a few examples among many others. All these findings, as well as the new emerging concepts on the psychological-immune link, gave scientific credibility to the postulated interaction between social, psychological, and biological factors in the production of illness (Fig 2.4). Thus, there is today a general agreement about the interaction between biological mechanisms and

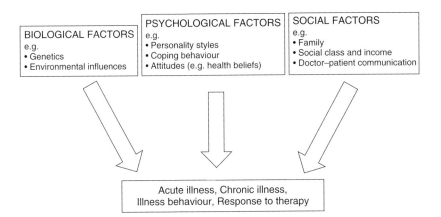

Fig 2.4 The biopsychosocial model of illness and healing is basically a model that considers biological, psychological and social factors as crucial determinants of both getting sick and responding to a treatment.

psychosocial influences, although many of these interactions are still little understood or completely unknown.

To recognize that the patient's psychological state may influence biological factors means to pose the patient, with his emotional, cognitive, and motivational experiences, at the centre of medical care. In the history of medicine this certainly represents an important step, as it was neglected in many medical cultures over the centuries. This does not mean that it was psychoneuroendocrinoimmunology that led to the patient-centred medical care, but it certainly posed some of the scientific bases for this approach. For example, a doctor-centred approach, whereby the doctor was supposed to have magical powers, was typical of many cultures, such as ancient Egypt and medieval Europe, whereas a more scientific and humanistic approach in the doctor–patient relationship was present in the Greek culture. Here there was a higher degree of humanism in dealing with the needs, well-being, and interests of people, and medical ethics was posed above the self-interests of class and status, as evidenced in the Hippocratic Oath:

> The regimen I adopt shall be for the benefit of my patients according to my ability and judgment, and not for their hurt or for wrong. Whatsoever house I enter, there will I go for the benefit of the sick, refraining from all wrongdoing or corruption, and especially from any seduction, of male or female, of bond free. Whatsoever things I see or hear concerning the life of men, in my attendance on the sick or even apart there from, which ought not be noised abroad, I will keep silence thereon, counting such things to be as sacred secrets. (Kaba and Sooriakumaran 2007)

The biopsychosocial approach has to do not only with the pathophysiology of illness, but also with possible management. It gave rise to a series of therapeutic interventions which are called, as a whole, mind-body medicine. Mind-body interventions are aimed at targeting those psychosocial factors that are supposed to be at the very origin of many diseases, although their effectiveness is often questioned. These include hypnosis, meditation, cognitive-behavioural therapy, relaxation, and imagery techniques.

The crucial role of psychosocial factors is also shown in the conventional therapeutic setting, whereby placebo effects with different mechanisms and in different systems can be found. Indeed, placebo effects derive from the psychosocial context around the patient and the therapy (see also Chapter 6). A positive context may lead to positive outcomes, the placebo effects, whereas a negative context may lead to negative outcomes, the nocebo effects (Benedetti 2008b).

The efforts to understand the mechanisms that are at the basis of the interaction between psychosocial and biological factors are shown by the recent explosion of placebo research. By using many sophisticated neurobiological approaches, several mechanisms have been identified and many new concepts have emerged (Benedetti 2008a, b; Enck et al. 2008; Price et al. 2008; Finniss et al. 2010). This neuroscientific approach is paying dividends and is giving credibility to old concepts that were waiting for scientific validation. In particular, the psychosocial influences on the therapeutic outcome, which are typical of placebo effects, have been described within a biological context that explains clinical practice in relation to many brain functions, thus putting psychosocial investigation into the neurobiological domain (see Chapter 6).

2.2.2 Medical concepts vary across cultures but the psychosocial component stays the same

The new insights into anatomy, physiology, and molecular biology over the centuries has led to modern scientific medicine, although this applies mainly to Western society. The intimate relationship between biology and medicine is at the very heart of the Western medical profession, and the molecular/cellular approach to the disease is often paralleled by the biopsychosocial approach which takes both patient and disease into consideration.

Many medical concepts change completely across different cultures worldwide. There are many medical approaches that neglect, completely or in part, the Western approach. According to the World Health Organization, in many African and Asian countries, about 80% of people use traditional medicine, that is, a kind of medical practice which has local origins and foundations. One of the most popular examples is represented by traditional Chinese medicine, which uses medical concepts in opposition to the Western medical world. For example, the concept of Qi (vital energy) is crucial in many medical practices such as acupuncture. Qi is said to flow along different channels of the body, which are called meridians, and many therapeutic approaches are aimed at interfering with Qi by restoring its normal flow through the body meridians. Acupuncture aims to interfere with the Qi flow by inserting a needle in different points of the skin. Although acupuncture can be effective in some conditions, the fundamental difference between the traditional Chinese approach and the Western medical approach resides in the explanation of the underlying mechanism and in the interpretation of acupuncture within a scientific and philosophical context. As shown in Fig 2.5, the effects that follow the insertion of an acupuncture needle into the skin can be seen within a Western context (A), which is based on key anatomical-physiological concepts, or a traditional Chinese context (B), which is mainly based on philosophical foundations. According to the first mechanistic interpretation, when the needle pierces the skin, it stimulates mechanoreceptors which activate inhibitory interneurons. These, in turn, inhibit pain transmission along the nociceptive pathway. According to the Chinese philosophical explanation, when the needle pierces the skin, it interferes with the Qi flow in a given meridian of the body. This induces a restoration of Qi flow, which had been lost and had caused illness.

From the perspective of the patient, either interpretations do not make a big difference. What matters is the efficacy of acupuncture. The study of the placebo effect in acupuncture treatments may help clarify this point. In 2005, a brain imaging study was performed that clearly showed the relative contribution of specific and placebo mechanisms of acupuncture (Pariente et al. 2005). In a single-blind, randomized crossover study in 14 patients suffering from painful osteoarthritis, three interventions were compared under positron emission tomography scans: (1) real acupuncture, (2) placebo Streitberger needle acupuncture, whereby the needle is pushed against the skin but it actually moves into the handle, giving the impression that it has pierced the skin, (3) overt placebo, whereby subjects are told that the needle would not pierce the skin and that it did not have therapeutic effectiveness. Real acupuncture was found to activate the ipsilateral insula to a greater extent compared with placebo. Interestingly, both real acupuncture and placebo Streitberger needle, in which there is the same expectation of therapeutic effect (placebo effect), produced a more powerful effect than overt placebo, in which there is no expectation of positive therapeutic outcome, in the right dorsolateral prefrontal cortex, anterior cingulate cortex, and midbrain. Therefore, acupuncture seems to have both specific effects in the insula and placebo effects in the dorsolateral and cingulate cortex, and in the midbrain.

Expectations about positive therapeutic outcomes may activate specific brain regions, and such expectations may sometimes be the real cause of the

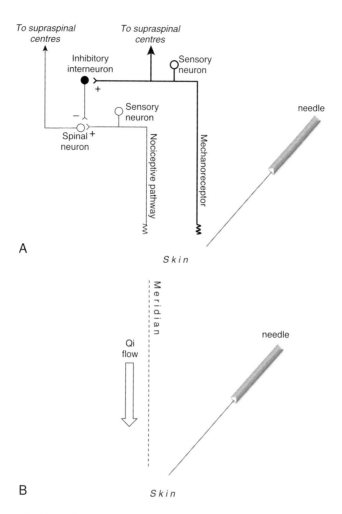

Fig 2.5 Mechanisms of acupuncture according to the Western medical knowledge (A) and to traditional Chinese medicine (B). According to Western medicine, the insertion of the needle causes activation of mechanoreceptors and inhibitory interneurons which, in turn, inhibit the afferent nociceptive signals (A). According to Chinese medicine, the insertion of the needle into a given meridian of the body restores a normal flow of the vital energy Qi (B).

clinical improvement. This is shown by some clinical trials whereby expectations were assessed. Bausell et al. (2005) conducted a study on acupuncture in which patients were asked which group they believed they belonged to (either placebo or real acupuncture), and found that those patients who believed they belonged to the real treatment group experienced larger clinical improvement than those patients who believed they belonged to the placebo group. Likewise, Linde et al. (2007) performed four randomized controlled trials in which real acupuncture was compared to placebo acupuncture in migraine, tension-type headache, chronic low back pain, and osteoarthritis of the knee. This study examined the effects of 864 patients' expectations on the therapeutic outcome, irrespective of which group the patients belonged to. The patients were asked whether they considered acupuncture to be an effective therapy in general and what they personally expected from it. In addition, after three acupuncture sessions, the patients were asked how confident they were that they would benefit from the treatment. The investigators found that those patients with higher expectations about acupuncture experienced larger clinical improvements than those with lower expectations, irrespective of the allocation to real acupuncture or placebo acupuncture. Thus it did not really matter whether the patients actually received the real or the sham procedure. What mattered was whether they believed in acupuncture and expected a benefit from it.

This represents a nice example of how both the Western and the traditional Chinese approach fail to explain the effects of needle insertion. The psychological component may play a crucial role here, and neither inhibitory interneurons along the nociceptive pathway nor the Qi flow, as shown in Fig 2.5, are the real explanations of acupuncture. The clinical improvement in those patients who receive a placebo is very complex and is attributable to plenty of factors, all of them embedded in the patient–healer relationship (Kaptchuk et al. 2009)

There are plenty of local traditional medical approaches all over the world, and each of them uses different concepts and approaches. Although all of them invoke philosophical and religious principles and possible underlying mechanisms, none of them is usually recognized by the Western medical approach. For example, Ayurvedic medicine is a system of traditional medicine native to India which is based on five great elements: earth, water, fire, air, and space. The balance of these elements is crucial and every effort should be made to keep them balanced. Siddha and Unani medicine are similar to Ayurveda and, accordingly, use similar philosophical principles. In Africa there are plenty of local medical practices, such as Muti in Southern Africa and Ifá in Western Africa, and most of them, if not all, are based on religious beliefs. The list is long worldwide, and even in Western societies traditional practices may be adopted. For example, in many rural areas of Western countries, people may have never seen a modern doctor and may rely on local traditions and irrational forms of cure.

Despite the high number of variations in medical practice across different cultures, the therapist–patient relationship is maintained across different Western and non-Western countries. Any patient is eager to find a solution to his discomfort and he tries to seek relief. To do this, he interacts with a doctor, and finally he receives a therapy. This is the sequence of events that characterizes any culture, irrespective of biomedical concepts, philosophical approaches, and medical practice. In the following section, these aspects will be further developed, and they will be treated in detail throughout this volume.

2.3 Medical practice meets neuroscience

2.3.1 Scientific medicine needs to include the study of the patient's and doctor's brain

Being a patient is a common situation across all cultures, regardless of medical beliefs and practices. Being a patient means to get sick and to try to suppress one's own discomfort, such as pain or nausea, or even anxiety and fear of the possible end of life. In this regard, the encounter with the healer is a fundamental step that virtually all patients will eventually face. With the emergence of scientific medicine, both in its biological and psychosocial aspects, a better understanding of the patient's behaviour would certainly be advantageous to the patient himself as well as to the therapist. In fact, the latter could improve his skills, particularly those that involve communication and social interaction, to his patient's advantage.

The recent advances of neurosciences come at an auspicious time, in which there is a strong need to increase our knowledge about the patient's behaviour as well as about all those psychological and social factors that impact on illness. Several key concepts in human behaviour that can be described through behavioural, cognitive, molecular neurosciences can indeed be applied to a variety of behavioural repertoires that characterize the condition of being a patient. For example, neurosciences can investigate the patient's brain when he gets sick as well as when he meets the therapist or receives a treatment. In this way, the patient–healer encounter can be put into the neurobiological domain, and this can shed light on some unanswered questions.

The same concepts hold true for the doctor's brain. Neurosciences can better understand those neural processes that take place in any individual who, by virtue of his profession, has to do with suffering and healing. The recent advances of neurosciences in the domain of emotions, empathy, and compassion, can be at the very heart of good medical practice and may help to create better health professionals.

It is important to realize that, although this neuroscientific approach necessarily involves biological, psychological, and social factors, it differs from the biopsychosocial model in many ways. In fact, to study the patient's (and doctor's) brain and behaviour means to study not so much illness, but rather how the patient reacts to illness. Whereas the biopsychosocial model investigates how biological factors merge with psychosocial factors in the production of illness, the study of the patient's brain has little to do with illness itself. Rather it deals with illness-initiated behaviour. In this sense, the patient's behaviour can be subdivided into different steps, each of which is amenable of a truly neuroscientific investigation.

2.3.2 To become and to be a patient involves four steps and relative brain processes

From a behavioural and neuroscientific viewpoint, to become and to be a patient involves at least four steps (Fig 2.6). In contrast to Fig 2.4, in which the general concept of the biopsychosocial model is depicted, Fig 2.6 shows these steps without considering illness itself, but only how illness triggers the patient's behaviour. In this way, the doctor-patient relationship can be fully integrated within the domain of neuroscience. It involves many physiological processes in the patient's brain, from the very beginning of illness to the therapeutic act. Indeed, in the next four chapters, these four steps will be expanded, and the patient's brain will be analyzed in detail from a neuroscientific perspective.

As a first step, a healthy subject feels sick and this occurs on the basis of sensory feedback arising from the body (Chapter 3). Interoceptive sensibility and awareness is critical to produce a feeling of sickness, and both bottom-up and top-down mechanisms take place. In fact, the bottom-up processes arising from the periphery to the central nervous system are modulated by top-down cognitive and affective influences. For example, attention and anxiety can induce different pain experiences in different individuals and in different circumstances. This is the step that initiates the subsequent patient's behaviour.

Second, the feeling of sickness, which involves the physical and psychological discomfort experienced by the subject, activates motivational and reward mechanisms that are aimed at suppressing the discomfort and at seeking pleasure (Chapter 4). The doctor and the therapy are powerful rewards, and the whole patient's reward circuitry is engaged while he seeks relief. To suppress illness-initiated discomfort is not different from the suppression of hunger and thirst.

Third, when the patient meets the doctor, and more in general, the healer, this interaction triggers some complex brain processes that have to do with trust and hope (Chapter 5). When the interaction is positive, all these mechanisms are enhanced. When it is negative, negative emotions, such as anxiety and depression, are induced. In the third step there are two actors, the patient and the doctor. The doctor's brain is also worthy of consideration, because both empathy and compassion mechanisms may get involved. The intricate interaction among trust and hope on the one hand, and empathic and compassionate behaviour on the other, may give rise to opposite outcomes, either positive or negative.

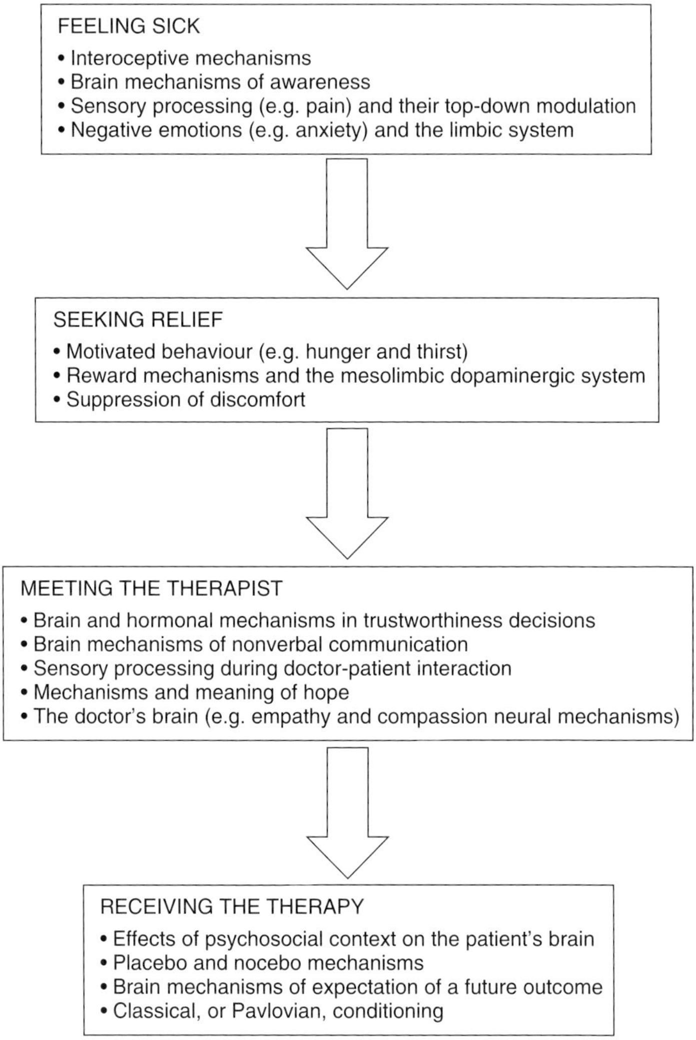

FEELING SICK
- Interoceptive mechanisms
- Brain mechanisms of awareness
- Sensory processing (e.g. pain) and their top-down modulation
- Negative emotions (e.g. anxiety) and the limbic system

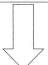

SEEKING RELIEF
- Motivated behaviour (e.g. hunger and thirst)
- Reward mechanisms and the mesolimbic dopaminergic system
- Suppression of discomfort

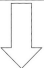

MEETING THE THERAPIST
- Brain and hormonal mechanisms in trustworthiness decisions
- Brain mechanisms of nonverbal communication
- Sensory processing during doctor-patient interaction
- Mechanisms and meaning of hope
- The doctor's brain (e.g. empathy and compassion neural mechanisms)

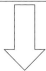

RECEIVING THE THERAPY
- Effects of psychosocial context on the patient's brain
- Placebo and nocebo mechanisms
- Brain mechanisms of expectation of a future outcome
- Classical, or Pavlovian, conditioning

Fig 2.6 In contrast to the biopsychosocial model of Fig 2.4, which has to do with the biological, psychological and social influences on illness, the study of the patient's brain and behaviour, or the neuroscience of the doctor-patient relationship, investigates the behaviour and the brain mechanisms that are initiated by illness. The four steps that are depicted in this scheme (feeling sick, seeking relief, meeting the therapist, receiving the therapy) can all be approached from a neuroscientific point of view. For each step, the main brain mechanisms that are involved are shown.

Fourth, the therapeutic act activates expectation and placebo mechanisms that are at the very heart of the therapeutic outcome (Chapter 6). The therapeutic act is a reward and, accordingly, may activate reward mechanisms. Plenty of other mechanisms may be at work here, such as classical conditioning or reduction of negative emotions (e.g. anxiety). The therapeutic act is the final step, and its neuroscientific investigation has been a valuable approach to better understand the action and meaning of many therapies.

References

Ader R and Cohen N (1975). Behaviorally conditioned immunosuppression. *Psychosomatic Medicine*, **37**, 333–40.

Atkinson RS and Boulton TB (1989). *The history of anaesthesia*. The Parthenon Publishing Group, London.

Bausell RB, Lao L, Bergman S, Lee WL and Berman BM (2005). Is acupuncture analgesia an expectancy effect? Preliminary evidence based on participants' perceived assignments in two placebo-controlled trials. *Evaluation & the Health Professions*, **28**, 9–26.

Benazzouz A and Hallett M (2000). Mechanism of action of deep brain stimulation *Neurology*, **55**(**S6**), S13–S17.

Benazzouz A, Gao DM, Ni ZG, Piallat B, Bouali-Benazzouz R and Benabid AL (2000). Effect of high-frequency stimulation of the subthalamic nucleus on the neuronal activities of the substantia nigra pars reticulate and ventrolateral nucleus of the thalamus in the rat. *Neuroscience*, **99**, 289–95.

Benedetti F (2008a). Mechanisms of placebo and placebo-related effects across diseases and treatments. *Annual Review of Pharmacology and Toxicology*, **48**, 33–60.

—— (2008b). *Placebo effects: understanding the mechanisms in health and disease*. Oxford University Press, Oxford.

Bergman H, Wichmann T, Karmon B and DeLong MR (1994). The primate subthalamic nucleus. II. Neuronal activity in the MPTP model of parkinsonism. *Journal of Neurophysiology*, **72**, 507–20.

Blandini F, Nappi G, Tassorelli C and Martignoni E (2000). Functional changes of the basal ganglia circuitry in Parkinson's disease. *Progress in Neurobiology*, **62**, 63–88.

Bernard C (1865). *An introduction to the study of experimental medicine*. Dover Publications 1957, New York, NY.

Bliss M (1982). *The discovery of insulin*. The University of Chicago Press, Chicago, IL.

Brent L (1997). *A history of transplantation immunology*. Academic Press, San Diego, CA.

Brown P (2003). Oscillatory nature of human basal ganglia activity: relationship to the pathophysiology of Pakinson's disease. *Movement Disorders*, **18**, 357–63.

Brown P, Oliviero A, Mazzone P, Insola A, Tonali P and Di Lazzaro V (2001). Dopamine dependency of oscillations between subthalamic nucleus and pallidum in Parkinson's disease. *Journal of Neuroscience*, **21**, 1033–8.

Bulloch W (1938). *The history of bacteriology*. Oxford University Press.

Collier HOJ (1984). The story of aspirin. In: MJ Parnham and J Bruinvels, eds. *Discoveries in pharmacology*, pp. 555–93. Elsevier, Amsterdam.

DeBakey ME (1985). Medical advances resulting from animal research. In: J Archibald, J Ditchfield and HC Rowsell, eds. *The contribution of laboratory animal science to the welfare of man and animals: past, present and future*, pp. XIX–XXVI. Gustav Fischer Verlag, New York, NY.

Dowling HF (1977). *Fighting infections*. Harvard University Press, Cambridge, MA.

Ehinger BEJ (1986). Animal experimentation ethics from an experimenter's point of view. *Acta Physiologica Scandinavica*, **554**, 69–77.

Elenkov IJ and Chrousos GP (1999). Stress hormones, Th1/Th2 patterns, pro/anti-inflammatory cytokines and susceptibility to disease. *Trends in Endocrinology and Metabolism*, **10**, 359–68.

Elenkov IJ, Wilder RL, Chrousos GP and Vizi ES (2000). The sympathetic nerve – an integrative interface between two supersystems: the brain and the immune system. *Pharmacological Reviews*, **52**, 595–638.

Enck P, Benedetti F and Schedlowski M (2008) New insights into the placebo and nocebo responses. *Neuron*, **59**, 195–206.

Engel G (1977). The need for a new medical model: a challenge for biomedicine. *Science*, **196**, 129–36.

Fink K, Meder W, Dooley DJ and Gothert M (2000). Inhibition of neuronal Ca^2+ influx by gabapentin and subsequent reduction of neurotransmitter release from rat neocortical slices. *British Journal of Pharmacology*, **130**, 900–6.

Finniss DG, Kaptchuk TJ, Miller F and Benedetti F (2010). Biological, clinical and ethical advances of placebo effects. *Lancet*, **375**, 686–95.

French RD (1975). *Antivivisection and medical science in Victorian society*. Princeton University Press, Princeton, NJ.

Gabka J and Vaubel E (1983). *Plastic surgery past and present*. Karger, Basel.

Gordon-Taylor G (1958). *Sir Charles Bell: his life and times*. Livingstone, Edinburgh.

Holzer P and Lembeck F (1983). Analgesia up to the twentieth century. In: MJ Parnham and J Bruinvels, eds. *Discoveries in pharmacology*, pp. 357–77. Elsevier, Amsterdam.

Kaba R and Sooriakumaran P (2007). The evolution of the doctor–patient relationship. *International Journal of Surgery*, **5**, 57–65.

Kaptchuk TJ, Shaw J, Kerr CE et al. (2009). 'Maybe I made up the whole thing': placebos and patients' experiences in a randomized controlled trial. *Culture, Medicine and Psychiatry*, **33**, 382–411.

Katafuchi T, Ichijo T, Take S and Hori T (1993). Hypothalamic modulation of splenic natural killer cell activity in rats. *Journal of Physiology*, **471**, 209–21.

Katafuchi T, Okada E, Take S and Hori T (1994). The biphasic changes in splenic natural killer cell activity following ventromedial hypothalamic lesions in rats. *Brain Research*, **652**, 164–8.

Kirsch I and Sapirstein G (1998). Listening to prozac but hearing placebo: a meta-analysis of antidepressant medication. *Prevention & Treatment*, Available at: http://journals.apa.org/prevention/volume1/pre0010002a.html

Levy R, Dostrovsky JO, Lang AE, Sime E, Hutchinson WD and Lozano AM (2001). Effects of apomorphine on subthalamic nucleus and globus pallidus internus neurons in patients with Parkinson's disease. *Journal of Neurophysiology*, **86**, 249–60.

Levy R, Hutchinson WD, Lozano AM and Dostrowsky JO (2000). High-frequency synchronization of neuronal activity in the subthalamic nucleus of parkinsonian patients. *Journal of Neuroscience*, **20**, 7766–75.

Levy R, Hutchinson WD, Lozano AM and Dostrowsky JO (2002). Synchronised neuronal discharge in the basal ganglia of parkinsonian patients is limited to oscillatory activity. *Journal of Neuroscience*, **22**, 2855–61.

Limousin P, Krack P, Pollak P et al. (1998). Electrical stimulation of the subthalamic nucleus in advanced Parkinson's disease. *New England Journal of Medicine*, **339**, 1105–11.

Linde K, Witt CM, Streng A et al. (2007). The impact of patient expectations on outcomes in four randomized controlled trials of acupuncture in patients with chronic pain. *Pain*, **128**, 264–71.

Livingston A (1983). The sleep of innocence. In: MJ Parnham and J Bruinvels, eds. *Discoveries in pharmacology*, Elsevier, Amsterdam.

Maltete D, Jodoin N, Karachi C et al. (2007). Subthalamic stimulation and neuronal activity in the substantia nigra in Parkinson's disease. *Journal of Neurophysiology*, **97**, 4017–22.

Maurice N, Thierry AM, Glowinski J and Deniau JM (2003). Spontaneous and evoked activity of substantia nigra pars reticulata neurons during high-frequency stimulation of the subthalamic nucleus. *Journal of Neuroscience*, **23**, 9929–36.

Nicoll C and Russell S (1990). Analysis of animal rights literature revels the underlying motives of the movement: ammunition for counter offensive by scientists. *Endocrinology*, **127**, 985–9.

Nini A, Feingold A, Slovin H and Bergman H (1995). Neurons in the globus pallidus do not show correlated activity in the normal monkey, but phase-locked oscillations appear in the MPTP model of parkinsonism. *Journal of Neurophysiology*, **74**, 1800–5.

Okamoto S, Ibaraki K, Hayashi S and Saito M (1996). Ventromedial hypothalamus suppresses splenic lymphocyte activity through sympathetic innervation. *Brain Research*, **739**, 308–13.

Olmstead JMD and Olmstead EH (1952). *Claude Bernard and the experimental method in medicine*. Henry Schuman, New York, NY.

Pariente J, White P, Frackowiak RSJ and Lewith G (2005). Expectancy and belief modulate the neuronal substrates of pain treated by acupuncture. *NeuroImage*, **25**, 1161–7.

Paton W (1994). *Man and mouse: animals in medical research*. Oxford University Press, Oxford.

Pavlov V and Tracey K (2005). The cholinergic anti-inflammatory pathway. *Brain, Behavior, and Immunity*, **19**, 493–9.

Phillips MT and Sechzer JA (1989). *Animal research and ethical conflict*. Springer, Heidelberg.

Price DD, Finniss DG and Benedetti F (2008). A comprehensive review of the placebo effect: recent advances and current thought. *Annual Review of Psychology*, **59**, 565–90.

Rosenbusch G, Oudkerk M and Ammann E (1995). *Radiology in medical diagnostics. Evolution of X-ray applications 1895–1995*. Blackwell Science, Oxford.

Ruesch H (1978). *The slaughter of the innocent*. Bantam Books, New York, NY.

Rupke NA (1987). *Vivisection in historical perspective*. Croom Helm, London.

Scheidemandel HHE (1976). Did George Washington die of quinsy? *Archives of Otolaringology*, **102**, 519.

Selwyn S (1986). The discovery of penicillin and cephalosporins. In: MJ Parnham and J Bruinvels, eds. *Discoveries in pharmacology*, pp. 283–301. Elsevier, Amsterdam.

Shi LH, Luo F, Woodward D and Chang JY (2006). Basal ganglia neural responses during behaviorally effective deep brain stimulation of the subthalamic nucleus in rats performing a treadmill locomotion test. *Synapse*, **59**, 445–57.

Singer W (1993). The significance of alternative methods for the reduction of animal experiments in the neurosciences. *Neuroscience*, **57**, 191–200.

Solomon GF and Moos RH (1964). Emotions, immunity, and disease: a speculative theoretical integration. *Archives of General Psychiatry*, **11**, 657–74.

Sternberg EM (1997a). Emotions and disease: from balance of humors to balance of molecules. *Nature Medicine*, **3**, 264–7.

—— (1997b). Neural-immune interactions in health and disease. *Journal of Clinical Investigation*, **100**, 2641–7.

Tai CH, Boraud T, Bezard E, Bioulac B, Gross C and Benazzouz A (2003). Electrophysiological and metabolic evidence that high-frequency stimulation of the subthalamic nucleus bridles neuronal activity in the subthalamic nucleus and the substantia nigra reticulata. *FASEB Journal,* **17**, 1820–30.

Tracey K (2002). The inflammatory reflex. *Nature*, **420**, 853–9.

Williams D, Tijssen M, Van Bruggen G et al. (2002). Dopamine dependent changes in the functional connectivity between basal ganglia and cerebral cortex in the human. *Brain,* **125**, 1558–69.

Chapter 3

Feeling sick: a combination of bottom-up and top-down events

Summary and relevance to the clinician

1) Feeling sick is a complex combination of events that may arise from damaged peripheral tissues as well as from their modulation by psychosocial factors. Therefore, the clinician must consider a symptom not so much as a single and isolated entity, but rather within the psychological and social context of the patient. The mere assessment of peripheral tissue damage considers bottom-up processes only, without taking the top-down modulation into consideration.

2) Interoceptive sensibility is at the very heart of the process of feeling sick. Whereas usually internal organs are not perceived in normal conditions, they may get access to consciousness in particular circumstances. This is due to the activation of receptors that project to a variety of subcortical and cortical regions. For example, several areas of the cerebral cortex are activated by interoceptive stimuli arising from the gastrointestinal and cardiovascular systems.

3) The insular cortex and the anterior cingulate cortex are key regions in interoceptive processing and in awareness. A peculiar feature of these areas in hominoid primates is the presence of clusters of large spindle-shaped neurons among the pyramidal neurons in layer 5, the so-called von Economo neurons. There is a phylogenetic progression of the von Economo neurons. In fact, they are present in adult humans, but progressively decrease in children, gorillas, and chimpanzees, and are completely lacking in macaque monkeys. Some studies have related the insula to agnosognosia, that is, the lack of awareness about a functional impairment, such that agnosognosic patients do not recognize their own illness.

4) Different emotional states, such as anxiety and depression, or different cognitive tasks, like attention and distraction, may have profound effects on interoceptive awareness, such that perceptions can be reported in different ways from time to time, and interoceptive-evoked brain activity may vary in different circumstances. For example, activation within right

insular and bilateral dorsal anterior cingulate gyrus during oesophageal stimulation is significantly greater with visual presentation of fearful than neutral faces.

5) Pain is a representative symptom and is better understood compared with other symptoms, like nausea and fatigue. Thus, its study helps us better understand bottom-up processes and top-down modulation. Pain is perceived differently in different individuals and in different circumstances, and these differences are attributable to both psychosocial and genetic factors. In order to understand the pain intensity of his patient, the clinician should assess not only the tissue damage, but also his psychological state. This may uncover possible emotion-induced amplification of pain.

6) The descending pain modulatory network is a complex series of cortical and subcortical regions which are interconnected by different neurochemical pathways, e.g. opioidergic, dopaminergic, serotoninergic. These neurotransmitters may inhibit and/or facilitate pain transmission.

7) Feeling sick does not necessarily mean physical suffering. For example, negative emotions, such as anxiety, may be induced by negative diagnoses of asymptomatic diseases or, otherwise, the subject may realize that the colour of his body is changing, as occurs in jaundice. Negative emotions are important in the process of feeling sick because they modulate the magnitude of a symptom, e.g. pain.

8) Negative emotions are processed in the limbic system and can be studied with both imaging techniques and intraoperative electrical stimulation. The latter is particularly interesting because it shows that the ongoing context is crucial in evoking emotional experiences. For example, the emotional responses in the ventral pole of the subthalamic nucleus can be better described as context-dependent rather that site-dependent.

9) The effect of anxiety on pain is one of the most studied. Anxiety-induced hyperalgesia is mediated, at least in part, by cholecystokinin (CCK). In fact, CCK antagonists can prevent it. In addition, expecting pain may induce both hyperalgesic and allodynic effects, and these are related to the enhancement of several subcortical and cortical areas. In the rostroventromedial medulla there are neurons that contain both CCK and opioid receptors and that might take part in the emotional modulation of pain.

10) Other negative emotions, such as anger and depression, impact on pain perception but the mechanisms are less understood compared with anxiety. The amplifying effect of depressive symptoms on pain is likely to be mediated by a functional deficit of the prefrontal cortex and the descending pain modulatory network. According to this perspective,

negative emotions-induced hypo-responsivity of the prefrontal cortex might provide the basis for the aggravation of pain.

11) Overall, the process of feeling sick is an intricate combination of bottom-up and top-down events that eventually initiates the seeking behaviour aimed at suppressing both physical discomfort and negative emotions, as described in the next chapter.

3.1 The patient feels sick through bottom-up and top-down processes

3.1.1 What is a symptom?

How one gets sick is not the purpose of this chapter. Instead, this chapter attempts to look at how one feels sick, regardless of the underlying pathology. Of course, there are plenty of symptoms in different medical conditions, and these reflect the organ or apparatus that is impaired or that is undergoing progressive damage. When one feels sick, he will eventually become a patient, that is, a person who is in need and in search of relief from his discomfort (Chapter 4).

It goes without saying that the concept of symptom is crucial in clinical practice, but it is also particularly interesting from a neuroscientific viewpoint for at least two reasons. First, a symptom emerges from signals arising along a sensory system, thus it can be treated and investigated as any other sensory modality. Second, by definition, a symptom must be perceived by the patient, and this perceptual experience can be analysed by using a neuroscientific approach. Perception of a symptom implies awareness, that is, the patient consciously recognizes that something is going wrong within his own body. In addition, behaviour often changes and these changes can be analysed in a number of ways.

There are a variety of symptoms that do not need to be described in detail here. For example, nausea, fever, itch, and the like may be perceived as signals of malfunctioning of the body. Although the pathways conveying these signals are more or less understood in different medical conditions, there is no need in this context to describe them all. Typically, pain is one of the most common symptoms and, accordingly, section 3.2 will be devoted to it. Today we know how several pathways convey pain signals from the periphery to higher brain centres, as well as these pain signals are modulated by a variety of psychological factors that may either enhance or reduce the global experience of pain. Compared to other symptoms such as nausea, pain processing and modulation are better understood, hence section 3.2 will describe pain in some detail as a representative symptom among many others.

Not only are symptoms experienced, but they usually change the behaviour of the sick. This is particularly important in special non-communicative populations of patients, who cannot report their symptoms to doctors, such as children and the demented elderly (see Chapter 7). Behavioural changes are also important in veterinary medicine, whereby symptoms and diseases must be inferred by behavioural observation only. Apart from specific behavioural changes that are adaptive in nature, like the limitation of movements to avoid pain, from an evolutionary perspective behavioural changes may have different meanings. For example, illness-induced impaired behaviour might be an important signal of need, whereby the animal benefits from signalling its infirmity, e.g. by soliciting parental care (Weary et al. 2009). In this regard, it is interesting to note that behaviour can often be interpreted as a signal of vigour, in which the healthy status of the individual is communicated to the other members of the social group. For example, from a mate choice perspective, females benefit by preferentially responding to healthy males.

Despite the occurrence of specific symptoms in specific conditions, it is important to realize that there are some common concepts that are shared by them all. The sensory experience giving rise to what we call symptom is built up from the periphery to the central nervous system according to bottom-up processes that convey a number of information to the brain. Simultaneously, the incoming sensory experience is shaped by top-down influences that make a symptom different from patient to patient. Therefore, the symptom experience of each patient is unique and is not comparable to others. Many factors can shape it, including cultural factors, as will be described in section 3.2 for pain. Thus the neuroscientific analysis of the sensory signals that build up a symptom gives us important information on both the mechanisms of the symptom itself and complex brain processes.

3.1.2 Detection of a symptom is a combination of interoception and other factors

Interoceptive sensibility, that is, the sensory inputs arising from internal organs, plays a fundamental role in the perception of different symptoms, yet it is not the only one. Pennebaker (1982) and Pennebaker and Hoover (1984) emphasized the distinction between visceral detection and visceral perception. While the former implies the use of physiological information only, the latter relies on both internal physiological information as well as on external environmental information. Age, sex, social and economic status all contribute to symptom perception. Not to mention expectations, which play a crucial role in the perception of many symptoms, such as pain. For example, expecting a painful event leads to hyperalgesia and exaggerated responses to a non-painful stimulus, and this will be addressed in detail in sections 3.2 and 3.3.3.

Interoceptive sensibility, or interoception, refers to the ability to detect the internal organs (Cameron 2002). In general, it only occurs in some

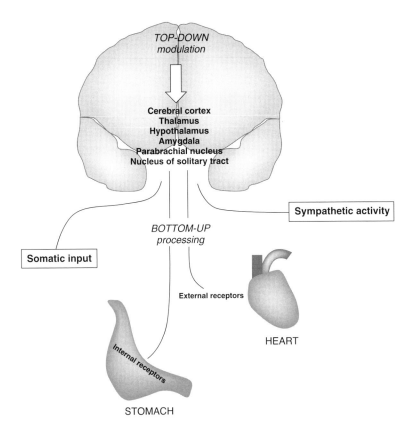

Fig 3.1 General organization of interoceptive sensibility and its modulation. The activity of the viscera can activate either receptors that are located in the surrounding tissue (external) or receptors that belong to the organ itself (internal). The afferent pathways from these receptors reach a variety of subcortical and cortical regions. Besides this bottom-up processing there is an important top-down modulation by a number of cognitive and affective factors. Interoceptive sensibility is also modulated by somatic inputs and by sympathetic activity, as well as by genetic factors.

special circumstances. For example, it is possible to detect the heart beating during intense physical exercise and the motility of the stomach when one is hungry. Normally, at rest, neither the heart nor the stomach can be detected. There are at least two mechanisms through which such perception arises (Fig 3.1). The first is an indirect mechanism, whereby the organ excites nearby receptors. For example, the increased cardiac activity during exercise increases the volume and the displacement of the heart during beating, thus stimulating different receptors in the pericardium, mediastinum, and even in the ribs. The second mechanism is direct, as there are some mechanoreceptors in the organ that are excited by the increased activity. For example, the distension of the stomach activates receptors that are located in the gastric wall.

The fibres from the receptors inside or surrounding the organ reach the spinal cord and ascend through a dedicated lamina-1 spinothalamocortical pathway that converge with vagal afferents to interoceptive centres, such as the nucleus of the solitary tract and different cortical regions, like the insula (Craig 2002). The nucleus of the solitary tract, which represents a very important region in visceral sensory processing receives from visceral afferent pathways that are distributed in different subnuclei: cardiovascular in the medial and dorsolateral, pulmonary in the ventral and ventrolateral, respiratory in the interstitial, and gastrointestinal in the parvocellular (Cameron 2002). Other regions are crucial for interoceptive integration (Fig 3.1), like the parabrachial nucleus, hypothalamus, thalamus, amygdale, and different cortical areas (see section 3.1.3).

This interoceptive sensibility and bottom-up processing, whereby information travels from the periphery to the central nervous system, is not sufficient to produce feelings of sickness. A top-down mechanism is also important (Fig 3.1) and the effects of expectancy, attention, and emotions represent nice examples. Symptoms can be built up in different ways. If a subject expects a specific negative outcome, he may experience real negative outcomes. In a meta-analysis performed by Amanzio et al. (2009), the rates of adverse events in the placebo arms of clinical trials were compared for three classes of anti-migraine drugs: non-steroid anti-inflammatory drugs (NSAID), triptans and anticonvulsants. It was found that the rate of adverse events in the placebo arms of trials with anti-migraine drugs was high and, most interestingly, that the adverse events in the placebo arms corresponded to those of the anti-migraine medication against which the placebo was compared. For example, anorexia and memory difficulties, which are typical adverse events of anticonvulsants, were also more frequent in the placebo arm of these trials. Of course, placebos are inert treatments, thus they lack intrinsic pharmacological properties. Nonetheless, the verbal instructions about the anti-migraine medications are capable of eliciting the very same adverse events in those patients who received a placebo, thus indicating that symptoms can be created on the basis of specific expectations. Therefore, before entering the double-blind arm of a treatment trial, the examiner's instructions about the possible adverse events associated with a specific anti-migraine drug may affect the outcomes in the placebo group. In particular, if the active treatment is presented as an anticonvulsant drug, the examiner may suggest that the patient will experience those adverse events that are specific to this pharmacological class, such as fatigue, anorexia, somnolence, and paraesthesia. On the other hand, if the treatment consists of NSAID, the suggested adverse events may be gastrointestinal symptoms and dry mouth.

The bottom-up processing and the top-down modulation in Fig 3.1 are crucial for generating a variety of symptoms, and their interaction is fundamental for their modulation. However, it should be noted that symptom perception is also influenced by other factors, such as somatic input. For example, somatic stimulation can affect awareness of visceral stimulation. It is possible to reduce awareness of gastric and duodenal distension by stimulating the hand electrically (Coffin et al. 1994). It is also possible to obtain an opposite effect, for example, to inhibit somatic nociceptive reflexes by gastric distension (Bouhassira et al. 1994). Gastrointestinal interoceptive awareness can also be influenced by sympathetic activity. In fact, by increasing sympathetic activity, Iovino et al. (1995) found increased perception of duodenal distension.

Besides the variety of cognitive and affective influences upon interoceptive sensibility, genetic differences, e.g. along the bottom-up processes, must not be forgotten. At different levels, both in the peripheral and the central nervous system, different phenotypes can be responsible for a lower or higher susceptibility to interoceptive stimulation.

3.1.3 Different brain regions respond to interoceptive stimuli

Brain imaging studies have greatly contributed to the understanding of interoceptive processing in the central nervous system. Many regions have been found to be activated by visceral stimulation. In particular, many studies have been performed by applying different types of stimuli to the gastrointestinal tract. For example, the mechanical stimulation of the oesophagus at different intensities, from the mildest stimulus that produces awareness to stronger stimuli, has been found to activate bilaterally the parietal operculum, the insula, and the primary somatosensory cortex (Aziz et al. 1997; Binkofski et al. 1998). The stimulation of the rectum by means of a rectal balloon has been found to increase cerebral blood flow particularly in pre-central motor areas, in the primary somatosensory cortex and in the thalamus, as well as to elicit evoked potentials that are correlated to the amount of distension (Rothstein et al. 1996).

In a study of gastric distension by Stephan et al. (2003), in which an intragastric balloon was inflated and deflated alternately during positron emission tomography scanning, it was found that four key regions were modulated by this mechanical stimulation: dorsal brainstem, left inferior frontal gyrus, bilateral insula, and right subgenual anterior cingulate cortex (Fig 3.2). Interestingly, the brainstem represents vagal projection zones for visceral afferent processing, whereas the inferior frontal gyrus processes food-related stimuli, and the distension of the stomach mimics the ingestion of a meal, thus simulating satiety. In addition, both the insula and subgenual anterior cingulate cortex

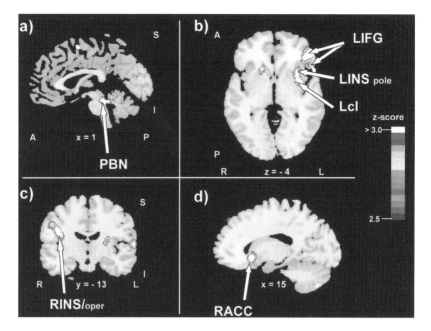

Fig 3.2 Positron emission tomography during stomach distention. Arrows point to areas with significant changes in regional cerebral blood flow in four a priori defined regions of interest involved in visceral sensation: (a) dorsal brain stem nuclei; (b) left inferior frontal gyrus; (b and c) insular cortex/claustrum; (d) subgenual anterior cingulate cortex. A, anterior; I, inferior; L, left; Lcl, left claustrum; LIFG, left inferior frontal gyrus; LINS, left insula; LINS pole, left insular pole; P, posterior; PBN, parabrachial nucleus; R, right; RACC, right anterior cingulate cortex; RINS/oper, right insula/operculum; S, superior; x, sagittal plane; y, coronal plane; z, horizontal plane. See colour plate 1.
Source: From Stephan et al. 2003 with permission from Springer and the Society for Surgery of the Alimentary Tract, Copyright 2003.

respond to emotional stimulation. Taken together, the results of this study show that the stomach projects via vagal afferent pathways to visceral cortical areas that also participate in emotional and affective processing.

Compared to the large number of gastrointestinal studies of interoception, there are fewer number of studies on other systems, such as the cardiovascular and respiratory systems. This is probably attributable to a somehow more difficult methodological approach as well as to a less clear-cut awareness of the heart, vessels, lungs, and respiratory tract. By using maximal inspiration, the Valsalva manoeuvre, and isometric handgrip to induce changes in heart rate, blood pressure, and respiratory function, King et al. (1999) found activations in the insular cortex, medial prefrontal cortex and thalamus. By measuring regional brain activity with functional magnetic resonance during an interoceptive task wherein subjects judged the timing of their own heartbeats, Critchley et al. (2004) observed enhanced activity in the insula, somatomotor cortex, supplementary motor area, and anterior cingulate cortex (Fig 3.3). In this study, there was a striking correlation between the activity in the right anterior insula and the interoceptive performance, such that the insula activity predicted subjects' accuracy in the heartbeat detection task. In addition, local grey matter volume of right anterior insular cortex correlated with both heartbeat detection accuracy and subjective ratings of interoceptive awareness.

3.1.4 The insula plays a crucial role in awareness

A common finding across the different studies investigating interoception is represented by the activation of the insular cortex. There is now compelling experimental evidence that the insula plays a crucial role in, and actually mediates, interoceptive awareness. Although both the anterior cingulate cortex and the insular cortex are typically activated during states of autonomic arousal, the former is related to contextual arousal states whereas the latter is responsible for the representation of different body states (Aziz et al. 2000; Critchley et al. 2000, 2001, 2002).

Besides its role in interoception, the current available evidence suggests that the insula is fundamental in human awareness. This evidence comes from several lines of research in different fields whereby awareness was investigated. For example, insula activation has been found during awareness of body movements, self-recognition, vocalization and music, emotional feelings, like maternal and romantic love, anger, fear, disgust, trust, and empathy. In addition, insula activation is also present during visual-auditory awareness, time perception, attention, perceptual decision making, and cognitive control (Craig 2009). Interestingly, in virtually all studies on emotions, there is a co-activation of the insular and anterior cingulate cortex, which is likely to be based on the dual projection of the lamina-1 spinothalamocortical tract to both regions (Craig 2002, 2009). Whereas the anterior insular cortex is a likely locus of awareness, the anterior cingulate cortex is likely to initiate behaviours.

As emphasized by Craig (2009), a peculiar feature of the anterior insular cortex and the anterior cingulate cortex in hominoid primates is the presence of clusters of large spindle-shaped neurons among the pyramidal neurons in layer 5. These are called von Economo neurons, and Craig proposed that they are the substrate for fast interconnections between the physically separated anterior insular and anterior cingulate cortices. These neurons may underlie the joint activity in the anterior insula and the anterior cingulate cortex. There is

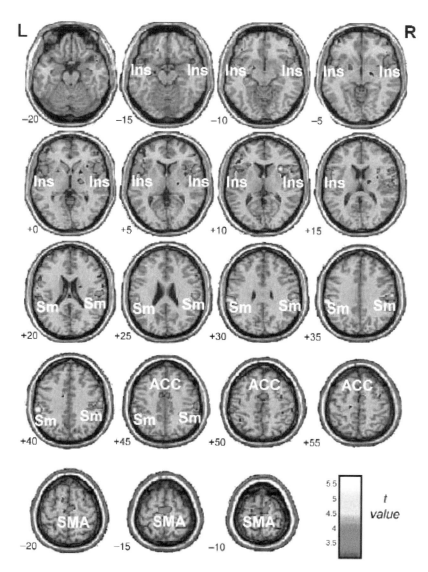

Fig 3.3 Functional magnetic resonance during interoceptive attention, whereby the subjects judge the timing of their own heartbeats. Note the activation in bilateral anterior insula (Ins), lateral somatomotor and adjacent parietal cortices (Sm), anterior cingulate (ACC), and supplementary motor cortices (SMA). See colour plate 3. Source: From Critchley et al. 2004 with permission from Nature Publishing Group, Copyright 2004.

a phylogenetic progression of the von Economo neurons. In fact, they are present in adult humans, but progressively decrease in children, gorillas, and chimpanzees, and completely lack in macaque monkeys (Nimchinsky et al. 1999).

A schematic organization of the human insula is represented in Fig 3.4, in which it can be seen that the primary interoceptive representation is located in the posterior-middle portion, whereas the anterior and ventral portion is occupied by motivational, social and cognitive functions. It is worth noting that the interoceptive representation reaches the anterior border of the insula in macaques, which do not have von Economo neurons, and that the most anterior insula contains von Economo neurons in humans. This suggests that the anterior insula evolved more recently. In other words, the anterior insula has no equivalent in monkeys (Craig 2009). According to Craig (2009), awareness is generated in the insula and the posterior-to-anterior progression of the information is crucial for generating it. In fact, the interoceptive representation in the posterior insula, which conveys homeostatic information from the whole body, are re-integrated in the mid-insula and associated to emotionally salient environmental stimuli. In this regard, it is worth noting that the mid-insula receives information from the nucleus accumbens, which represents an important region for reward and emotional integration (Menon and Levitin 2005).

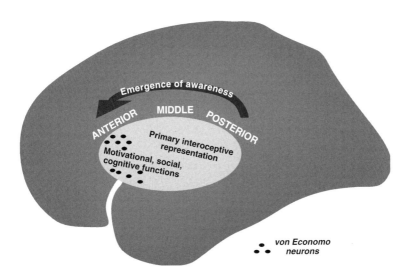

Fig 3.4 Organization of the human insula. The primary interoceptive representation is located in the posterior-middle portion, whereas the anterior and ventral portion is occupied by motivational, social, and cognitive functions. Note that the von Economo neurons, which are completely lacking in macaques, are located mainly in the most anterior part in humans. According to Craig (2009), the posterior-to-anterior progression of the information is crucial for generating awareness.

The progression of information processing to the anterior insula, wherein motivational and social functions are represented, is the final step in this posterior-to-anterior emergence of awareness. Albeit interesting, this model needs validation and further research into insula physiology will be necessary.

Some clinical studies have related the insula to anosognosia, that is, the lack of awareness about a functional impairment, such that anosognosic patients do not recognize their own illness. For example, anosognosia for hemiplegia has been found to be associated to a damage in the right mid-insula (Karnath et al. 2005; Spinazzola et al. 2008). Interestingly, patients with frontotemporal dementia and degeneration of the von Economo neurons in the insula show a loss of emotional awareness (Seeley et al. 2006).

3.1.5 Interoceptive awareness undergoes a top-down modulation

As shown in Fig 3.1, the interoceptive signals arising from the peripheral receptors undergo a top-down modulation by a variety of emotional, motivational, cognitive, and social factors. Therefore, interoceptive sensibility is not always the same, but rather it can increase or decrease according to the type of modulation. Different emotional states, such as anxiety and depression, or different cognitive tasks, like attention or distraction, may have profound effects on interoceptive awareness, such that perceptions can be reported in different ways from time to time. Gastrointestinal function is particularly amenable to top-down influences. For example, irritable bowel syndrome and non-cardiac chest pain are affected by many psychosocial factors which can modulate the perception of the symptoms (Whitehead et al. 1988; Ho et al. 1998).

In a study by Phillips et al. (2003), the brain responses to non-painful oesophageal stimulation was studied in association with emotional stimuli. Either neutral or fearful facial expressions were presented to healthy volunteers while undergoing distension of the oesophagus with a balloon and during scanning with functional magnetic resonance imaging. In this way, both subjective sensations of oesophageal distension and brain responses could be recorded. Activation within right insular and bilateral dorsal anterior cingulate gyrus was found to be significantly greater during oesophageal stimulation with fearful than with neutral faces. In addition, anxiety and discomfort were measured after presentation of faces depicting either low, moderate, or high intensities of fear. Anxiety and discomfort, as well as activation within the left dorsal anterior cingulate gyrus and bilateral anterior insulae, were greater with high-intensity compared with low-intensity expressions. Therefore, visceral stimulation occurring in a negative emotional context is associated with altered brain responses in the anterior cingulate gyrus and insula, which indicates a modulatory effect of emotional context upon interoceptive sensibility.

There are many other regions that process emotional expressions and that are linked to specific emotional responses. For example, whereas expressions of disgust have been found to activate the insula and the ventral striatum (Phillips et al. 1997; Sprengelmeyer et al. 1998), expressions of fear have been found to affect the amygdala (Breiter et al. 1996; Morris et al. 1996; Phillips et al. 1997). Although a few data are available to date, the top-down modulation of interoceptive sensibility is likely to be a complex phenomenon that involves many neural systems and that is associated with specific types of modulation. For example, positive emotions may affect brain responses to visceral stimulation in a completely different way compared to negative emotions. This opposite action of a positive and negative emotional/cognitive context is well known for pain modulation and will be described in section 3.2.

3.2 Bottom-up and top-down processes contribute to the global experience of pain

3.2.1 Pain experience is built up from the periphery to the central nervous system

Pain can be considered a representative symptom for many reasons. First, it is one of the most common symptoms across a variety of medical and surgical conditions. Second, its mechanisms are much better understood compared with other symptoms, like nausea, itch, tiredness, fatigue, and such like. Third, it undergoes an important top-down modulation that can be investigated by using sophisticated biological tools. Therefore, the investigation of pain is particularly interesting for a better understanding of its bottom-up processes from the periphery to the higher centres as well as their top-down modulation by a number of psychological factors.

Usually, when a tissue is damaged, the nerve terminals of the nociceptors may be activated by a variety of factors, such as the mechanical damage itself and the release of endogenous substances. These generate afferent signals in the peripheral and central nociceptive pathways that reach different regions of the brain. To distinguish between bottom-up and top-down events along the pain pathways, it is useful to talk about nociception whenever we refer to all those biophysical and biochemical events that take place from the nociceptors to the higher centres, whereas the word pain is better suited to indicate the global experience of pain, which comes from a combination of nociception (bottom-up) and all the psychologically activated modulatory effects (top-down).

It is common practice to differentiate nociceptive pain, whereby the peripheral nociceptors are activated by a number of physical and chemical factors, from neuropathic pain, in which the damage is not so much at the level of the peripheral tissue, but rather at the level of the nervous system itself, be it peripheral like a nerve trunk or central such as the spinal cord. In addition, somatic pain is different from visceral pain, for the former comes from superficial tissues such as the skin and muscles, whereas the latter originates from the viscera, i.e. the internal organs. These subdivisions are useful to understand the bottom-up processes which underlie the nociceptive transmission from the peripheral structures to the brain.

A schematic diagram depicting the principal structures that are involved in the bottom-up processes from the periphery to the higher centres is shown in Fig 3.5. The receptors responsible for the initiation of pain signals in the periphery are free nerve endings located in most of the body structures and can be associated to two groups of primary afferent fibres, Aδ and C. Unmyelinated, thin (0.4–1.2 μm in diameter) and slowly conducting (0.5–2 m/s) C fibres are activated mainly by a class of receptors called polymodal, for they are responsive to all modalities, i.e. mechanical, thermal, chemical. Their response increases monotonically with stimulus intensity and their receptive field is very small, in the range of a few squared millimetres. By contrast, myelinated, medium-calibre (2–6 μm) and medium-conducting (12–30 m/s) Aδ fibres are classically linked to two main types of receptors: type I and type II mechano-heat nociceptors. Type I are high-threshold mechanoreceptors showing long latency, slow adaptation, and relatively large receptive fields, whereas type II display smaller receptive fields and respond rapidly with a quick adaptation (Treede et al. 1991). Both types are also sensitive to heat (Treede et al. 1995). In addition to Aδ and C fibres, myelinated, large (>10 μm in diameter), fast conducting (30–100 m/s) Aβ fibres can also be involved in nociception. These fibres are excited by weak mechanical stimuli, thus they are termed 'low-threshold', in opposition to 'high-threshold' nociceptors. In normal conditions, they convey touch and other non-noxious information, but they can become responsible for the phenomenon of mechanical allodynia, i.e. the perception of a normally innocuous mechanical stimulus as painful, after tissue injury and/or nerve lesion. By applying noxious heat stimuli on the hairy skin of human subjects, a double pain sensation can be evoked: a pricking acute and very brief impression ('first' pain) is followed after some delay by a dull burning feeling ('second' pain). Substantial evidence links the former to the activity of Aδ type II and the second to that of polymodal C receptors.

Discharge in nociceptive primary afferent fibres does not automatically imply pain perception. By correlating microneurographic recordings with psychophysical curves in human subjects, it was observed that activation is possible at levels of mechanical stimulus intensity below pain threshold. Also, the pain level induced by the same electrical activity of a C fibre can differ by varying stimulus modality (heat or pressure). As with any sensory system, final perception and

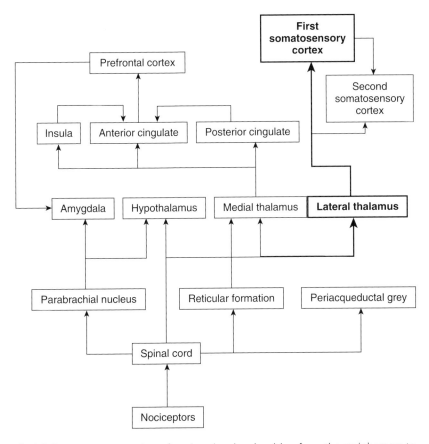

Fig 3.5 Bottom-up processing of nociceptive signals arising from the periphery up to the higher centres. Pathways and regions in bold represent the lateral pain system, which is responsible for sensory-discriminative functions, whereas the remaining pathways and regions represent the medial pain system, which has to do with the emotional component of pain, e.g. unpleasantness and suffering. Note that only the main regions and pathways are shown and, in addition, some overlapping between the lateral and medial system may be present.

evaluation of the stimulus depends on signal processing and integration at subsequent stages, and phenomena like spatial summation or co-activation of other fibres may also play a role (Van Hees and Gybels 1981).

The cell body of the primary afferent fibres is located in the dorsal root ganglia (and in the Gasserian ganglion of the trigeminal nerve). Glutamate is their main neurotransmitter, but often the same presynaptic terminals also release a number of neuropeptides, such as substance P (Willis and Coggeshall 1991). Many attempts have been made to further characterize nociceptive neurons on the basis of their receptor expression, growth factor sensitivity, neurotransmitter and neuromodulator content. For example, a class of neurons containing fluoride-resistant acid phosphatase (FRAP) or peptides (somatostatin and substance P) have been identified (Nagy and Hunt 1982). A second population of neurons, positive to somatostatin and substance P, containing the calcitonin-gene-related peptide (CGRP) and expressing the tyrosine kinase trkA receptor with high affinity for the nerve growth factor (NGF) has also been identified (Silverman and Kruger 1990; Averill et al. 1995), thus showing the high level of complexity of the bottom-up processes from the periphery to the central nervous system. It has been suggested that the two systems provide parallel pathways for the processing of nociceptive information (Hunt and Rossi 1985) and that both cell populations can play a role in the development of chronic pain states, maybe selectively in inflammatory conditions and neuropathic states, respectively (Snider and McMahon 1998).

These processes are plastic and may change in different conditions, for example during development as well as after injury. In fact, during embryogenesis and early postnatal life, the large majority of murine small diameter dorsal root ganglion cells expresses trkA and requires NGF for survival but, as the animal matures, many of these neurons change their trophic factor dependency, down-regulating trkA and up-regulating receptors for the glial cell line-derived neurotrophic factor (GDNF) (Silos-Santiago et al. 1995; Molliver et al. 1997). Similarly, after peripheral axotomy, primary sensory neurons modify neuropeptide expression, down-regulating substance P and CGRP and up-regulating tyrosine and galanin (Hokfelt et al. 1994). There is now compelling evidence of the role of different neurotrophic factors in regulating short- and long-term changes in nociceptor sensitivity and dorsal horn excitability. For example, in many inflammatory conditions, NGF levels increase and its administration in the experimental setting (in animals and humans) provokes sensory abnormalities, like thermal hyperalgesia, which are prevented by anti-NGF antibodies (Lewin et al. 1993; Petty et al. 1994; Woolf et al. 1994; Mendell et al. 1999).

The specificity theory, which considers specific bottom-up processes in the genesis of pain as a separate modality that is encoded and transmitted along a specific channel, finds solid evidence in the existence of high-threshold somatic nociceptors, which are excited only by stimuli intense enough to threaten the integrity of the skin. However, the pattern theory, which postulates the existence of intensity-receptors, still finds support for the visceral district. Here, both specific nociceptors and intensity-receptors have been found in different apparatuses and even in the same organ (Cervero and Jänig 1992; Sengupta and Gebhart 1995).

The central branches of the nociceptive dorsal root ganglion neurons enter the dorsal horn and make synaptic contacts with second-order projecting neurons, interneurons or motoneurons (for spinal reflexes). The grey matter of the spinal cord is classically subdivided cytoarchitectonically into 10 laminae, numbered from I to X, where laminae I to VI make up the dorsal horn, VII to IX the ventral horn, and lamina X is situated around the central canal (Rexed 1952). Nociceptive input is mainly concentrated in laminae I, II, V, VI, and X. Second-order projecting neurones belong to two classes: nociceptive-specific and wide-dynamic range cells. The former receive information only from Aδ and C fibres, whereas the latter receive inputs from nociceptive and Aβ fibres, thus encompassing a much wider range of stimulus intensities (Price and Dubner 1977).

Since the mid-1960s, when the gate control theory of pain was first published (Melzack and Wall 1965), the dorsal horn and its circuitry has become the subject of intense study and hot debate. The theory put forward a model whereby pain impulses could be filtered and modified upon entering the spinal cord (the 'gate'), so that, depending on the simultaneous arrival of nociceptive and non-nociceptive signals and the ensuing balance of activation/ inhibition of inhibitory interneurons, noxious information could gain more or less access to ascending pathways. The theory had its most forceful and lasting impact in the emphasis it posed on the function of the central nervous system as an active dynamic modulator of incoming signals, both in the enhancing and suppressing directions (Melzack 1999). The dorsal horn thus gained consideration as a state-dependent sensory processor, which could be set in different modes (or states), its output being drastically altered by pathological conditions (Woolf 1994).

A substantial increase of the nociceptive output from the dorsal horn occurs in central sensitization, whereby an exaggerated response to painful stimuli can be observed (hyperalgesia). Whereas in peripheral sensitization the pain threshold is decreased by the sensitized Aδ and C high-threshold afferent fibres, in central sensitization low-intensity stimuli can attain the status of pain through the Aβ mechanoreceptors in virtue of the processing at the dorsal horn level (Torebjörk et al. 1992; Treede et al. 1992). The investigation of the anatomical, physiological, and biochemical substrates of these phenomena make the dorsal horn, particularly the first synapse in the pain pathway, one of the hottest spot in pain physiology.

3.2.2 There is not a single pain centre but a distributed system

Spinal cord nociceptive projection neurons convey information upward to the brainstem and diencephalic regions, and hence to the cortex (Willis 1985;

Bonica 1990; Willis and Coggeshall 1991; Willis and Westlund 1997; Yaksh 1998). The spinothalamic tract is the most important ascending pain system, especially in primates and humans, although its role is not exclusively devoted to the conduction of nociceptive information, carrying also temperature and proprioceptive signals. It is formed by fibres originating mainly in the contralateral side, although an uncrossed ipsilateral component has also been described. The fibres are somatotopically arranged, so that the caudal ones are located more laterally and those from progressively more rostral segments join in medioventrally. In the lateral thalamus, the main projection target is the ventral posterior lateral nucleus (VPL), both in its caudal (VPL$_c$) and oral (VPL$_o$) parts. Other projection sites include the ventral posterior inferior nucleus (VPI) and the medial part of posterior thalamus (POm). Nociceptive fibres coming from the trigeminal system convey discriminative information to the thalamic ventral posterior medial nucleus (VPM), forming a trigeminothalamic tract. In the medial thalamus, fibres terminate in the intralaminar nuclear group, especially the central lateral (CL) and parafascicular (PF) nuclei, and in the medial dorsal nucleus (MD), without somatotopic organization.

The spinothalamic pathway is not the only ascending nociceptive system. The spinoreticular and spinomesencephalic tracts carry nociceptive information from the spinal cord to the reticular formation and the midbrain. Collaterals or terminals of ascending fibres contact neurons in a variety of regions, like the caudal medulla, the medial reticular formation, and parabrachial region. In the midbrain, relay stations include the periaqueductal grey (PAG) and the cuneiform nucleus. The majority of fibres follow a crossed path, but ipsilateral projections have also been reported. These pathways represent the anatomical substrate of circuits subserving general functions such as aversive behaviour, arousal, activation of autonomic reflexes. Of relevance to human pain transmission is the dorsal column pathway, which has recently been implicated in visceral nociception (Willis and Westlund 2001).

In Fig 3.5, the intricate organization of the nociceptive pathways and areas from the spinal cord to the higher centres is shown. Part of the spinothalamic tract, the lateral thalamus and its cortical projections to the first somatosensory area (SI) is usually considered to be crucial for pain perception. Electrophysiological recordings and behavioural experiments performed in awake and anaesthetized monkeys, have shown that a variable percentage of ventroposterolateral and ventroposteromedial cells of the lateral thalamus respond to noxious stimuli. These neurons belong to both 'nociceptive specific' and 'wide dynamic range' types, are somatotopically ordered and have small contralateral receptive fields, as do the second-order dorsal horn neurons projecting to these nuclei (Kenshalo et al. 1980; Bushnell and Duncan

1987; Apkarian and Shi 1994). From these nuclei in the lateral thalamus, fibres reach the ipsilateral first SI, whose neurons have been demonstrated to have the same cellular properties as the thalamic neurons (Kenshalo and Isensee 1983; Kenshalo and Douglass 1995). This system, which is shown in bold in Fig 3.5, encodes the sensory-discriminative aspects of pain sensation and is called 'lateral system'.

Parallel and complementary to this lateral pain system, a 'medial system' exists (Treede et al. 1999), whose functions deal with the affective-emotional component of pain, i.e. those aspects regarding its unpleasantness, its negative hedonic quality, and the negative emotions associated with it. Without this emotional aspect, which in one word can be called 'suffering', the pain experience is incomplete and can hardly be defined as such. In Fig 3.5, some of the main regions involved in the medial pain system are shown, e.g. the medial thalamus, the insula and the parietal operculum, the prefrontal and orbito frontal, as well as the anterior and posterior cingulate cortices. Many of these areas are strongly connected with one another and with many other regions of the limbic system, i.e. the ensemble of paleocortical and subcortical structures involved in the global processing of emotions (Papez 1937; MacLean 1990). In contrast to the lateral pain system, here the somatotopic organization is generally lacking, suggesting a role in nonspecific arousal rather than its precise spatial and temporal localization.

It is clear from this brief description of the bottom-up nociceptive processes that there is not a pain centre in which the final pain experience emerges, but rather there is a distributed system that is made up of an intricate network of cortical and subcortical areas, each with some specific functions. This network is often referred to as the 'pain matrix'. Although today we know that different areas of the cerebral cortex belong to this matrix, the idea that the cerebral cortex is involved in the perception of pain is relatively recent. In fact, an early report by Head and Holmes (1911) attributed it only to the thalamus, because even extensive lesions of the cortex never appeared to be associated with changes in pain sensation, and electrical stimulation of the somatosensory cortex during surgery had never been reported to elicit pain (Penfield and Boldrey 1937). In 1951, a study by Marshall evidenced localized loss of pain sensation in patients with parietal lesions (Marshall 1951), and in the 1980s the first nociceptive neurons were recorded in the monkey's first somatosensory area (Kenshalo and Isensee 1983).

Today, the role of the cortex in pain perception is well established. The first and second somatosensory areas appear to be activated simultaneously by pain stimuli, suggesting a preserved direct access of information from thalamus to the second somatosensory cortex and hence to temporal lobe limbic structures involved in learning and memory. The high correlation between stimulus intensity and activity in the contralateral first somatosensory area is not paralleled in the second somatosensory area, where bilateral sharp activation above threshold seems to reflect more the all-or-none recognition of the noxious stimulus rather than its discriminative evaluation (Timmermann et al. 2001).

Human brain imaging studies have been fundamental to better clarify the pain matrix. Following painful stimulation, activation of different cortical regions has been found, such as the first and second somatosensory areas (SI and SII), the anterior cingulate cortex, the insular cortex, and the prefrontal cortex (Davis et al. 1998; Hudson 2000), although some discrepancies are present, such as activations in some studies and de-activations in some others (Bushnell et al. 1999). One explanation for such variation might be the influence of cognitive and affective modulation on the activity of several brain regions (see section 3.2.4).

Whereas the first somatosensory cortex is classically associated to the lateral pain system and the sensory-discriminative component of pain (Fig 3.5), encoding stimulus spatial, temporal, and intensity information, the second somatosensory and the insular cortices have almost constantly been implicated in pain representation: parasylvian lesions can modify pain perception and parasylvian seizures can be painful (Greenspan et al. 1999; Scholz et al. 1999). A potential sensory-discriminative role for these areas is uncertain and still open to discussion. Anatomical data in primates (Apkarian and Shi 1994; Craig et al. 1994) and magnetoencephalographic data in humans (Ploner et al. 1999, 2000) suggest a direct access of nociceptive information to both secondary somatosensory and insular cortex, rather than an indirect pathway via the first somatosensory cortex. Moreover, the insula may also be part of circuits subserving pain affect. In the Schilder-Stengel syndrome, patients with insular lesions suffer from pain asymbolia, whereby pain sensation is normal, but their reaction is anomalous, with inadequate emotional responses and lack of withdrawal (Berthier et al. 1988).

Another cortical area which is also part of the limbic system and which is constantly activated by painful stimuli is the anterior portion of the cingulate gyrus. The cingulate cortex has been proposed to be divided in two distinct regions, on the basis of different cytoarchitecture and connections: an anterior 'executive' portion, engaged in multiple motor functions including those related to affect, and a posterior 'evaluative' portion, involved in visuospatial and mnestic functions (Vogt et al. 1992). The anterior portion can be further subdivided into an 'affect' and a 'cognition' division. The former, extensively connected with the amygdala and the periaqueductal grey, is implicated in the assignment of the emotional content to stimuli and in the evaluation of their motivational value, and takes part in the regulation of endocrine and autonomic functions. The latter, with rich connections to the striatum, contributes to motor control and cognitive response selection, including appropriate pain responsiveness (Devinsky et al. 1995). Imaging studies show that pain-related activity in the anterior cingulate cortex can be selectively modulated by cognitive factors (Petrovic and Ingvar 2002). Interestingly, an illusion of pain, such as the noxious cold produced by a thermal grid with alternated innocuous hot and cold bars, is sufficient to activate it (Craig et al. 1996). In addition, many cognitive/affective manipulations, such as attention, distraction, expectation, and placebo, influence its activity (Longe et al. 2001; Petrovic et al. 2002; Porro et al. 2002) (see section 3.2.4).

Rather than being localized in a pain centre, pain thus appears to be a highly distributed system, whereby the awareness of the different pain components arise from the contribution of many regions, with information processed in a parallel rather than in a serial way (Coghill et al. 1999).

3.2.3 Pain experience changes across individuals and circumstances

Bottom-up mechanisms are not enough to generate the global experience of pain. A painful stimulus can be perceived in different ways in different circumstances, and different individuals may perceive pain differently in the same circumstance. Indeed, pain perception undergoes a complex modulation by a variety of psychological, social, and demographic factors. For example, there is compelling evidence of racial and ethnic differences in pain perception. In a study by Riley et al. (2002), higher levels of unpleasantness and negative affect as well more pain behaviour was found in African-American chronic pain patients compared to whites, whereas no differences in pain intensity reports were found. Likewise, differences in pain perception are present across ages, and these have to do with affect and behaviour rather than intensity and unpleasantness (Riley et al. 2000). The fact that race, ethnicity, and age are related to affect and behaviour of pain suggests that different psychological and social factors may be at work here, such as the different meaning that is attributed to pain in different cultures and ages (Riley and Wade 2004). However, it should be pointed out that genetic factors might be involved as well (see below).

Substantial differences in emotional responses, like depression, anxiety, anger, fear, and frustration, to chronic pain can also be found in females and males. Whereas chronic pain females mainly show frustration, emotional responses in males are characterized by anxiety (Riley et al. 2001). Personality factors have also been found to be related to pain experience. For example, both neuroticism and extraversion have been described as good predictors of pain behaviour and suffering (Wade et al. 1992).

Besides these, race, age, sex, and personality inter-individual differences, the global experience of pain shows a huge variability within the single individual. These intra-individual variations reflect different psychological and social contexts. In other words, the very same noxious stimulus can be experienced differently in different circumstances. It is common clinical practice that directed attention and distraction can be manipulated in a number of ways to reduce pain. For example, music (Kwekkeboom 2003), cartoon movies (Landolt et al. 2002), virtual reality (Hoffman et al. 2000) are all good distracters that have been found to decrease pain in a variety of clinical settings.

One of the main problems to understand the mechanisms of distraction-induced analgesia in the clinical setting is represented by the fact that the presentation of music or a video also alters mood, arousal, and vigilance. Conversely, emotional factors can be controlled in the experimental setting in order to separate emotional from attentional influences. At least two experimental paradigms have been used in the laboratory: spatial attention and cross-modal attention. In the first case, the subject has to attend to two different locations on the body, such as two painful thermal stimuli. In these conditions, subjects are less accurate in detecting a stimulus change if it occurs outside his attentional focus (Bushnell et al. 1985). Similar attentional effects can be found by adopting a cross-modal attention paradigm, whereby subjects have to shift their attention from a painful stimulus to another sensory stimulus, like a sound, and vice versa (Bushnell et al. 1999). In this case, when the subjects attend to a noxious heat stimulus, the primary somatosensory cortex shows the largest attention-related modulation, but lesser effects can also be observed in the anterior cingulate and insular cortices. Conversely, when the subjects attend to an auditory stimulus, a significant reduction in the primary somatosensory cortex activity occurs (Fig 3.6).

Pain experience is also known to be powerfully affected by emotions, whose mechanisms will be described in more detail in section 3.3. For example, hypnotically induced emotional feelings have been found to have a powerful influence on hot water experimental pain. Negative emotions, like sadness–depression, anger–frustration, fear–anxiety, increase both pain intensity and unpleasantness. Conversely, positive emotions, such as relaxation, expected relief, satisfaction, decrease intensity and unpleasantness (Rainville 2004).

It is not easy to separate cultural, cognitive, and emotional factors from genetic variability. Although some studies on ethnic differences in pain perception have been pursued, it is not yet clear whether inter-race differences are mainly attributable to cultural differences or rather to genetic factors. For example, studies of transgenic knockout mice clearly show the existence of at least 102 genes whose knockdown alters pain or analgesic sensitivity, although generally the promising

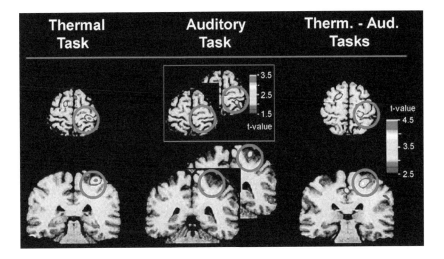

Fig 3.6 The effects of attention on pain processing. When subjects attend to a noxious heat stimulus (left), the primary somatosensory cortex enhances its activity. Conversely, when the subjects attend to an auditory stimulus (centre), a significant reduction of the primary somatosensory cortex activity occurs. Differences in pain-related activity during the two attentional conditions are revealed by subtracting positron emission tomography data recorded during the auditory task from that recorded during the heat-discrimination task (right). See colour plate 2. Source: From Bushnell et al. 1999 with permission of the National Academy of Science USA, Copyright 1999.

targets identified in animals have failed so far to demonstrate clinical efficacy in human trials (LaCroix-Fralish and Mogil 2009). Although genetic association studies of pain have been performed in humans, and at least 23 genes have been found to be associated with experimental pain, clinical pain, or analgesia (excluding headache and migraine genes), it should be noted that there are still open controversies and, most importantly, these studies still remain unreplicated (LaCroix-Fralish and Mogil 2009). Therefore, although inter-individual pain variability may involve both a cultural and genetic component, the latter must be treated with great caution and certainly needs further research and more powerful association studies in human subjects.

3.2.4 A complex neural network is responsible for the top-down modulation of pain

During the past few decades we have learnt that a neural network exists in the brain that is capable of modulating the afferent nociceptive inputs in a variety of ways, from inhibition to facilitation, thereby influencing the global experience of pain in different situations and in different individuals. The pioneering stimulation of periaqueductal grey was shown to produce powerful analgesia in the rat (Reynolds 1969), and stereospecific binding sites in the central nervous system for opioids were then discovered (Pert and Snyder 1973), followed by the identification of endogenous enkephalins (Hughes 1975). Today we know that endogenous opioid neuropeptides are not the only modulators of pain, and in fact many neurotransmitters have been identified that contribute to the intricate modulatory network of nociception (Millan 2002). This network, in turn, represents the biological substrate of the top-down modulation of pain, as occurs in stress-induced analgesia (Willer and Albe-Fessard 1980; Fanselow 1994) and placebo-induced analgesia (Benedetti 2008; Eippert et al. 2009a, b). Several other contexts may be important for the activation of this modulatory network (Fields and Basbaum 1999; Price 1999).

The neuroanatomical organization of the neural circuits that modulate pain is shown in Fig 3.7A. It is characterized by a hierarchical series of descending pathways from the cerebral cortex to sub-cortical regions, like the hypothalamus, amygdala, periacqueductal grey and nucleus of the solitary tract, down to the parabrachial nucleus, the dorsoreticualr nucleus, the rostroventromedial medulla, and the spinal cord (Fields and Basbaum 1999; Millan 2002; Fields 2004). Although the characterization of this descending network mostly relies on experiments performed in animals, there are several lines of evidence, both indirect and direct, that the same pain-modulatory system is present in humans. First, the descending circuitry is highly conserved across different mammalian species, from rodents and cats (Abols and Basbaum 1981) to nonhuman primates (Manning et al. 2001). Second, studies performed by means of positron emission tomography and the radioactive opioid ^{11}C-diprenorphine in humans, confirm previous animal findings about the distribution of endogenous opioids, including regions that belong to the descending pain modulatory system (Jones et al. 1991; Willoch et al. 1999, 2004). Third, some regions in the human cerebral cortex and in the brainstem are affected by both a placebo, which is known to activate endogenous opioid systems, and the rapidly acting opioid agonist remifentanil. In particular, these regions include the anterior cingulate cortex, the orbitofrontal cortex, the lower pons/medulla, and the periacqueductal grey, thus suggesting that the descending anterior cingulate/preiacqueductal grey/rostroventromedial medulla pain-modulating circuit is activated in humans in both placebo and opioid analgesia (Petrovic et al. 2002). In addition, this descending pain control network not only reaches the brainstem (Eippert et al. 2009a), but it also goes down to the spinal cord, thus affecting the early nociceptive processing (Eippert et al. 2009b). Fourth, stimulation of different areas in the

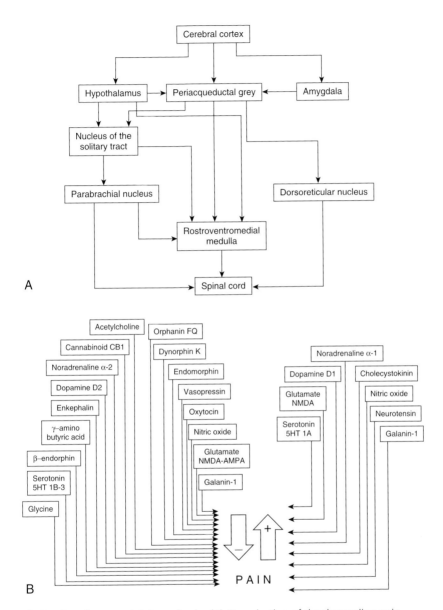

Fig 3.7 Top-down modulation of pain. (A) Organization of the descending pain modulatory network, with the principal regions and pathways. (B) The main neurotransmitters-neuromodulators that are involved in pain modulation, either inhibiting or facilitating pain transmission.

human brain, included the cerebral cortex and the peracqueductal grey, produce analgesia, and this effect is exploited in the clinical setting to treat a variety of painful conditions (Kumar et al. 1997).

As far as the neurochemistry of the pain modulatory network is concerned, the opioid system is one of the best described. Opioid receptors can be found throughout the brain, brainstem, and spinal cord (Pfeiffer et al. 1982; Wamsley et al. 1982; Atweh and Kuhar 1983; Sadzot et al. 1991; Fields and Basbaum 1999; Fields 2004). These receptors may exert analgesic effects through different mechanisms (Jensen 1997), such as modulation at the spinal level and/or control of cortical and brainstem regions. The modulation of the spinal cord is one of the best described (Fields and Basbaum 1999; Fields 2004). The opioid system in the brainstem is constituted of different regions, like the periacqueductal grey, the parabrachial nuclei, and the rostroventromedial medulla (Fields and Basbaum 1999; Fields 2004). Although the opioid receptors are less characterized in the cortex, autoradiographic studies indicate high concentrations of opioid receptors in the cingulate cortex and prefrontal cortex (Wamsley et al. 1982; Pfeiffer et al. 1982; Sadzot et al. 1991) and one of the highest levels of opioid receptor binding has been found in the anterior cingulate cortex (Vogt et al. 1993). Positron emission tomography with the radioactive opioid ^{11}C-diprenorphine, confirm previous animal and human autoradiography findings (Jones et al. 1991; Willoch et al. 1999, 2004). In addition, opioid receptor agonists, such as remifentanil and fentanyl have been shown to act on several regions known to be involved in pain-processing and containing high concentrations of opioid receptors (Firestone et al. 1996; Adler et al. 1997; Casey et al. 2000; Wagner et al. 2001; Petrovic et al. 2002).

Many other neurotransmitters and neuromodulators have been found to modulate pain, as shown in Fig 3.7B. Not only is pain inhibited but it is also facilitated by a variety of endogenous neurochemical systems (Millan 2002). It is difficult to identify a specific action for many neurotransmitters, for they may act as both inhibitory and facilitatory agents. For example, dopaminergic, noradrenergic, and serotoninergic systems may be both inhibitory and facilitatory, probably depending on at least two factors. First, the receptor that is involved is crucial (Fig 3.7B), such as the dopaminergic D1 and D2, the noradrenergic α-1 and α-2, the serotoninergic 1B and 1A (Millan 2002). Second, different combinations of different neurotransmitters may shift the balance from inhibition to facilitation, and vice versa.

Although it is not always clear when and how these systems are activated, different psychological and social factors are likely to represent the adequate stimuli for their activation. A subtle and finely tuned psychosocial modulation is likely to affect these networks in different circumstances and in different individuals. In the previous section, we have seen that attention, distraction, social differences across ethnic groups, ages, and sexes, are all factors that may affect these neurochemical systems. Today, one of the best models that helps us understand these intricate psychological-neurochemical interactions is represented by placebo analgesia and nocebo hyperalgesia (Benedetti 2008), whereby several complex psychosocial factors may activate different neurotransmitters and different systems (see also section 3.3.3 and Chapter 6).

3.3 Emotions influence the perception of symptoms

3.3.1 Feeling sick does not necessarily mean physical suffering

Although physical suffering represents one of the most common situations that make a subject feel sick, the subjective sensation of symptoms like pain, nausea, dyspnoea, and the like, is not always present. For example, a subject may notice that the colour of his own body is changing, as in the case of jaundice, or that a body part is losing its shape, as occurs with a deforming tumour. In these cases, there is no physical suffering but rather psychological suffering, whereby negative emotions, like fear and anxiety, make a subject feel sick. Likewise, an individual may realize that something is going wrong within his own body by sheer chance, without any sensory feedback (i.e. without any symptom). This is quite common whenever a radiological or blood examination uncovers asymptomatic pathologies. Again, in these cases also, negative diagnoses lead to negative emotions. In order for a subject to feel sick, psychological suffering is not very different from physical suffering. Negative emotions trigger the seeking behaviour that will be described in Chapter 4 in the same way as physical suffering does.

Therefore, during the process of feeling sick, several events may take place. First, feeling sick may depend on the occurrence of physical suffering like pain. Second, the subject may detect something unusual through his own senses, such as his own body changing colour, and this in turn leads to fear and anxiety. Third, the subject learns from instrumental examinations that something within his own body does not work properly, and again this induces fear and anxiety. In all these cases, negative emotions are at the very heart of the process of feeling sick. Even in the case of physical suffering (e.g. pain), fear and anxiety about the origin and the cause of the pain take the same form as with negative diagnoses. Pain itself has an important emotional component (see section 3.2), although it differs from an emotion in that it requires the presence of a bodily sensation with qualities like those reported during tissue-damaging stimulation (Price 1999; Rainville 2004).

The important role of negative emotions in the process of feeling sick resides not so much in the fact that fear, anxiety, and depression are normal components of illness, but rather in the fact that they may influence the symptom itself. Catastrophizing about pain and fear of pain may have dramatic effects on the global pain experience (Asmudson et al. 2004). Pain perception can be modulated in a number of ways by negative emotions, so that the patient's report of his own pain is tightly related to his negative emotions. Therefore, whenever the magnitude of a symptom is assessed, this must be considered as inseparable from the patient's negative emotions.

3.3.2 Positive and negative emotions are processed in the limbic system

Positive and negative emotions can be described from different perspectives. For example, they can be conceptualized in terms of opposite subjective experiences, like pleasure on the one hand and discomfort on the other, or otherwise they can be viewed as opposite action tendencies, whereby approaching behaviour characterizes positive emotions whereas avoidance behaviour represents negative emotions. The level of arousal can be considered as well, with calmness and relaxation as the main components of positive emotional states and alertness and excitation as the main characteristics of negative emotional states. While excitement involves urges to move, depression is associated with lack of desire to move, and whereas satisfaction is associated with calmness and warmth, anxiety is associated with inner tension in the viscera (Price et al. 1985). Many overlaps do exist though, for example high arousal levels are often shared by both negative and positive emotions, such as fear and happiness, respectively. Indeed, rather than two opposite emotional states only, positive and negative, several discrete emotional states have been recognized and described over the last centuries, from Darwin (1872) to MacLean (1970, 1990) and to Ekman (1999), just to mention a few notable authors.

Several discrete emotions have been recognized such as happiness, surprise, sadness, anger, disgust, and fear. These are better described as representing subsets of positive and negative emotional states, and both positive and negative emotions can be further subdivided into subgroups of basic, general, and specific emotions. For example, basic emotions are deprivation of food and water or satisfaction by sex; general emotions are sadness, fear or happiness and enthusiasm; specific emotions are bad/nice sound or disgusting/good taste. Different emotional states have been found to be related to specific changes in viscerosomatic activity, starting from the classical James-Lange theory of emotions to more recent studies (Ekman et al. 1983; Levenson et al. 1990; Vernet-Maury et al. 1999; Rainville 2004). Cognitive factors have been found to be involved as well, whereby evaluative processes are crucial in the emotional state that is experienced, while viscerosomatic activity would contribute only to the level of arousal but not to the quality of the emotion (Schacter and Singer 1962).

Different areas of the limbic system are involved in emotional processing and have been found to be activated during the evocation of specific emotions, like happiness, sadness, fear, anger, and disgust (Lane et al. 1997; Damasio et al. 2000). For example, Damasio et al. (2000) found that the activity in the anterior cingulate cortex increases in anger and sadness and decreases in happiness. Interestingly, many of these areas belong to the pain neuromatrix, such as the anterior cingulate cortex, the insula, the parietal operculum, the hypothalamus, the amygdala, and some loci in the brainstem. This shared network by emotion and pain emphasizes that common physiological processes may be at work here, and points out to the importance of the emotional component of the pain experience (Rainville 2004). In this regard, it is worth noting that changes in pain unpleasantness are related to changes in anterior cingulate cortex activity (e.g. Rainville et al. 1997).

Different human limbic regions are sensitive to electrical stimulation. Their activation by passing electrical current through implanted electrodes may elicit subjective emotional experiences. For example, different portion of the subthalamic region, such as the associative-limbic portion of the subthalamic nucleus has been reported to produce emotion-related responses, such as euphoria and hypomania (Ghika et al. 1999) and mirthful laughter (Krack et al. 2001), and its long-lasting stimulation may have important effects on mood, either positive or negative (Berney et al. 2002; Funkiewiez et al. 2003; Schneider et al. 2003). In addition, the stimulation of the substantia nigra pars reticulata has been found to induce acute depression (Bejjani et al. 1999; Kumar et al. 1999).

Brain stimulation studies must be interpreted with caution, at least as far as the anatomical localization is concerned. In fact, the stimulation of a site may activate, either orthodromically or antidromically, distant regions, thus making it difficult to localize a given emotional experience. Despite these neuroanatomical limitations, some interesting findings have emerged. In general, studies on the stimulation of the limbic system indicate that the particular responses evoked are not related to specific electrode locations, but rather to the subject's psychological traits and concerns. In other words, limbic stimulation appears to produce effects that are dependent on the ongoing context (Halgren 1982; Benedetti et al. 2004; Lanotte et al. 2005). For example, the emotional responses in the ventral pole of the subthalamic nucleus can be better described as context-dependent rather that site-dependent. In fact, the stimulation of the subthalamic nucleus ventral pole and the adjacent substantia nigra pars reticulata evokes emotional and autonomic responses that vary according to the experimental condition, e.g. expected versus unexpected stimulation (Benedetti et al. 2004).

3.3.3 Anxiety about pain activates brain circuits that increase the pain

Understanding how negative emotions impact on the perception of a symptom, such as pain, is of paramount importance, and good medical practice should consider this influence as a crucial point in the doctor–patient relationship. For this reason, some details will be given here for anxiety and pain, one of the most studied topics in this regard. In general, negative emotions are good predictors of pain-related behaviour, according to the rule 'the more intense the negative emotional state, the more intense the pain'. In fact, the majority of studies using mood induction on experimentally induced pain found that positive mood reduces pain perception whereas negative mood increases pain perception. Many strategies to induce positive or negative mood have been used, such as exposure to film scenes, reading depressive or elative statements, listening to different types of music, smelling pleasant and unpleasant odours, and the presentation of various emotive pictures (Wiech and Tracey 2009).

Negative emotions that are induced by telling a subject that a painful stimulation will be delivered shortly, may result in either amplification of pain if a mild pain stimulus is delivered (hyperalgesia) or even in the perception of pain when a tactile stimulus is applied (allodynia). A study by Colloca et al. (2008) used a nocebo procedure, whereby verbal suggestions of painful stimulation were given to healthy volunteers before administration of either tactile or low-intensity painful electrical stimuli. This study clearly showed that these anxiogenic verbal suggestions are capable of turning tactile stimuli into pain as well as low-intensity painful stimuli into high-intensity pain. Therefore, by defining hyperalgesia as an increase in pain sensitivity and allodynia as the perception of pain in response to innocuous stimulation, nocebo suggestions of a negative outcome can produce both hyperalgesic and allodynic effects.

Sawamoto et al. (2000) found that expectation of painful stimulation amplifies perceived unpleasantness of innocuous thermal stimulation. These psychophysical findings were correlated to enhanced transient brain responses to the non-painful thermal stimulus in the anterior cingulate cortex, the parietal operculum and posterior insula (Fig 3.8). This enhancement consisted in both a higher intensity signal change (in the anterior cingulate cortex) and a larger volume of activated voxels (in the parietal operculum and posterior insula). Therefore, expecting a

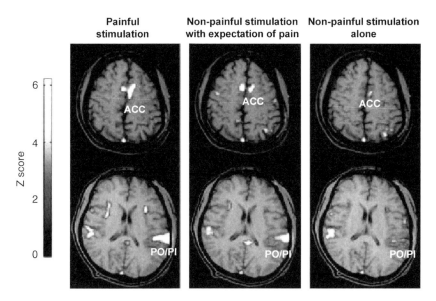

Fig 3.8 The effects of expecting pain on pain processing. Some areas of the pain matrix, such as the anterior cingulate cortex (ACC), the parietal operculum (PO), and posterior insula (PI), enhance their activity in response to non-painful stimulation when expecting pain (centre). The level of activation is almost similar to that following a real painful stimulation (left). By contrast, non-painful stimulation alone induces significant smaller activations (right). See colour plate 4.
Source: From Sawamoto et al. 2000, with permission from The Society for Neuroscience, Copyright 2000.

painful stimulus enhances both the subjective unpleasant experience of an innocuous stimulus and the objective responses in some brain regions.

Overall, expectations of a negative outcome, in this case the increase of pain, may result in the amplification of pain (Koyama et al. 1998; Price 2000; Dannecker et al. 2003), and several brain regions, like the anterior cingulate cortex, the prefrontal cortex, the insula, and the hippocampus have been found to be activated during the anticipation of pain in a variety of studies (Chua et al. 1999; Hsieh et al. 1999; Ploghaus et al. 1999, 2001; Porro et al. 2002, 2003; Koyama et al. 2005; Lorenz et al. 2005; Keltner et al. 2006). These effects are opposite to those elicited by positive expectations, whereby subjects expect pain reduction. In some studies, in which both positive and negative outcomes have been investigated with the same experimental approach, the modulation of both subjective experience and brain activation has been found. For example, in the study by Koyama et al. (2005), as the magnitude of expected pain increased, activation increased in the thalamus, insula, prefrontal cortex, and anterior cingulate cortex. By contrast, expectations of decreased pain reduced activation of pain-related brain regions, like the primary somatosensory cortex, the insular cortex and anterior cingulate cortex. In a different electroencephalographic study in which source localization analysis was performed, Lorenz et al. (2005) found a modulation of the electrical dipole in the secondary somatosensory cortex by nocebo-like and placebo-like suggestions. The dipole was modulated in the same direction of expectations, shrinking when pain decrease was expected and expanding when pain increase was anticipated.

In a similar study by Keltner et al. (2006), it was found that the level of expected pain intensity alters perceived pain intensity along with the activation of different brain regions. By using two visual cues, each conditioned to one of two noxious thermal stimuli (high and low), the authors showed that subjects reported higher pain when the noxious stimulus was preceded by the high-intensity visual cue. By comparing the brain activations produced by the two visual cues, these authors found significant differences in the ipsilateral caudal anterior cingulate cortex, the head of the caudate, the cerebellum, and the contralateral nucleus cuneiformis.

The link between negative emotions and pain increase has also been studied with a pharmacological approach, in order to identify possible neurotransmitters that are involved in anxiety-induced pain increase. By using an anxiogenic nocebo procedure, whereby an inert treatment is given along with verbal suggestions of pain worsening, Benedetti et al. (1997) gave proglumide, a nonspecific cholecystokinin (CCK) antagonist for both CCK-A and CCK-B receptors, or CCK-1 and CCK-2 according to the new classification (Noble et al. 1999), to postoperative patients during a post-surgical manipulation. Anxiety(nocebo)-induced hyperalgesia was found to be prevented by proglumide in a dose-dependent manner, thus suggesting that this effect is mediated by CCK. Whereas a dose as low as 0.05 mg was ineffective, a dose increase up to 0.5 mg and 5 mg proved to be effective. As CCK is also involved in anxiety mechanisms, it was hypothesized that proglumide affected anticipatory anxiety of the impending pain (Benedetti and Amanzio 1997; Benedetti et al. 1997). This effect was not antagonized by naloxone, thus indicating that it is not opioid-mediated.

In order to overcome some ethical limitations that were present in this clinical study, a similar experimental approach was used in healthy subjects. By investigating experimental ischemic arm pain, Benedetti et al. (2006) performed a detailed neuropharmacological study of anxiety(nocebo)-induced hyperalgesia. It was found that the oral administration of an inert substance, along with verbal suggestions of hyperalgesia, induced hyperalgesia and hyperactivity of the hypothalamic-pituitary-adrenal axis, as assessed by means of adrenocorticotropic hormone (ACTH) and cortisol plasma concentrations. Both nocebo-induced hyperalgesia and hypothalamus-pituitary-adrenal hyperactivity were blocked by the benzodiazepine, diazepam, thereby suggesting an involvement of anxiety. By contrast, the administration of the mixed CCK type-A/B receptor antagonist, proglumide, blocked nocebo hyperalgesia completely, but had no effect on hypothalamus-pituitary-adrenal hyperactivity, which suggests a specific involvement of CCK in the hyperalgesic but not in the anxiety component of the nocebo effect. Both diazepam and proglumide did not show analgesic properties on baseline pain, as they acted on the anxiety-induced pain increase only. These data indicate a close relationship between anxiety and nocebo hyperalgesia, but they also indicate that proglumide does not act by blocking anticipatory anxiety of the impending pain, as previously hypothesized (Benedetti and Amanzio 1997; Benedetti et al. 1997), but rather it interrupts a CCKergic link between anxiety and pain (Fig 3.9).

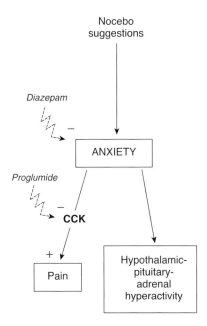

Fig 3.9 Negative verbal suggestions of pain worsening (nocebo) induce anxiety which, in turn, affects both the hypothalamus-pituitary adrenal axis and pain mechanisms. The link between anxiety and pain is represented by cholecystokinin (CCK), which has a facilitating effect on pain. Benzodiazepines, like diazepam, can block anxiety, thus preventing both hypothalamic-pituitary-adrenal hyperactivity and hyperalgesia. CCK antagonists, like proglumide, block the CCKergic anxiety-pain link only. Therefore, CCK antagonists do not inhibit pain per se but rather the anxiety-pain link.
Source: From Benedetti et al. 2006 with permission from The Society for Neuroscience, Copyright 2006.

Similar mechanisms are present in animals. For example, in a social-defeat model of anxiety in rats, it was shown that CI-988, a selective CCK-B receptor antagonist, prevents anxiety-induced hyperalgesia, with an effect that is similar to that produced by the anxiolytic drug, chlordiazepoxide (Andre et al. 2005). Similarly, other studies that used selective CCK-A and CCK-B receptor antagonists in animals and humans have shown the important role of CCKergic systems in the modulation of anxiety and in the link between anxiety and hyperalgesia (Benedetti and Amanzio 1997; Hebb et al. 2005). The pro-nociceptive and anti-opioid action of CCK has been documented in the brainstem in animals. For example, it has been shown that CCK is capable of reversing opioid analgesia by acting at the level of the rostroventromedial medulla, a region that plays a key role in pain modulation (Mitchell et al. 1998; Heinricher et al. 2001). It has also been shown that CCK activates pain-facilitating neurons within the rostroventromedial medulla (Heinricher and Neubert 2004).

In the rostroventromedial medulla of the rat there are neurons expressing both μ-opioid receptors and CCK-2 (or CCK-B according to the old classification) receptors. Over 80% of these cells co-express both receptors, whereas about 15% express only CCK-2, and very few cells express μ-opioid receptors only (Fig 3.10). Selective lesions of CCK-2 and μ-opioid expressing cells do not alter the basal sensory thresholds but abolish the hyperalgesia induced by microinjection of CCK into the rostroventromedial medulla, which suggests that these CCK-2/μ-opioid co-expressing rostroventromedial neurons facilitate pain and can be directly activated by CCK input to the rostroventromedial medulla (Zhang et al. 2009). The balance between opioid and CCK activity in these neurons might contribute to the affective/cognitive modulation of pain, although further research on this should be pursued in humans.

Whereas in anxiety-induced hyperalgesia the anxiety is about the pain itself, in stress-induced analgesia the anxiety is about a stressor that shifts the attention from the pain itself, e.g. towards a threatening stimulus in the environment (Colloca and Benedetti 2007). Therefore, directed attention plays a key role, as shown in Fig 3.11. In the case of anxiety-induced hyperalgesia, whereby attention is focused on the impending pain, the biochemical link between this anticipatory anxiety and the pain increase is represented by the CCKergic systems. Conversely, in stress-induced analgesia, a general state of arousal stems from a stressful situation in the environment, so that attention is now focused on the environmental stressor. In this case, there is experimental evidence that analgesia results from the activation of the endogenous opioid systems (Willer and Albe-Fessard 1980; Terman et al. 1986; Flor and Grusser 1999).

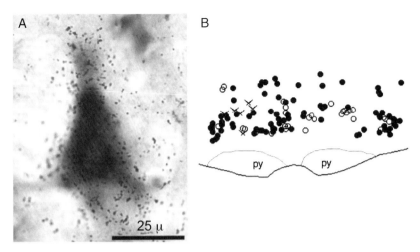

Fig 3.10 Double hybridization histochemistry for CCK-2 (or CCK-B according to the old classification) and μ-opioid receptors transcripts in the rostroventromedial medulla of the rat. (A) A pyramidal neuron in the rostroventromedial medulla labelled for both CCK-2 (silver grains) and μ-opioid (dark blue) receptors. (B) Map of neurons co-labelled for CCK-2 and μ-opioid receptors (closed circles), CCK-2 receptors only (open circles), and μ-opioid receptors only (crosses) in the rostroventromedial medulla. Note that most neurons co-express both μ-opioid and CCK-2 receptors. py, pyramid. See colour plate 5.
Source: From Zhang et al. 2009, with permission from Oxford University Press, Copyright 2009.

It is worth noting that the CCK and opioid neuromodulatory systems can modulate emotional states and other external signals as well, such as visual stimuli. In fact, the CCK agonist pentagastrin has been found to increase the rating of unpleasantness for both neutral and unpleasant pictures, and to decrease the rating of pleasantness for neutral pictures. By contrast, the opioid agonist remifentanil increases the pleasantness for neutral pictures. These findings indicate that CCK and opioids modulate how external stimuli, and not only noxious stimuli, are emotionally perceived (Gospic et al. 2008).

3.3.4 Anger and depression influence pain perception

Compared to anxiety, much less is known about the neurobiological mechanisms that link other negative emotions, like anger and depression, to pain and other symptoms. Anger affects pain more severely when it is directed at oneself than when directed at others, such as health care providers (Okifuji et al. 1999). Therefore, as we have seen for anxiety-induced hyperalgesia and stress-induced analgesia in the previous section, in this case also, the target of the

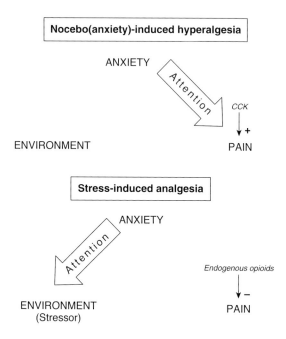

Fig 3.11 Whereas in nocebo(anxiety)-induced hyperalgesia attention is focused on the pain and cholecystokinin (CCK) induces pain facilitation, in stress-induced analgesia attention is directed to a stressor in the environment and endogenous opioids inhibit the pain.
Source: From Colloca and Benedetti 2007 with permission from Wolters Kluwer Health and Lippincott Williams & Wilkins, Copyright 2007.

emotion is important. Anger has been found to induce more consistent changes in pain unpleasantness rather than pain intensity (Huynh Bao and Rainville 2003; Rainville 2004). In addition, anger activates some regions of the brain that are also involved in pain processing, like the anterior cingulate cortex, the amygdale, and the brainstem (Damasio et al. 2000). There is also some experimental evidence that the endogenous opioid systems are involved in anger-associated changes in pain. In fact, a reduction in endogenous opioid activity has been found during anger (Bruehl et al. 2002, 2003).

There is also a clear-cut link between depression and pain. A high degree of co-morbidity between chronic pain and depression is widely recognized (Vimpari et al. 1995; Feinmann 1999; Korszun 2002; Mongini et al. 2007), and there is compelling evidence that depressed pain-free individuals are on average two times more likely to develop chronic musculoskeletal pain than non-depressed pain-free individuals (Magni et al. 1994; Carroll et al. 2004; Larson et al. 2004). It should be noted, however, that patients suffering from major depression can show normal or even reduced sensitivity to noxious stimuli applied to the skin (Bar et al. 2003, 2006, 2007; Dickens et al. 2003; Lautenbacher et al. 1994), but show hyperalgesia for deep somatic pain (Bar et al. 2005), which indicates a high degree of variability in this population of patients. Neuroimaging studies in patients with major depression disorder have shown higher activation levels in left ventrolateral thalamus, the right ventrolateral prefrontal cortex, and the dorsolateral prefrontal cortex (Bar et al. 2007), and increased activation in the right amygdala and decreased activation in periaqueductal grey, rostral anterior cingulate, and prefrontal cortices (Strigo et al. 2008). In addition, Giesecke et al. (2005) found that fibromyalgia patients with major depression showed bilateral amygdala activation and a signal increase in the anterior insula following painful stimulation, whereas fibromyalgia patients without depressive symptoms showed no changes. Likewise, Schweinhardt et al. (2008) found an activation cluster in the medial prefrontal cortex of rheumatoid arthritis patients that correlated with the degree of depressive symptoms.

A lack of descending inhibition (see section 3.2.4) might be one of the mechanisms which is responsible for these effects (Julien et al. 2005; Klauenberg et al. 2008), but the activation of descending facilitatory pathways may also occur, and indeed studies in animals have identified a descending facilitatory projection from the periaqueductal grey to the rostral ventral medulla inducing pro-nociceptive effects (Carlson et al. 2007) (see also the previous section 3.3.3). Key regions in this descending pain modulatory network are prefrontal, anterior cingulate, and insular cortices, amygdala, hypothalamus, and brainstem structures like the periaqueductal grey, rostral ventromedial medulla, dorsolateral pons/tegmentum, and the descending projections to the spinal dorsal horn, although the prefrontal cortex is likely to play a major role (Tracey and Mantyh 2007; Wiech and Tracey 2009). According to this perspective, a negative emotions-induced hypo-responsivity of the prefrontal cortex might provide the basis for the aggravation of pain. In other words, the prefrontal hypo-responsivity might be triggered by negative emotions (Wiech and Tracey 2009). Interestingly, Wager et al. (2008) found evidence that the activation of the prefrontal cortex leads to a reduction in negative emotion by influencing those structures that are directly involved in emotional experiences.

References

Abols IA and Basbaum AI (1981). Afferent connections of the rostral medulla of the cat: a neural substrate for midbrain-medullary interactions in the modulation of pain. *Journal of Comparative Neurology*, **201**, 285–97.

Adler LJ, Gyulai FE, Diehl DJ, Mintun MA, Winter PM and Firestone LL (1997). Regional brain activity changes associated with fentanyl analgesia elucidated by positron emission tomography. *Anesthesiology and Analgesia*, **84**, 120–6.

Amanzio M, Latini Corazzini L, Vase L and Benedetti F (2009). A systematic review of adverse events in placebo groups of anti-migraine clinical trials. *Pain*, **146**, 261–69.

Andre J, Zeau B, Pohl M, Cesselin F, Benoliel JJ and Becker C (2005). Involvement of cholecystokininergic systems in anxyety-induced hyperalgesia in male rats: behavioral and biochemical studies. *Journal of Neuroscience*, **25**, 7896–904.

Apkarian AV and Shi T (1994). Squirrel monkey lateral thalamus. I. Somatic nociresponsive neurons and their relation to spinothalamic terminals. *Journal of Neuroscience*, **14**, 6779–95.

Asmudson G, Vlaeyen J and Crombez G (2004). *Understanding and treating fear of pain.* Oxford University Press, Oxford.

Atweh F and Kuhar MJ (1983). Distribution and physiological significance of opioid receptors in the brain. *British Medical Bulletin*, **39**, 47–52.

Averill S, McMahon SB, Clary DO, Reichardt LF and Priestley JV (1995). Immunocytochemical localization of trkA receptors in chemically identified subgroups of adult rat sensory neurons. *European Journal of Neuroscience*, **7**, 1484–94.

Aziz Q, Anderson JLR, Valind S et al. (1997). Identification of human brain loci processing esophageal sensation using positron emission tomography. *Gastroenterology*, **113**, 50–9.

Aziz Q, Schnitzler A and Enck P (2000). Functional neuroimaging of visceral sensation. *Journal of Clinical Neurophysiology*, **17**, 604–12.

Bar KJ, Brehm S, Boettger MK, Boettger S, Wagner G and Sauer H (2005). Pain perception in major depression depends on pain modality. *Pain*, **117**, 97–103.

Bar KJ, Brehm S, Boettger MK, Wagner G, Boettger S and Sauer H (2006). Decreased sensitivity to experimental pain in adjustment disorder. *European Journal of Pain*, **10**, 467–71.

Bar KJ, Greiner W, Letsch A, Kobele R and Sauer H (2003). Influence of gender and hemispheric lateralization on heat pain perception in major depression. *Journal of Psychiatric Research*, **37**, 345–53.

Bär KJ, Wagner G, Koschke M, Boettger S, Boettger MK, Schlösser R et al. (2007). Increased prefrontal activation during pain perception in major depression. *Biological Psychiatry*, **62**, 1281–7

Bejjani BP, Damier P, Arnulf I, Thivard L, Bonnet AM, Dormont D et al. (1999). Transient acute depression induced by high-frequency deep-brain stimulation. *New England Journal of Medicine*, **340**, 1476–80.

Benedetti F (2008). Placebo effects: understanding the mechanisms in health and disease. Oxford University Press, Oxford.

Benedetti F and Amanzio M (1997). The neurobiology of placebo analgesia: from endogenous opioids to cholecystokinin. *Progress in Neurobiology*, **52**, 109–25.

Benedetti F, Amanzio M, Casadio C, Oliaro A and Maggi G et al. (1997). Blockade of nocebo hyperalgesia by the cholecystokinin antagonist proglumide. *Pain*, **71**, 135–40.

Benedetti F., Amanzio M, Vighetti S and Asteggiano G (2006). The biochemical and neuroendocrine bases of the hyperalgesic nocebo effect. *Journal of Neuroscience*, **26**, 12014–22.

Benedetti F, Colloca L, Lanotte M, Bergamasco B, Torre E and Lopiano L (2004). Autonomic and emotional responses to open and hidden stimulations of the human subthalamic region. *Brain Research Bulletin*, **63**, 203–11.

Berney A, Vingerhoets F, Perrin A, Guex P, Villemure JG, Burkhard PR et al. (2002). Effect on mood of subthalamic DBS for Parkinson's disease. *Neurology*, **59**, 1427–9.

Berthier M, Starkstein S and Leiguarda R (1988). Asymbolia for pain: a sensory-limbic disconnection syndrome. *Annals of Neurology*, **24**, 41–9.

Binkofski F, Schnitzler A, Enck P et al. (1998). Somatic and limbic cortex activation: a functional magnetic resonance imaging study. *Annals of Neurology*, **44**, 811–5.

Bonica JJ, ed (1990). *The management of pain*. 2nd ed. Lea and Febiger, Philadelphia.

Bouhassira D, Chollet R, Coffin M et al. (1994). Inhibition of a somatic nociceptive reflex by gastric distension in humans. *Gastroenterology*, **107**, 985–92.

Breiter HC, Etcoff NL, Whalen PJ et al. (1996). Response and habituation of the human amygdala during visual processing of facial expression. *Neuron*, **17**, 875–87.

Bruehl S, Burns JW, Chung OY, Ward P and Johnson B (2002). Anger and pain sensitivity in chronic low back pain patients and pain-free controls: the role of endogenous opioids. *Pain*, **99**, 223–33.

Bruehl S, Chung OY, Burns JW and Biridepalli S (2003). The association between anger expression and chronic pain intensity: evidence for partial mediation by endogenous opioid dysfunction. *Pain*, **106**, 317–24.

Bushnell MC and Duncan GH (1987). Mechanical response properties of ventroposterior medial thalamic neurons in the alert monkey. *Experimental Brain Research*, **67**, 603–14.

Bushnell MC, Duncan GH, Dubner R, Jones RL and Maixner W (1985). Attentional influences on noxious and innocuous cutaneous heat detection in humans and monkeys. *Journal of Neuroscience*, **5**, 1103–10.

Bushnell MC, Duncan GH, Hofbauer RK, Ha B, Chen JI and Carrier B (1999). Pain perception: is there a role for primary somatosensory cortex? *Proceedings of the National Academy of Science USA*, **96**, 7705–9.

Cameron OG (2002). *Visceral sensory neuroscience*. Oxford University Press, Oxford, UK.

Carlson JD, Maire JJ, Martenson ME and Heinricher MM (2007). Sensitization of pain-modulating neurons in the rostral ventromedial medulla after peripheral nerve injury. *Journal of Neuroscience*, **27**, 13222–31.

Carroll LJ, Cassidy JD and Cote P (2004). Depression as a risk factor for onset of an episode of troublesome neck and low back pain. *Pain*, **107**, 134–9.

Casey KL, Svensson P, Morrow TJ, Raz J, Jone C and Minoshima S (2000). Selective opiate modulation of nociceptive processing in the human brain. *Journal of Neurophysiology*, **84**, 525–33.

Cervero F and Jänig W (1992). Visceral nociceptors: a new world order? *Trends in Neurosciences*, **15**, 374–8.

Chua P, Krams M, Toni I, Passingham R and Dolan R (1999). A functional anatomy of anticipatory anxiety. *Neuroimage*, **9**, 563–71.

Coffin B, Azpiroz F and Malagelada JR (1994). Somatic stimulation reduces perception of gut distension in humans. *Gastroenterology*, **107**, 1636–42.

Coghill RC, Sang CN, Maisog JM and Iadarola MJ (1999). Pain intensity processing within the human brain: a bilateral, distributed mechanism. *Journal of Neurophysiology*, **82**, 1934–43.

Colloca L and Beneetti F (2007). Nocebo hyperalgesia: how anxiety is turned into pain. *Current Opinion in Anaesthesiology*, **20**, 435–9.

Colloca L, Sigaudo M and Benedetti F (2008). The role of learning in nocebo and placebo effects. *Pain*, **136**, 211–8.

Craig AD (2002). How do you feel? Interoception: the sense of the physiological condition of the body. *Nature Reviews Neuroscience*, **3**, 655–66.

Craig AD (2009). How do you feel–now? The anterior insula and human awareness. *Nature Reviews Neuroscience*, **10**, 59–70.

Craig AD, Bushnell MC, Zhang ET and Blomqvist A (1994). A thalamic nucleus specific for pain and temperature sensation. *Nature*, **372**, 770–3.

Craig AD, Reiman EM, Evans A and Bushnell MC (1996). Functional imaging of an illusion of pain. *Nature*, **384**, 258–60.

Critchley HD, Corfield DR, Chandler M, Mathias CJ and Dolan RJ (2000). Cerebral correlates of peripheral cardiovascular arousal: a functional neuroimaging study. *Journal of Physiology*, **523**, 259–70.

Critchley HD, Mathias CJ and Dolan RJ (2001). Neural correlates of first and second-order representation of bodily states. *Nature Neuroscience*, **4**, 207–12.

Critchley HD, Mathias CJ and Dolan RJ (2002). Fear-conditioning in humans: the influence of awareness and arousal on functional neuroanatomy. *Neuron*, **33**, 653–63.

Critchley HD, Wiens S, Rothstein P, Ohman A and Dolan RJ (2004). Neural systems supporting interoceptive awareness. *Nature Neuroscience*, **7**, 189–95.

Damasio AR, Grabowski TJ, Bechara A, Damasio H, Ponto LL, Parvizi J et al. (2000). Subcortical and cortical brain activity during the feeling of self-generated emotions. *Nature Neuroscience*, **3**, 1049–56.

Dannecker EA, Price DD and Robinson ME (2003). An examination of the relationships among recalled, expected, and actual intensity and unpleasantness of delayed onset muscle pain. *Journal of Pain*, **4**, 74–81.

Darwin C (1872). *The expression of emotions in man and animals.* Appleton, New York.

Davis KD, Kwan CL, Crawley AP and Mikulis DJ (1998). Functional MRI study of thalamic and cortical activations evoked by cutaneous heat, cold, and tactile stimuli. *Journal of Neurophysiology*, **80**, 1533–46.

Devinsky O, Morrell MJ and Vogt BA (1995). Contributions of anterior cingulate cortex to behaviour. *Brain*, **118**, 279–306.

Dickens C, McGowan L and Dale S (2003). Impact of depression on experimental pain perception: a systematic review of the literature with meta-analysis. *Psychosomatic Medicine*, **65**, 369–75.

Eippert F, Bingel U, Schoell ED et al. (2009a). Activation of the opioidergic descending pain control system underlies placebo analgesia. *Neuron*, **63**, 533–43.

Eippert F, Finsterbusch J, Bingel U and Buchel C (2009b). Direct evidence for spinal cord involvement in placebo analgesia. *Science*, **326**, 404.

Ekman P (1999). Facial expressions. In: Dalgleish T and Power M, eds. *Handbook of cognition and emotion*, pp 301–20. John Wiley & Sons, New York.

Ekman P, Levenson RW and Friesen WV (1983). Autonomic nervous system activity distinguishes among emotions. *Science*, **221**, 1208–10.

Fanselow MS (1994). Neural organization of the defensive behavior system responsible for fear. *Psychonomic Bulletin & Review*, **1**, 429–38.

Feinmann C (1999). *The mouth, the face and the mind*. Oxford University Press, Oxford.

Fields H (2004). State-dependent opioid control of pain. *Nature Reviews Neuroscience*, **5**, 565–75.

Fields HL and Basbaum AI (1999). Central nervous system mechanisms of pain modulation. In: Wall PD and Melzack R, ed. *Textbook of Pain Livingstone*, pp. 309–29. Churchill, Edinburgh.

Firestone LL, Gyulai F, Mintun M, Adler LJ, Urso K and Winter PM (1996). Human brain activity response to fentanyl imaged by positron emission tomography. *Anesthesia and Analgesia*, **82**, 1247–51.

Flor H and Grusser SM (1999). Conditioned stress-induced analgesia in humans. *European Journal of Pain*, **3**, 317–24.

Funkiewiez A, Ardouin C, Krack P et al. (2003). Acute psychotropic effects of bilateral subthalamic nucleus stimulation and levodopa in Parkinson's disease. *Movement Disorders*, **18**, 524–30.

Ghika J, Vingerhoets F, Albanese A and Villmeure JG (1999). Bipolar swings in mood in a patient with bilateral subthalamic deep brain stimulation (DBS) free of antiparkinsonian medication. *Parkinsonism & Related Disorders*, **5** (Suppl. 1), 104.

Giesecke T, Gracely RH, Williams DA, Geisser ME, Petzke FW and Clauw DJ (2005). The relationship between depression, clinical pain, and experimental pain in a chronic pain cohort. *Arthritis and Rheumatism*, **52**, 1577–84.

Gospic K, Gunnarsson T, Fransson P, Ingvar M, Lindefors N and Petrovic P (2008). Emotional perception modulated by an opioid and a cholecystokinin agonist. *Psychopharmacology*, **197**, 295–307.

Greenspan JD, Lee RR and Lenz FA (1999). Pain sensitivity alterations as a function of lesion location in the parasylvian cortex. *Pain*, **81**, 273–82.

Halgren E (1982). Mental phenomena induced by stimulation in the limbic system. *Human Neurobiology*, **1**, 251–60.

Head H and Holmes G (1911). Sensory disturbances from cerebral lesions. *Brain*, **34**, 102–254.

Hebb ALO, Poulin J-F, Roach SP, Zacharko RM and Drolet G (2005). Cholecystokinin and endogenous opioid peptides: interactive influence on pain, cognition, and emotion. *Progress in Neuro-Psychopharmacology & Biological Psychiatry*, **29**, 1225–38.

Heinricher MM and Neubert MJ (2004). Neural basis for the hyperalgesic action of cholecystokinin in the rostral ventromedial medulla. *Journal of Neurophysiology*, **92**, 1982–9.

Heinricher MM, McGaraughty S and Tortorici V (2001). Circuitry underlying antipioid actions of cholecystokinin within the rostral ventromedial medulla. *Journal of Neurophysiology*, **85**, 280–6.

Ho KY, Kang JY, Yeo B and Ng WL (1998). Non-cardiac, non-oesophgeal chest pain: the relevance of psychological factors. *Gut*, **43**, 105–10.

Hoffman HG, Doctor JN, Patterson DR, Carrougher GJ and Furness TA III (2000). Virtual reality as an adjunctive pain control during burn wound care in adolescent patients. *Pain*, **85**, 305–9.

Hokfelt T, Zhang X and Wiesenfeld-Hallin Z (1994). Messenger plasticity in primary sensory neurons following axotomy and its functional implications. *Trends in Neurosciences*, **17**, 22–30.

Hsieh JC, Stone-Elander S and Ingvar M (1999). Anticipatory coping of pain expressed in the human anterior cingulated cortex: a positron emission tomography study. *Neuroscience Letters*, **26**, 262, 61–4.

Hudson AJ (2000). Pain perception and response: central nervous system mechanisms. *Canadian Journal of Neurological Sciences*, **27**, 2–16.

Hughes J (1975). Search for the endogenous ligand of the opiate receptor. *Neurosciences Research Program Bulletin*, **13**, 55–8.

Hunt SP and Rossi J (1985). Peptide- and non-peptide-containing unmyelinated primary afferents: the parallel processing of nociceptive information. *Philosophical Transactions of the Royal Society of London B: Biological Sciences*, **308**, 283–9.

Huynh Bao QV and Rainville P (2003). Modulation of experimental pain by emotion induced using hypnosis. *Pain Research and Management*, Suppl. **8**, 35B.

Iovino P, Azpiroz F, Domingo E and Malagelada JR (1995). The sympathetic nervous system modulates perception and reflex responses to gut distension in humans. *Gastroenterology*, **108**, 680–6.

Jensen TS (1997). Opioids in the brain: supraspinal mechanisms in pain control. *Acta Anaesthesiologica Scandinavica*, **41**, 123–32.

Jones AK, Qi LY, Fujirawa T et al. (1991). In vivo distribution of opioid receptors in man in relation to the cortical projections of the medial and lateral pain systems measured with positron emission tomography. *Neuroscience Letters*, **126**, 25–8.

Julien N, Goffaux P, Arsenault P and Marchand S (2005). Widespread pain in fibromyalgia is related to a deficit of endogenous pain inhibition. *Pain*, **114**, 295–302.

Karnath HO, Baier B and Nagele T (2005). Awareness of the functioning of one's own limbs mediated by the insular cortex? *Journal of Neuroscience*, **25**, 7134–8.

Keltner JR, Furst A, Fan C, Redfern R, Inglis B and Fields HL (2006). Isolating the modulatory effect of expectation on pain transmission: a functional magnetic imaging study. *Journal of Neuroscience*, **26**, 4437–43.

Kenshalo DR Jr, Giesler GJ Jr, Leonard RB and Willis WD (1980). Responses of neurons in primate ventral posterior lateral nucleus to noxious stimuli. *Journal of Neurophysiology*, **43**, 1594–614.

Kenshalo DR and Douglass DK (1995). The role of the cerebral cortex in the experience of pain. In: B Bromm, JE Desmedt, eds. *Pain and the brain: from nociception to cognition*. pp. 21–34. Raven Press, New York.

Kenshalo DR and Isensee O (1983). Responses of primate SI cortical neurons to noxious stimuli. *Journal of Neurophysiology*, **50**, 1479–96.

King AB, Menon RS, Hachinski V and Cechetto DF (1999). Human forebrain activation by visceral stimuli. *Journal of Comparative Neurology*, **41**, 572–82.

Klauenberg S, Maier C, Assion HJ et al. (2008). Depression and changed pain perception: hints for a central disinhibition mechanism. *Pain*, **140**, 332–43.

Korszun A (2002). Facial pain, depression and stress–connections and directions. *Journal of Oral Pathology and Medicine*, **31**, 615–9.

Koyama T, McHaffie JG, Laurienti PJ and Coghill RC (2005). The subjective experience of pain: where expectations become reality. *Proceedings of the National Academy of Sciences of the United States of America*, **102**, 12950–5.

Koyama T, Tanaka YZ and Mikami A (1998). Nociceptive neurons in the macaque anterior cingulate activate during anticipation of pain. *Neuroreport*, **9**, 2663–7.

Krack P, Kumar R, Ardouin C, Dowsey PL, McVicker JM, Benabid AL et al. (2001). Mirthful laughter induced by subthalamic nucleus stimulation. *Movement Disorders*, **16**, 867–75.

Kumar R, Krack P and Pollak P (1999). Transient acute depression-induced by high-frequency deep-brain stimulation. *New England Journal of Medicine*, **341**, 1003–4.

Kumar K, Toth C and Nath RK (1997). Deep brain stimulation for intractable pain: a 15-year experience. *Neurosurgery*, **40**, 736–46.

Kwekkeboom KL (2003). Music versus distraction for procedural pain and anxiety in patients with cancer. *Oncology Nursing Forum*, **30**, 433–40.

LaCroix-Fralish ML and Mogil JS (2009). Progress in genetic studies of pain and analgesia. *Annual Review of Pharmacology and Toxicology*, **49**, 97–121.

Landolt MA, Marti D, Widmer J and Meuli M (2002). Does cartoon movie distraction decrease burned children's pain behavior? *Journal of Burn Care and Rehabilitation*, **23**, 61–5.

Lane RD, Reiman EM, Ahern GL, Schwartz GE and Davidson RJ (1997). Neuroanatomical correlates of happiness, sadness, and disgust. *American Journal of Psychiatry*, **154**, 926–33.

Lanotte M, Lopiano L, Torre E, Bergamasco B, Colloca L and Benedetti F (2005). Expectation enhances autonomic responses to stimulation of the human subthalamic limbic region. *Brain, Behavior and Immunity*, **19**, 500–9.

Larson SL, Clark MR and Eaton WW (2004). Depressive disorder as a long-term antecedent risk factor for incident back pain: a 13-year follow-up study from the Baltimore Epidemiological Catchment Area sample. *Psychological Medicine*, **34**, 211–9.

Lautenbacher S, Roscher S, Strian D, Fassbender K, Krumrey K and Krieg JC (1994). Pain perception in depression: relationships to symptomatology and naloxone-sensitive mechanisms. *Psychosomatic Medicine*, **56**, 345–52.

Levenson RW, Ekman P and Friesen WV (1990). Voluntary facial action generates emotion-specific autonomic nervous system activity. *Psychophysiology*, **27**, 363–84.

Lewin GR, Ritter AM and Mendell LM (1993). Nerve growth factor-induced hyperalgesia in the neonatal and adult rat. *Journal of Neuroscience,* **13**, 2136–48.

Longe SE, Wise R, Bantick S et al. (2001). Counter-stimulatory effects on pain perception and processing are significantly altered by attention: an fMRI study. *Neuroreport,* **12**, 2021–5.

Lorenz J, Hauck M, Paur RC et al. (2005). Cortical correlates of false expectations during pain intensity judgments—a possible manifestation of placebo/nocebo cognitions. *Brain, Behavior and Immunity*, **19**, 283–95.

MacLean PD (1970). The triune brain, emotion, and scientific bias. In: FO Schmitt, ed. *The neurosciences*, pp. 336–48. Rockefeller University, New York, NY.

—— (1990). *The triune brain in evolution: role in paleocerebral functions*. Plenum Press, New York.

Magni G, Moreschi C, Rigatti-Luchini S and Merskey H (1994). Prospective study on the relationship between depressive symptoms and chronic musculoskeletal pain. *Pain*, **56**, 289–97.

Manning BH, Merin NM, Meng ID and Amaral DG (2001). Reduction in opioid- and cannabinoid-induced antinociception in rhesus monkeys after bilateral lesions of the amygdaloid complex. *Journal of Neuroscience*, **21**, 8238–46.

Marshall J (1951). Sensory disturbances in cortical wounds with special reference to pain. *Journal of Neurology, Neurosurgery and Psychiatry*, **14**, 187–204.

Melzack R (1999). From the gate to the neuromatrix. *Pain,* Suppl **6**, S121–6.

Melzack R and Wall PD (1965). Pain mechanisms: a new theory. *Science*, **150**, 971–9.

Mendell LM, Albers KM and Davis BM (1999). Neurotrophins, nociceptors, and pain. *Microscopical Research and Technology*, **45**, 252–61.

Menon V and Levitin DJ (2005). The rewards of music listening response and physiological connectivity of the mesolimbic system. *Neuroimage*, **28**, 175–84.

Millan MJ (2002). Descending control of pain. *Progress in Neurobiology*, **66**, 355–474.

Mitchell JM, Lowe D and Fields HL (1998). The contribution of the rostral ventromedial medulla to the antinociceptive effects of systemic morphine in restrained and unrestrained rats. *Neuroscience,* **87**, 123–33.

Molliver DC, Wright DE, Leitner ML et al. (1997). IB4-binding DRG neurons switch from NGF to GDNF dependence in early postnatal life. *Neuron,* **19**, 849–61.

Mongini F, Ciccone G, Ceccarelli M, Baldi I and Ferrero L (2007). Muscle tenderness in different types of facial pain and its relation to anxiety and depression: a cross-sectional study on 649 patients. *Pain*, **131**, 106–11.

Morris JS, Frith CD, Perrett DI, Rowland D, Young AW, Calder AJ et al. (1996). A differential neural response in the human amygdala to fearful and happy facial expressions. *Nature*, **383**, 812–5.

Nagy JI and Hunt SP (1982). Fluoride-resistant acid phosphatase-containing neurones in dorsal root ganglia are separate from those containing substance P or somatostatin. *Neuroscience,* **7**, 89–97.

Nimchinsky EA, Gilissen E, Allman JM, Perl DP, Erwin JM and Hof PR (1999). A neuronal morphologic type unique to humans and great apes. *Proceedings of the National Academy of USA*, **96**, 5268–73.

Noble F, Wank SA, Crawley JN, Bradwejn J, Seroogy KB, Hamon M et al. (1999). International Union of Pharmacology. XXI. Structure, disribution, and functions of cholecystokinin receptors. *Pharmacological Reviews*, **51**, 745–81.

Okifuji A, Turk DC and Curran SL (1999). Anger in chronic pain: investigations of anger targets and intensity. *Journal of Psychosomatic Research*, **47**, 1–12.

Papez JW (1937). A proposed mechanism of emotions. *Archives of Neurology and Psychology*, **38**, 725–43.

Penfield W and Boldrey E (1937). Somatic motor and sensory representation in cerebral cortex of man as studied by electrical stimulation. *Brain*, **60**, 389–443.

Pennebaker JW (1982). *The psychology of physical symptoms*. Springer-Verlag, New York, NY.

Pennebaker JW and Hoover CW (1984). Visceral perception versus visceral detection: disentangling methods and assumptions. *Biofeedback & Self Regulation*, **9**, 339–52.

Pert CB and Snyder SH (1973). Opiate receptor: demonstration in nervous tissue. *Science*, **179**, 1011–3.

Petrovic P and Ingvar M (2002). Imaging cognitive modulation of pain processing. *Pain*, **95**, 1–5.

Petrovic P, Kalso E, Petersson KM and Ingvar M (2002). Placebo and opioid analgesia— imaging a shared neuronal network. *Science*, **295**, 1737–40.

Petty BG, Cornblath DR, Adornato BT, Chaudhry V, Flexner C, Wachsman M et al. (1994). The effect of systemically administered recombinant human nerve growth factor in healthy human subjects. *Annals of Neurology*, **36**, 244–6.

Pfeiffer A, Pasi A, Mehraein P and Herz A (1982). Opiate receptor binding sites in human brain. *Brain Research*, **248**, 87–96.

Phillips ML, Gregory LJ, Cullen S, Coen S, Ng V, Andrew C et al. (2003). The effect of negative emotional context on neural and behavioural responses to oesophageal stimulation. *Brain*, **126**, 669–84.

Phillips ML, Young AW, Senior C, Brammer M, Andrew C, Calder AJ et al. (1997). A specific neural substrate for perceiving facial expressions of disgust. *Nature*, **389**, 495–8.

Ploghaus A, Narain C, Beckmann CF, Clare S, Bantick S, Wise R et al. (2001). Exacerbation of pain by anxiety is associated with activity in a hippocampal network. *Journal of Neuroscience*, **21**, 9896–903.

Ploghaus A, Tracey I, Gati JS et al. (1999). Dissociating pain from its anticipation in the human brain. *Science*, **284**, 1979–81.

Ploner M, Schmitz F, Freund HJ and Schnitzler A (1999). Parallel activation of primary and secondary somatosensory cortices in human pain processing. *Journal of Neurophysiology*, **81**, 3100–4.

Ploner M, Schmitz F, Freund HJ and Schnitzler A (2000). Differential organization of touch and pain in human primary somatosensory cortex. *Journal of Neurophysiology*, **83**, 1770–6.

Porro CA, Baraldi P, Pagnoni G et al. (2002). Does anticipation of pain affect cortical nociceptive systems? *Journal of Neuroscience*, **22**, 3206–14.

Porro CA, Cettolo V, Francescato MP and Baraldi P (2003). Functional activity mapping of the mesial hemispheric wall during anticipation of pain. *Neuroimage*, **19**, 1738–47.

Price DD (1999). *Psychological mechanisms of pain and analgesia*. IASP Press, Seattle, WA.

—— (2000). Psychological and neural mechanisms of the affective dimension of pain. *Science*, **288**, 1769–72.

Price DD and Dubner R (1977). Neurons that subserve the sensory-discriminative aspects of pain. *Pain*, **3**, 307–38.

Price DD, Barrell JE and Barrell JJ (1985). A quantitative-experiential analysis of human emotions. *Motivation and Emotion*, **9**, 19–38.

Rainville P (2004). Pain and emotions. In: DD Price and MC Bushnell, eds. *Psychological methods of pain control: basic science and clinical perspectives*, pp. 117–41. IASP Press, Seattle, WA.

Rainville P, Duncan GH, Price DD, Carrier B and Bushnell MC (1997). Pain affect encoded in human anterior cingulate but not somatosensory cortex. *Science*, **277**, 968–71.

Rexed B (1952). The cytoarchitectonic organization of the spinal cord in the rat. *Journal of Comparative Neurology*, **96**, 415–66.

Reynolds DV (1969). Surgery in the rat during electrical analgesia induced by focal brain stimulation. *Science*, **164**, 444–5.

Riley JL and Wade JB (2004). Psychological and demographic factors that modulate the different stages and dimensions of pain. In: DD Price and MC Bushnell, eds. *Psychological methods of pain control: basic science and clinical perspectives*, pp. 19–41. IASP Press, Seattle, WA.

Riley JL III, Robinson ME, Wade JB, Myers CD and Price DD (2001). Sex differences in negative emotional response to chronic pain. *Journal of Pain*, **2**, 354–9.

Riley JL III, Wade JB, Robinson ME and Price DD (2000). The stages of pain processing across the adult lifespan. *Journal of Pain*, **1**, 162–70.

Riley JL III, Wade JB, Myers CD, Sheffield D, Papas RK and Price DD et al. (2002). Racial/ethnic differences in the experience of chronic pain. *Pain*, **100**, 291–8.

Rothstein RD, Stecker M, Reivich M, Alavi A, Ding XS, Jaggi J et al. (1996). Use of positron emission tomography and evoked potentials in the detection of cortical afferents from the gastrointestinal tract. *American Journal of Gastroenterology*, **91**, 2372–6.

Sadzot B, Price JC, Mayberg HS et al. (1991). Quantification of human opiate receptor concentration and affinity using high and low specific activity and diprenorphine and positron emission tomography. *Journal of Cerebral Blood Flow and Metabolism*, **11**, 204–19.

Sawamoto N, Honda M, Okada T, Hanakawa T, Kanda M, Fukuyama H et al. (2000). Expectation of pain enhances responses to nonpainful somatosensory stimulation in the anterior cingulated cortex and parietal operculum/posterior insula: an event-related functional magnetic resonance imaging study. *Journal of Neuroscience*, **20**, 7438–45.

Schacter S and Singer JE (1962). Cognitive, social, and physiological determinants of emotional state. *Psychological Reviews*, **69**, 379–99.

Schneider F, Habel U, Volkmann J, Regel S, Kornischka J, Sturm V et al. (2003). Deep brain stimulation of the subthalamic nucleus enhances emotional processing in Parkinson's disease. *Archives of General Psychiatry*, **60**, 296–302.

Scholz J, Vieregge P and Moser A (1999). Central pain as a manifestation of partial epileptic seizures. *Pain*, **80**, 445–50.

Schweinhardt P, Kalk N, Wartolowska K, Chessell I, Wordsworth P and Tracey I (2008). Investigation into the neural correlates of emotional augmentation of clinical pain. *Neuroimage*, **40**, 759–66.

Seeley WW, Carlin DA, Allman JM et al. (2006). Early frontotemporal dementia targets neurons unique to apes and humans. *Annals of Neurology*, **60**, 660–7.

Sengupta JN and Gebhart GF (1995). Mechanosensitive afferent fibers in the gastrointestinal and lower urinary tracts. In: GF Gebhart, ed. *Visceral pain. Progress in pain research and management*, vol.**5**, pp. 75–98. IASP Press, Seattle, WA.

Silos-Santiago I, Molliver DC, Ozaki S, Smeyne RJ, Fagan AM, Barbacid M et al. (1995). Non-TrkA-expressing small DRG neurons are lost in TrkA deficient mice. *Journal of Neuroscience,* **15**, 5929–42.

Silverman JD and Kruger L (1990). Selective neuronal glycoconjugate expression in sensory and autonomic ganglia: relation of lectin reactivity to peptide and enzyme markers. *Journal of Neurocytology,* **19**, 789–801.

Snider WD and McMahon SB (1998). Tackling pain at the source: new ideas about nociceptors. *Neuron*, **20**, 629–32.

Spinazzola L, Pia L, Folegatti A, Marchetti C and Berti A (2008). Modular structure of awareness for sensorumotor disorders: evidence from anosognosia for emiplegia and anosognosia for hemianaesthesia. *Neuropsychologia*, **46**, 915–26.

Sprengelmeyer R, Rausch M, Eysel UT and Przuntek H (1998). Neural structures associated with recognition of facial expressions of basic emotions. *Proceedings of the Royal Society of London B: Biological Sciences*, **265**, 1927–31.

Stephan E, Pardo JV, Faris PL, Hartman BK, Kim SW, Ivanov EH et al. (2003). Functional neuroimaging of gastric distension. *Journal of Gastrointestinal Surgery*, **7**, 740–9.

Strigo A, Simmons AN, Matthews SC, Craig AD and Paulus MP (2008). Association of major depressive disorder with altered functional brain response during anticipation and processing of heat pain. *Archives of General Psychiatry*, **65**, 1275–84.

Terman GW, Morgan MJ and Liebeskind JC (1986). Opioid and non-opioid stress analgesia from cold water swim: importance of stress severity. *Brain Research*, **372**, 167–71.

Timmermann L, Ploner M, Haucke K, Schmitz F, Baltissen R and Schnitzler A (2001). Differential coding of pain intensity in the human primary and secondary somatosensory cortex. *Journal of Neurophysiology*, **86**, 1499–503.

Torebjörk HE, Lundberg LE and LaMotte RH (1992). Central changes in processing of mechanoreceptive input in capsaicin-induced secondary hyperalgesia in humans. *Journal of Physiology*, **448**, 765–80.

Tracey I and Mantyh PW (2007). The cerebral signature for pain perception and its modulation. *Neuron*, **55**, 377–91.

Treede RD, Kenshalo DR, Gracely RH and Jones AK (1999). The cortical representation of pain. *Pain*, **79**, 105–11.

Treede RD, Meyer RA, Raja SN and Campbell JN (1992). Peripheral and central mechanisms of cutaneous hyperalgesia. *Progress in Neurobiology*, **38**, 397–421.

Treede RD, Meyer RA and Campbell JN (1991). Classification of primate A-fibre nociceptors according to their heat response properties. *Pflügers Archives*, Suppl 1, **418**, R42.

Treede RD, Meyer RA, Raja SN and Campbell JN (1995). Evidence for two different heat transduction mechanisms in nociceptive primary afferents innervating monkey skin. *Journal of Physiology*, **483**, 747–58.

Van Hees J and Gybels J (1981). C nociceptor activity in human nerve during painful and non painful skin stimulation. *Journal of Neurology, Neurosurgery and Psychiatry*, **44**, 600–7.

Vernet-Maury E, Alaoui-Ismaili O, Dittmar A, Delhomme G and Chanel J (1999). Basic emotions induced by odorants: a new approach based on autonomic pattern results. *Journal of the Autonomic Nervous System*, **75**, 176–83.

Vimpari SS, Knuuttila ML, Sakki TK and Kivela SL (1995). Depressive symptoms associated with symptoms of the temporomandibular joint pain and dysfunction syndrome. *Psychosomatic Medicine*, **57**, 439–44.

Vogt BA, Finch DM and Olson CR (1992). Functional heterogeneity in cingulate cortex: the anterior executive and posterior evaluative regions. *Cerebral Cortex*, **2**, 435–43.

Vogt BA, Sikes RW and Vogt LJ (1993). Anterior cingulate cortex and the medial pain system. In Vogt BA and Gabriel M, eds. *Neurobiology of cingulate cortex and limbic thalamus: a comprehensive handbook*, pp. 313–44. Birkhäuser, Boston, MA.

Wade JB, Dougherty LM, Hart RP, Rafii A and Price DD (1992). A canonical correlation analysis of the influence of neuroticism and extraversion on chronic pain, suffering, and pain behaviour. *Pain*, **51**, 67–73.

Wager TD, Davidson ML, Hughes BL, Lindquist MA and Ochsner KN (2008). Prefrontal-subcortical pathways mediating successful emotion regulation. *Neuron*, **59**, 1037–50.

Wagner KJ, Willoch F, Kochs EF, Siessmeier T and Tölle TR (2001). Dose-dependent regional cerebral blood flow changes during remifentanil infusion in humans. *A positron emission tomography study. Anesthesiology*, **94**, 732–9.

Wamsley JK, Zarbin MA, Young WS and Kuhar MJ (1982). Distribution of opiate receptors in the monkey brain: an autoradiographic study. *Neuroscience*, **7**, 595–613.

Weary DM, Huzzey JM and von Keyserlingk (2009). Using behaviour to predict and identify ill health in animals. *Journal of Animal Sciences*, **87**, 770–7.

Whitehead WE, Bosmajian L, Zonderman AB, Costa PT Jr and Schster MM (1988). Symptoms of psychological distress associated with irritable bowel syndrome. Comparison of community and medical clinic samples. *Gastroenterology*, **95**, 709–14.

Wiech K and Tracey I (2009). The influence of negative emotions on pain: behavioral effects and neural mechanisms. *Neuroimage*, **47**, 987–94.

Willer JC and Albe-Fessard D (1980). Electrophysiological evidence for a release of endogenous opiates in stress-induced 'analgesia' in man. *Brain Research*, **198**, 419–26.

Willis WD (1985). *The pain system.* Karger, Basel.

Willis WD and Coggeshall RE (1991). *Sensory mechanisms of the spinal cord.* 2nd ed. Plenum Press, New York.

Willis WD Jr and Westlund KN (1997). Neuroanatomy of the pain system and of the pathways that modulate pain. *Journal of Clinical Neurophysiology,* **14**, 2–31.

Willis WD Jr and Westlund KN (2001). The role of the dorsal column pathway in visceral nociception. *Current Pain and Headache Reports,* **5**, 20–6.

Willoch F, Schindler F, Wester HJ et al. (2004). Central poststroke pain and reduced opioid receptor binding within pain processing circuitries: a [11C]diprenorphine PET study. *Pain,* **108**, 213–20.

Willoch F, Tolle TR and Wester HJ (1999). Central pain after pontine infarction is associated with changes in opioid receptor binding: a PET study with 11C-diprenorphine. *American Journal of Neuroradiology,* **20**, 686–90.

Woolf CJ (1994). The dorsal horn: state-dependent sensory processing and the generation of pain. In: PD Wall, R Melzack, eds. *Textbook of pain.* 3rd ed. pp. 101–12. Churchill-Livingstone, Edinburgh.

Woolf CJ, Safieh-Garabedian B, Ma QP, Crilly P and Winter J (1994). Nerve growth factor contributes to the generation of inflammatory sensory hypersensitivity. *Neuroscience,* **62**, 327–31.

Yaksh TL (1998). Physiologic and pharmacologic substrates of nociception and nerve injury. In: MJ Cousins, PO Bridenbaugh, eds. *Neural blockade in clinical anesthesia and management of pain.* 3rd ed. pp. 727–80. Lippincott-Raven Publishers, Philadelphia, PA.

Zhang W, Gardell S, Zhang D, Xie JY, Agnes RS, Badghisi H et al. (2009). Neuropathic pain is maintained by brainstem neurons co-expressing opioid and cholecystokinin receptors. *Brain,* **132**, 778–87.

Chapter 4

Seeking relief: the activation of motivational and reward circuits

Summary and relevance to the clinician

1) This chapter is aimed at analysing why and how the patient starts seeking relief. By asking this apparently simple question, the act of seeking relief is analysed in terms of motivated behaviour, whereby motivation mechanisms are at work in order to trigger the appropriate behavioural repertoire, whose final step is the suppression of discomfort.

2) Basic motivations, like hunger, thirst, and thermoregulation lead to the appropriate behaviours in order to placate the discomfort deriving from a lack of food and water as well as from excessive cold and hot temperatures. The behavioural repertoires that are activated in these conditions are basically characterized by the search of a means to get food or water, or to find a cold/warm place. Different specific biological mechanisms do exist for each of these motivated behaviours.

3) Although sex can be considered a motivated behaviour in all respects, it is quite different compared to hunger, thirst, and thermoregulation. In fact, whereas a lack of food/water intake may be harmful to health and critical for survival, the lack of sexual activity does not lead to any harm to health. Therefore, in the case of sex, motivation can be better conceptualized as aimed at getting a pleasant reward. There are motivated behaviours other than sex that aim to seek pleasure, like self-administration of drugs of abuse and gamble.

4) The distinction between suppressing discomfort and getting a reward is not always straightforward. When one wants to suppress his own discomfort from hunger, he is actually seeking the reward of food, which is itself the means leading to hunger suppression. The mesolimbic dopaminergic system is at the very heart of this seeking behaviour, and can be identified as a motivation/reward system. The main regions of this system are the ventral tegmental area, the nucleus accumbens, and the prefrontal cortex. The mesolimbic dopaminergic system is involved in many forms of reward, from

alimentary stimuli and food intake to sexual arousal and sexual activity, and from drugs of abuse and euphoria-inducing drugs to monetary incentives and gamble.

5) Seeking relief from sickness is a motivated behaviour in all respects. When a patient feels sick, he starts seeking relief, in the same way as when he is hungry or thirsty. Cultural differences play a crucial role when adopting a given behavioural repertoire. What the sick does first is to rely on the healer who, he believes, is capable of suppressing the pathological process. It is important to realize that, for the sake of this chapter, the ability, competence, and skills of the healer do not matter. What counts is the patient's behaviour, regardless of the healer whom he refers to.

6) Seeking relief from sickness is more similar to hunger and thirst than to sexual behaviour. In fact, like hunger and thirst, a lack of search of relief may be harmful to health and critical for survival. In this sense, seeking relief from sickness can be conceptualized as a powerful mechanism of survival.

7) There is compelling experimental evidence that the mesolimbic dopaminergic system may be activated when a subject expects clinical amelioration. Most, if not all, of this evidence comes from the placebo literature, whereby an inert medical treatment is administered along with verbal suggestions of improvement. In at least three medical conditions, Parkinson's disease, depression, and pain, the activation of the mesolimbic dopaminergic system has been found to be activated when expecting clinical improvement.

8) By considering the sickness-suppressing-motivated behaviour and the involvement of the motivation/reward neural network, the clinician must consider himself as a powerful reward, thus any effort should be directed to enhance the reward mechanisms. It will become clear in Chapter 6 that a therapy can, at least in some circumstances, be conceptualized as a reward.

4.1 Suppressing discomfort and seeking pleasure

4.1.1 Motivation is aimed at regulating internal states and at getting a reward

Motivation is a term that emerged from the need to explain the huge variability of behavioural responses. In fact, whereas in a simple reflex there is a good correlation between the intensity of the stimulus and the magnitude of the response, in more complex behavioural responses such correlation is lacking. In other words, the same stimulus does not always produce the same response.

For example, an alimentary stimulus may produce huge responses in some conditions, but no responses in some other circumstances.

Motivation is characterized by a set of factors that trigger, maintain, and orient behaviour. The concept of motivation can be better explained by considering homeostasis, i.e. the fact that a given system or physiological parameter is in equilibrium in normal circumstances (Hull 1951). For example, the temperature of the body is within a given homeostatic range in normal conditions (36–37°C in humans). Likewise, liquids and some nutritional substances, such as lipids and glycids, are maintained within a given homeostatic range. Any perturbation of this homeostasis leads to a tension of the organism, which is called drive, or motivation. This drive forces humans and animals to start the appropriate action, like looking for a warmer place, water, or food, so as to restore the normal homeostatic equilibrium. As soon as homeostasis returns to normal, the motivated behaviour ends.

Although these basic motivated behaviours are triggered by physical and chemical needs, e.g. the need to reintroduce liquids or lipids into the organisms, external stimuli or incentives may play a critical role in a variety of situations (Bolles 1975). For example, money is a powerful incentive to motivated behaviour in most individuals and, similarly, high scores are potent incentives for many students. By considering both internal states and external incentives, motivation can be better understood as a state of the brain, rather than a mere physical-chemical need of some tissues of the body (Stellar and Stellar 1985). On the basis of these considerations, it is clear that motivation has at least three main functions. First, it directs behaviour towards specific objectives. Second, it increases arousal, thus it forces the organism to act. Third, it organizes a coherent behavioural sequence which is appropriate to achieve the objective.

The general organization of motivated behaviour can be summarized as shown in Fig 4.1A. Either an increase or decrease in the variable to be controlled, e.g. body temperature or food/water intake, is revealed through receptors that send afferent signals to the control system. This in turn compares these changes with a reference value and, accordingly, adjusts the physiological variable. There are at least two mechanisms through which this adjustment takes place. First, some completely unconscious mechanisms, such hormone secretion, are activated that make the variable return to a normal value. Second, a behavioural repertoire is triggered, e.g. looking for some water, that restores the normal homeostatic range. External stimuli, or incentives, always operate upon the control system and may trigger motivated behaviour even in the absence of changes in the variable to be controlled, e.g. drinking even though there was no depletion of water in the body.

Although the organization of Fig 4.1A can explain many motivated behaviours such as termoregulation, hunger and thirst, it fails to account for other types of motivation. For example, in motivated sexual behaviour there appears to be no variable to be controlled. In other words, in sex there appears to be no homeostatic need of any tissue in the body. If one does not eat or drink, a harm to health may derive, whereas no harm to health is present if one does not have sexual activity. Figure 4.1B is a very simple model whereby a behavioural repertoire may produce pleasure, and the more intense the pleasure is, the more that behaviour is activated. In this case, there is no physiological variable to be controlled, but the motivated behaviour originates from the fact that it leads to a reward, i.e. pleasure. It is worth emphasizing that the model of Fig 4.1B may apply not only to sex but to hunger and thirst as well. In fact, sometimes food intake is not triggered by a real need, but rather by the search for pleasure, such as taste and flavour.

Motivation and reward are thus intimately related. The two schemas in Fig 4.1A and B are somehow similar, for they both trigger motivated behaviours. However, whereas the former is aimed at suppressing discomfort, e.g. too cold/too hot, hunger, and thirst, the latter is aimed at seeking a pleasant reward. Nonetheless, a straightforward distinction between discomfort suppression and reward search is not easy to make. For example, trying to suppress discomfort involves a reward, because being discomfort-free can be certainly considered a form of reward. Likewise, it turns out that reward search, be it sex or money, is certainly aimed at placating a negative internal state. In the last few decades, there have been substantial advances in the understanding of the neurobiological mechanisms of motivation and reward. These have clarified many unanswered questions and, particularly, have put motivated behaviour, once in the domain of psychological and behavioural sciences, into the realm of the neuroscientific approach.

4.1.2 Suppressing discomfort from hunger, thirst, and thermal variations

Specific mechanisms that are based on the model of Fig 4.1A have been identified for specific motivated behaviours. For example, the mechanisms that are aimed at suppressing hunger and thus stimulate food intake are very complex, involving both neural and hormonal regulatory factors, and are still a matter of debate. Here, the variable to be controlled is food intake, in order to guarantee the appropriate intake of different nutritional substances, such as lipids, glycids, and proteins. If 2-deoxyglucose is injected into the rabbit hepatic portal system, it replaces glucose in the liver, thereby inducing glucose depletion. After a few minutes, the rabbits start eating three-fold compared to controls, thus suggesting that glucose signals arising from the liver are critical to trigger

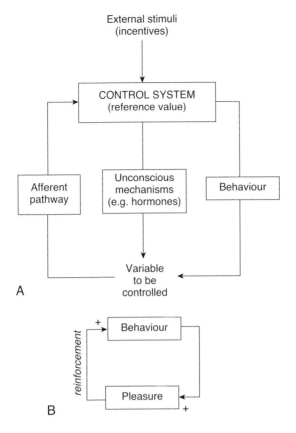

Fig 4.1 Motivated behaviour can be explained in at least two ways. (A) Suppressing discomfort. Changes in a variable to be controlled, e.g. body temperature or food/water intake, are detected by some receptors that send afferent signals to the control system. This compares these changes with a reference value and, accordingly, restores the normal value of the variable through both unconscious mechanisms, such as hormone secretion, and the activation of a behavioural act, e.g. looking for some water. External stimuli, or incentives, may trigger motivated behaviour even in the absence of changes in the variable to be controlled, e.g. drinking in the absence of liquids depletion. (B) Seeking pleasure. A given behaviour, e.g. the sexual act, may produce pleasure, thus motivated behaviour originates from the fact that it leads to a reward (sexual pleasure). The more intense the pleasure is, the more that behaviour is activated. Note that in this case there is no physiological variable to be controlled.

food intake (Novin et al. 1973). A similar effect has been found by blocking the metabolism of fatty acids (Ritter and Taylor 1990). The afferent pathway that conveys the information about glucose and fatty acids depletion travels along vagal afferents up to the nucleus of the solitary tract. The control system for the regulation of food intake is made up of different hypothalamic nuclei. Notably, the paraventricular nucleus secretes neuropeptide Y when there is glucose and fatty acids depletion. Its injection into the paraventricular nucleus of the rat leads to a two-fold increase in the frequency of food intake (Stanley et al. 1986). This occurs even if milk has been added with a bitter substance, which suggests a dramatic increase in motivation, despite the aversive taste of the milk (Flood and Morley 1991).

Once the behavioural repertoire has been initiated, the organism starts eating and introducing nutritional substances until a stop signal tells the control system that the eating behaviour must be stopped. An important stop signal is represented by the distension of the gastric wall which, in turn, activates mechanoreceptors (Olson et al. 1993). A second signal is represented by cholecystokinin (CCK). If an obese receives an injection of CCK, he reduces the intake of food (Pi-Sunyer et al. 1982), and this effect can be eliminated by cutting the vagal nerve (Smith et al. 1985). Other two stop signals are represented by insulin and leptin. In particular, leptin is an hormone produced by adipose cells, whose blood concentration is proportional to the amount of body fat. Its concentration is four-fold higher in obese than in normal people (Considine et al. 1996). Leptin acts on the hypothalamus reducing the secretion of neuropeptide Y in the paraventricular nucleus (Woods et al. 2000). Similarly, blood levels of insulin are proportional to the level of body fat and insulin reduces the secretion of neuropeptide Y in the hypothalamus (Schwartz and Seeley 1997). Ghrelin has also been found to be involved in feeding behaviour (Palmiter 2007).

All these mechanisms are embedded in the model of Fig 4.1A. It should be pointed out however that, for the sake of this volume, they are oversimplified. For example, the control system for food intake also includes the lateral hypothalamus, the ventromedial hypothalamus, as well as the arcuate nucleus of the hypothalamus. It is also worth noting that the model of Fig 4.1B may also apply to hunger. In this case, eating is not so much a physiological need attributable to the depletion of nutritional substances, but rather it assumes the role of hedonistic need, whereby one seeks pleasure through different tastes and flavours. In this regard, it is useful to remember that the sensation of empty stomach plays an important role in starting food intake, even if the stomach has long been known to be unnecessary to induce hunger (Ingelfinger 1944). Food intake is in this case only aimed at suppressing the uncomfortable local abdominal feeling of emptiness, without a real hunger sensation. Indeed, midbrain dopamine neurons have long been implicated in mediating reward and motivation in feeding behaviour. In fact, hormones implicated in regulating the homeostatic system, like insulin and leptin, also inhibit directly dopamine neurons, whereas ghrelin activates them (Palmiter 2007) (see also section 4.1.4).

Thirst mechanisms are also embedded in the model of Fig 4.1A and B. There are two types of thirst: hypovolumetric and osmotic. In hypovolumetric thirst, the extracellular volume of liquids decreases and this decrease is detected by pressure receptors (Fitzsimons and Moore-Gillon 1980). An important afferent pathway is represented by two hormones, renin and angiotensin. Whereas renin is necessary for the production of angiotensin, the injection of angiotensin into the subfornical organ in the brain induces the increase of water intake, and lesions of the subfornical organ abolish this effect (Simpson et al. 1978). In osmotic thirst, osmolarity is increased, for example, because of an increase of sodium chloride in extracellular fluids. The organum vasculosum lamina terminalis (OVLT) detects the increase in osmolarity and, accordingly, triggers liquids intake (Thrasher and Keil 1987). As for hunger, thirst can be merely hedonistic (Fig 4.1B), without any need to introduce liquids into the organism. For example, water intake can be aimed only at placating the uncomfortable sensation of dry mouth.

The model of Fig 4.1 also applies to thermoregulation. The afferent pathway is represented by thermoreceptors that are localized in different parts of the body, whereas the preoptic area of the hypothalamus is a thermostat that contains neurons sensitive to positive and negative variations of temperature (Nakashima et al. 1987). In this case, motivated behaviour aims to seek either warm or cold places.

4.1.3 Seeking pleasure from sex

What drives, orients, and maintains behaviour in hunger, thirst, and thermal variations is the suppression of discomfort, and this avoids harm to the organism. This is not so clear in other conditions, where a real discomfort may not be present, and where there is no harm to the individual. For example, differently from hunger and thirst, the absence of sex is not dangerous to health. However, it should be noted that whereas sex is not important for the survival of the single individual, it is crucial for the survival of the species. The pleasure that derives from the sexual act thus warrants repeated sexual activity across the individuals belonging to a given species. The model represented in Fig 4.1B seems to be appropriate for sex. In other words, sexual behaviour leads to pleasure which, in turn, acts as a reinforcement on the sexual behavioural repertoire itself, thereby stimulating the repetition of the act many times.

Besides sexual hormones, which may initiate and maintain sexual behaviour, many brain regions take part to the sexual act and these have been analysed in great detail, particularly in animals. The medial preoptic area of the hypothalamus and the medial amygdala have been found to be hyperactive when animals make sex spontaneously, and the stimulation of the medial preoptic area increases the frequency of the sexual intercourses in rodents

(Bloch et al. 1993, 1996; Pfaus et al. 1993) whereas the stimulation of the medial amygdala induces dopamine release (Matuszewich et al. 2000; Dominguez and Hull 2001). Gender-specific regions have also been found. For example, the sexually dimorphic nucleus of the hypothalamus is important for sexual activity in males (de Jonge et al. 1989), whereas the ventromedial nucleus of the hypothalamus is crucial for sexual behaviour in females (Pfaff and Sakuma 1979). Given the important role of dopamine in reward mechanisms (see section 4.1.4), it is interesting to note that dopaminergic activity increases during the sexual act (Mas et al. 1995) and that dopamine blockade in the medial preoptic area by means of antagonists reduces sexual activity (Warner et al. 1991). In humans, dopaminergic drugs have been found to stimulate sexual behaviour (Meston and Frohlich 2000).

Masters and Johnson (1966) have identified four phases of sexual activity. First, excitation is a period of increasing attention that aims to prepare the sexual act. Second, a plateau is reached, in which sexual attention is constantly high. Third, orgasm is that short-lasting phase where the peak of pleasure is reached. Fourth, resolution occurs, whereby attention decreases. These four phases are followed by a refractory period that may last minutes, hours, and even days, depending on the individual. Interestingly, whereas the intensity of hunger and thirst depends on the time lag from the latest meal or drink, the temporal factor in sex is not as important as for hunger and thirst. Sensory stimuli (visual, auditory, or tactile) play a much more important role to initiate another sexual act. In addition, the refractory period can be shortened in males if the partner changes, the so-called Coolidge effect. During the Coolidge effect, dopamine is released in the nucleus accumbens when the male copulates with the first female, then decreases to normal levels, but it is released again at high levels in the presence of a new female (Fiorino et al. 1997).

The distinction between the suppression of discomfort and the search of pleasure is not straightforward. It is clear that discomfort increases as the time lag from the latest meal or drink increases. Thus hunger and thirst are themselves uncomfortable sensations that can vary in intensity over time and that need to be placated by adopting the appropriate behaviour. By contrast, what drives the sexual act is not so much an increased discomfort from the latest sexual act, but rather an increased drive to get a pleasant reward. Nevertheless, it is also true that, if the sexual act is not consumed, an intense uncomfortable sensation often arises, and this needs to be eventually placated. For this reason, suppression of discomfort and search of pleasure are in many cases overlapping, or they even represent the same thing. By suppressing discomfort, one receives a reward, and by seeking a pleasant reward one actually wants to suppress the discomfort that might derive from not reaching that objective.

4.1.4 Reward-seeking behaviours involve the mesolimbic dopaminergic system

In the previous section we have seen that in motivated behaviours such as hunger and sex dopamine appears to play an important role. It increases during sexual activity (Mas et al. 1995) and is modulated by hormones implicated in food intake, e.g. insulin, leptin, and ghrelin (Palmiter 2007). Indeed, the mesolimbic dopaminergic system has been found to be activated in a number of reward-seeking behaviours, such that today it is better known as the motivation/reward dopaminergic system.

In the 1950s, Olds and Milner (1954) paved the road to the understanding of both the anatomy and physiology of the motivation/reward system. In their classical experiment, they implanted an electrode in several regions of the rat brain. The electrode was connected to a stimulator that could be activated by pressing a lever within the cage. Thus the rat, which was free to move around the cage, had the possibility to press the lever and to stimulate himself whenever he wanted. After a first period of wandering in his cage, he randomly pressed the lever, thus self-delivering an electrical stimulation. After a short period of learning, his behaviour changed completely. The rat started pressing the lever many times per minute, reducing dramatically the time spent for feeding, drinking, and grooming behaviour. This effect is called intracranial electrical self-stimulation. Sometimes it is so powerful that the health conditions of some rats deteriorate because of the suppression of both feeding and drinking behaviour.

The key questions that emerged from this and other experiments were mainly two: why rats stimulate themselves and which brain areas induce the self-stimulation effect. As to the first question, the most plausible explanation is that rats stimulate themselves repeatedly and compulsively because they experience a pleasant sensation. For this reason, the electrical self-stimulation is called positive reinforcement, or otherwise reward. In other words, the activation of these centres by electrical stimulation induces pleasure, thus the animals adopt a motivated behaviour that aims to repeatedly seek a reward. In support of the fact that animals feel a pleasant sensation there are several studies in humans. From the early studies in humans by Heath (1963) to more recent human studies (e.g. Benedetti et al. 2004; see also section 3.3.2), it has been found that the intraoperative stimulation of several limbic areas may produce pleasant sensations and even compulsive self-stimulation. For example, patients may report a general feeling of pleasure, such as happiness, or more specific pleasurable sensations, like sexual orgasm.

As to the second question, i.e. which regions produce these effects, many sites have been discovered over the past years. Their stimulation elicits the self-stimulation phenomenon, thereby indicating that these regions are involved in motivation/reward mechanisms (Corbett and Wise 1980; Fibiger et al. 1987; Nakahara et al. 1989). The most powerful effects can be obtained by stimulating the septal area, some regions of the hypothalamus, like the lateral hypothalamus, the medial forebrain bundle, and the ventral tegmental area. The general organization that has emerged from these and other studies is represented in Fig 4.2 in a simplified form. The ventral tegmental area sends a dopaminergic projection to the nucleus accumbens as well as to other regions, such as the amygdala. The nucleus accumbens, in turn, projects to the prefrontal cortex.

Many drugs of abuse act at the level of this network, thereby producing pleasure (Hoebel et al. 1983; Bozarth and Wise 1984; Wise and Rompre 1989). Their action on the mesolimbic dopaminergic system is the basis of addiction, whereby a compulsive behaviour, in this case the repeated self-administration of a drug, is aimed at seeking a reward. For example, heroin and nicotine act at the level of the ventral tegmental area, whose dopaminergic neurons also express opioid and cholinergic nicotinic receptors, whereas cocaine acts on the nucleus accumbens, prolonging dopaminergic activity (Wise 1996).

Lesion studies have clearly shown that damage to the motivation/reward system as shown in Fig 4.2 abolish both electrical self-stimulation and drug self-administration. For example, the lesion of the ventral tegmental area

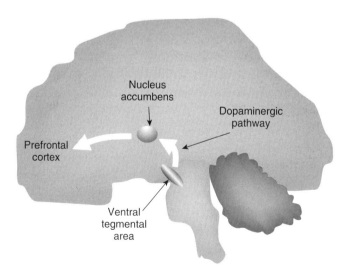

Fig 4.2 The mesolimbic dopaminergic system. In this simplified schema, the main regions are the ventral tegmental area that sends a dopaminergic projection to the nucleus accumbens which, in turn, projects to the prefrontal cortex.

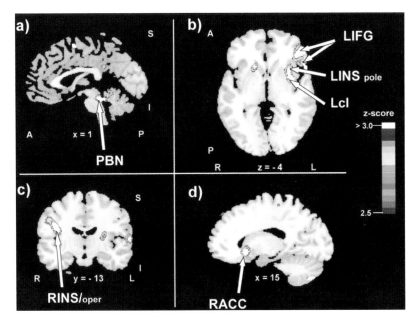

Plate 1 Positron emission tomography during stomach distention. Arrows point to areas with significant changes in regional cerebral blood flow in four a priori defined regions of interest involved in visceral sensation: (a) dorsal brain stem nuclei; (b) left inferior frontal gyrus; (b and c) insular cortex/claustrum; (d) subgenual anterior cingulate cortex. A, anterior; I, inferior; L, left; Lcl, left claustrum; LIFG, left inferior frontal gyrus; LINS, left insula; LINS pole, left insular pole; P, posterior; PBN, parabrachial nucleus; R, right; RACC, right anterior cingulate cortex; RINS/oper, right insula/operculum; S, superior; x, sagittal plane; y, coronal plane; z, horizontal plane. See p.60. Source: From Stephan et al. 2003 with permission from Springer and the Society for Surgery of the Alimentary Tract, Copyright 2003.

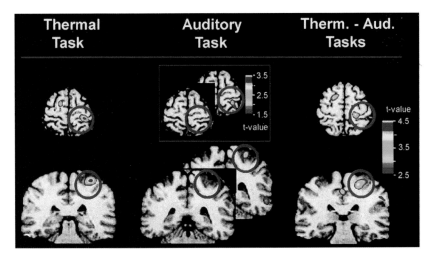

Plate 2 The effects of attention on pain processing. When subjects attend to a noxious heat stimulus (left), the primary somatosensory cortex enhances its activity. Conversely, when the subjects attend to an auditory stimulus (centre), a significant reduction of the primary somatosensory cortex activity occurs. Differences in pain-related activity during the two attentional conditions are revealed by subtracting positron emission tomography data recorded during the auditory task from that recorded during the heat-discrimination task (right). See p.75. Source: From Bushnell et al. 1999 with permission of the National Academy of Science USA, Copyright 1999.

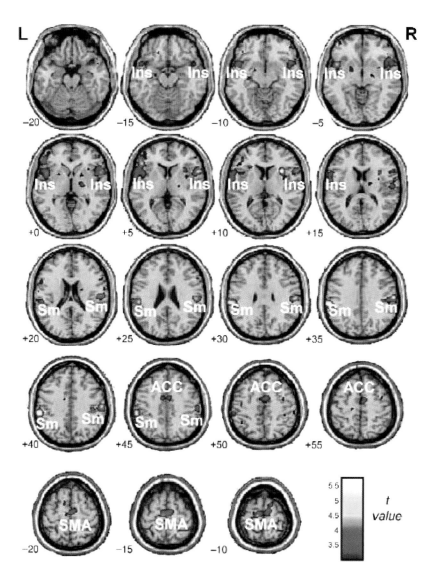

Plate 3 Functional magnetic resonance during interoceptive attention, whereby the subjects judge the timing of their own heartbeats. Note the activation in bilateral anterior insula (Ins), lateral somatomotor and adjacent parietal cortices (Sm), anterior cingulate (ACC), and supplementary motor cortices (SMA). See p.62.
Source: From Critchley et al. 2004 with permission from Nature Publishing Group, Copyright 2004.

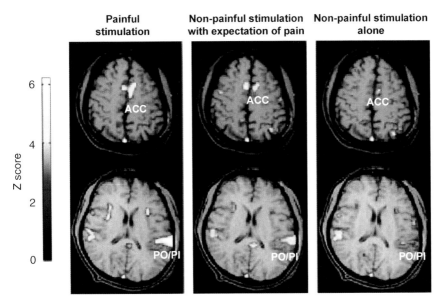

Plate 4 The effects of expecting pain on pain processing. Some areas of the pain matrix, such as the anterior cingulate cortex (ACC), the parietal operculum (PO), and posterior insula (PI), enhance their activity in response to non-painful stimulation when expecting pain (centre). The level of activation is almost similar to that following a real painful stimulation (left). By contrast, non-painful stimulation alone induces significant smaller activations (right). See p. 83.
Source: From Sawamoto et al. 2000, with permission from The Society for Neuroscience, Copyright 2000.

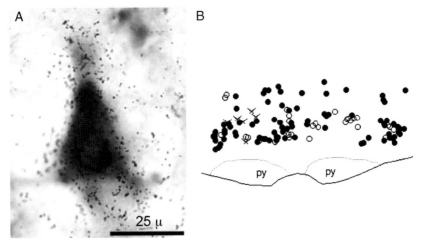

Plate 5 Double hybridization histochemistry for CCK-2 (or CCK-B according to the old classification) and μ-opioid receptors transcripts in the rostroventromedial medulla of the rat. (A) A pyramidal neuron in the rostroventromedial medulla labelled for both CCK-2 (silver grains) and μ-opioid (dark blue) receptors. (B) Map of neurons co-labelled for CCK-2 and μ-opioid receptors (closed circles), CCK-2 receptors only (open circles), and μ-opioid receptors only (crosses) in the rostroventromedial medulla. Note that most neurons co-express both μ-opioid and CCK-2 receptors. py, pyramid. See p.87.
Source: From Zhang et al. 2009, with permission from Oxford University Press, Copyright 2009.

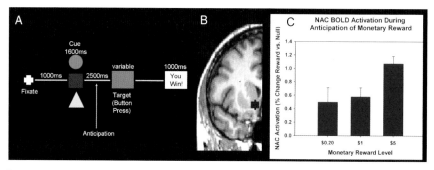

Plate 6 Activation of the nucleus accumbens by monetary reward. (A) Experimental design showing the Monetary Incentive Delay task. A cue representing a monetary value is followed by an anticipation phase and a neutral target requiring button press. The cue could be one of seven types, representing three different levels of monetary gain ($0.20, $1, and $5), a null condition ($0), or three levels of monetary loss ($-$0.20, $-$1, $-$5). (B) Functional magnetic resonance image showing nucleus accumbens activation. (C) Percent change in the nucleus accumbens magnetic resonance signal from low ($0.20) to intermediate ($1) to high ($5) monetary reward trials. Note that the brain responses are proportional to the reward value. NAC, nucleus accumbens. See p. 112.
Source: From Scott et al. 2007 with permission from Elsevier and Cell Press, Copyright 2007.

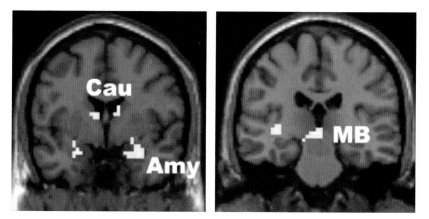

Plate 7 Subjects who receive oxytocin show no change in their trusting behaviour after they learned that their trust had been breached several times while control subjects (who did not receive oxytocin) decrease their trust. This difference in trust adaptation is associated with a specific reduction in activation in the amygdala, the midbrain regions, and the caudate nucleus in subjects receiving oxytocin. Amy, amygdala; Cau, caudate nucleus; MB, midbrain. See p.137.
Source: From Baumgartner et al. 2008 with permission from Elsevier and Cell Press, Copyright 2008.

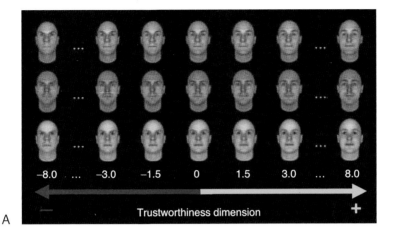

A

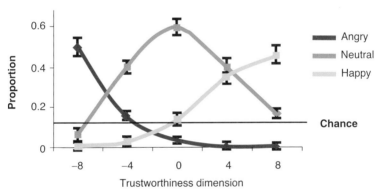

B

Plate 8 (A) Examples of faces with trustworthiness features that range from negative (i.e. untrustworthiness) to positive (total trustworthiness). The faces in the centre column were randomly generated and then their features were exaggerated to decrease (left three columns) and increase (right three columns) their perceived trustworthiness. (B) Categorization of faces as angry, happy, and neutral as a function of their trustworthiness. The x-axis represents the extent of exaggeration of facial features in standard deviation units. As the facial features become more exaggerated, the neutral categorization approaches chance, and this is particularly clear on the negative end of the continuum. As the facial features become more exaggerated in the negative direction (−8), the faces are mostly classified as angry, whereas when the trustworthy facial features become more exaggerated in the positive direction (+8), the faces are mostly classified as happy. See p.130.

Source: From Todorov 2008 with permission from John Wiley & Sons and the New York Academy of Sciences, Copyright 2008.

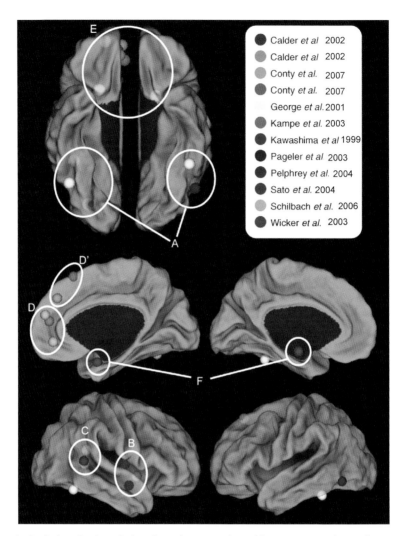

Plate 9 Cortical and subcortical regions that are activated by eye contact (mutual eye gaze that connects people together) in different studies. (A) Fusiform gyrus, particularly in the right hemisphere. (B) Anterior part of the right superior temporal sulcus. (C) Posterior part of right superior temporal sulcus. (D) Right medial prefrontal cortex (in two studies averted gaze was more effective than direct gaze (D'). (E) Orbitofrontal cortex. (F) Right and left amygdala. See p. 144

Source: From Senju and Johnson 2009 with permission from Elsevier and Cell Press, Copyright 2009.

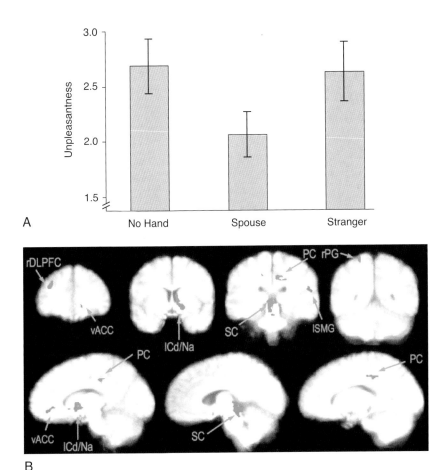

Plate 10 (A) Effect of hand-holding on unpleasantness about threat of an electric shock. Whereas there is no difference between the no-hand condition and holding a stranger's hand, a significant reduction in unpleasantness is present when holding the spouse's hand. (B) Threat-responsive regions affected by hand-holding condition. Green clusters indicate attenuation in the right dorsolateral prefrontal cortex (rDLPFC), left caudate–nucleus accumbens (lCd/Na), and superior colliculus (SC) when hoding the spouse's hand. Blue clusters indicate attenuation in the ventral anterior cingulate cortex (vACC), posterior cingulate (PC), right postcentral gyrus (rPG), and left supramarginal gyrus (lSMG) associated with both spouse and stranger hand-holding. See p.150.
Source: Adapted from Coan et al. 2006 with permission from
John Wiley & Sons and the Association for Psychological Science, Copyright 2006.

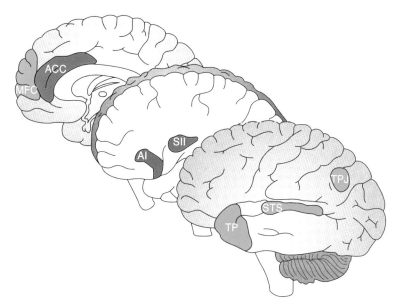

Plate 11 Brain regions typically involved in understanding others on the basis of cognitive perspective taking (green) and empathic emotional abilities (orange). MFC, medial prefrontal cortex; ACC, anterior cingulate cortex; AI, anterior insula; SII, secondary somatosensory cortex; TP, temporal poles; STS, superior temporal sulcus; TPF, temporo-parietal junction. See p.159.

Source: From Hein and Singer 2008 with permission from Elsevier, Copyright 2008.

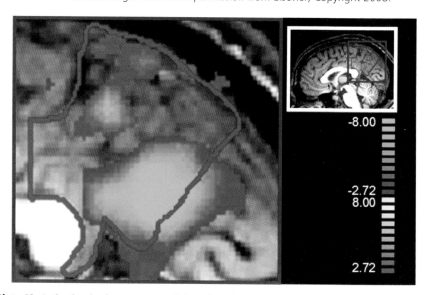

Plate 12 Activation in the posteromedial cortices (outlined in pink) for admiration for virtue and compassion for social pain (blue/green) versus admiration for skill and compassion for physical pain (orange/yellow). The red box frames the location of the magnified view. Note the clear separation between the anterosuperior sector activated by admiration for skill and compassion for physical pain, and the posteroinferior activated by admiration for virtue and compassion for social pain. See p.163.

Source: From Immordino-Yang et al. 2009 with permission from the National Academy of Sciences USA, Copyright 2009.

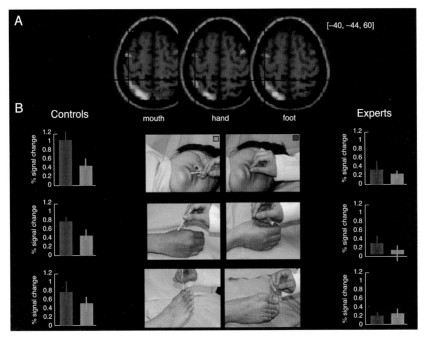

Plate 13 Regions within the somatosensory cortex when watching different body parts being pricked by a needle or touched by a Q-tip in experienced acupuncturists (experts) and in naive subjects (controls). (A) Watching different body parts (from left to right: mouth region, hand, foot) elicits differential activations around the somatosensory cortex. (B) The somatosensory activations are modulated by the expertise of the participants and the level of pain inferred. In controls, watching the body parts pricked by a needle (red columns) was associated with stronger signal than was watching a Q-tip (orange columns). In experts, the Q-tip and needle resulted in similar signal changes in the somatosensory cortex. See p.165.

Source: From Cheng et al. 2007 with permission by Elsevier, Copyright 2007.

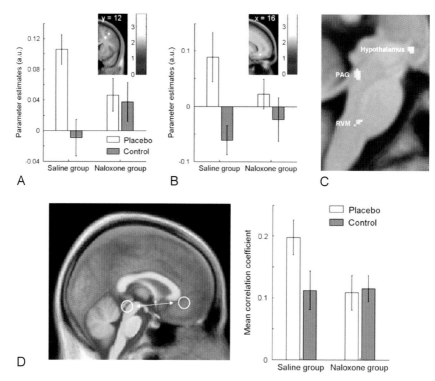

Plate 14 Activations of (A) the dorsolateral prefrontal cortex (DLPFC) and (B) the subgenual rostral anterior cingulate cortex (rACC) are significantly stronger under placebo compared to control in the saline group. This difference is strongly reduced in the naloxone group. (C) The sagittal slice shows placebo-enhanced responses in the hypothalamus, the periaqueductal grey (PAG), and the rostroventromedial medulla (RVM), all of which are significantly reduced by naloxone. (D) The midline sagittal slice depicts the approximate location of rACC and PAG. The intraindividual coupling between rACC and PAG is significantly stronger under placebo than under control in the saline group, whereas this difference is abolished in the naloxone group. Error bars indicate SEM. See p.195.

Source: From Eippert et al. 2009a with permission from Elsevier and Cell Press, Copyright 2009.

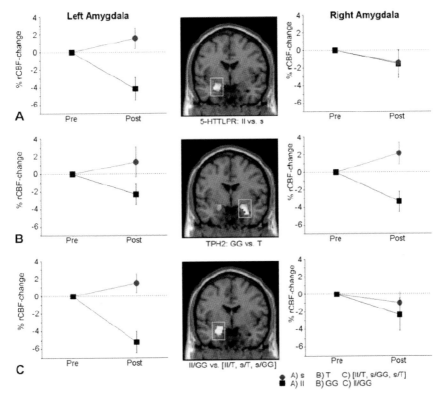

Plate 15 Changes in functional magnetic resonance imaging activity in the left and right amygdala after placebo administration during public speaking in different genetic subgroups. A significantly greater reduction of amygdala activity from pre- to post-placebo treatment was observed in the following: (A) long allele (ll) homozygotes compared with short (s) allele carriers of the serotonin transporter gene (5-HTTLPR), (B) G allele (GG) homozygotes compared with T allele carriers of the TPH2 G-703T polymorphism; and (C) long and G allele homozygous patients (ll/GG group) compared with patients carrying s and/or T alleles (ll/T, s/GG, s/T group). See p.205.

Source: From Furmark et al. 2008, with permission from the Society for Neuroscience, Copyright 2008.

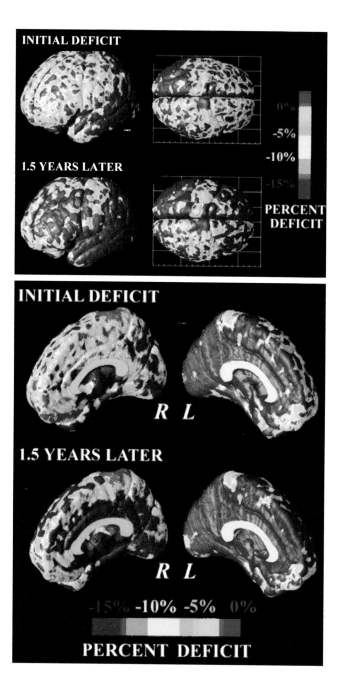

Plate 16 Average percentage loss of grey matter in Alzheimer's disease. Note the heavy loss in the frontal and temporal regions (top panel) as well of the medial portion of the hemispheres (bottom panel). Also note the asymmetric deficits and the relative sparing of the sensorimotor regions with virtually no grey matter loss (blue). See p.236.
Source: From Thompson et al. 2003 with permission from the Society for Neuroscience, Copyright 2003.

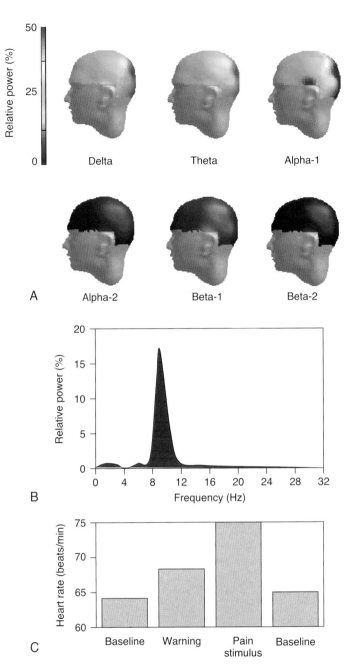

Plate 17 Alzheimer patient with mild-moderate cognitive impairment (MMSE = 21), and with stimulus detection = 3 mA, and pain threshold = 19 mA. (A) 3D mapping of the distribution of the relative powers of the delta, theta, alpha-1, alpha-2, beta-1, and beta-2 bands over the scalp. (B) Mean relative power spectrum obtained by averaging the relative powers of all the 19 electrodes. (C) Heart rate responses to warning (pain anticipation) and to pain stimulation. Note the normal electroencephalogram with an alpha-1 peak in the occipital and posterior parietal region, and the heart rate response to both warning and pain. See p.239.

Source: From Benedetti et al. 2004 with permission from the International Association for the Study of Pain, Copyright 2004.

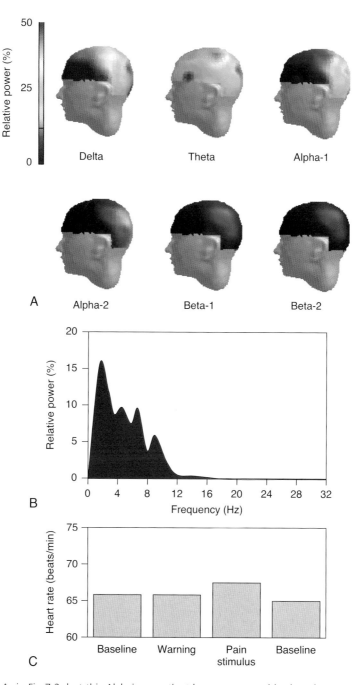

Plate 18 As in Fig 7.2, but this Alzheimer patient has severe cognitive impairment (MMSE =9), and stimulus detection = 4 mA, and pain threshold = 20 mA. Note the distribution of the delta and theta frequencies on the frontal, temporal, and parietal regions, and the small alpha-1 activity in the occipital region (A). Also note the prevalence of delta and theta rhythms (below 8 Hz) in the spectrum (B), the absence of the heart rate response to warning and the small heart rate response to pain (C). See p.240
Source: From Benedetti et al. 2004 with permission from the International Association for the Study of Pain, Copyright 2004.

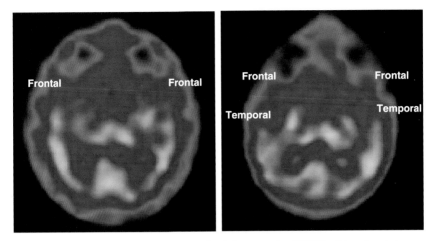

Plate 19 Single Photon Emission Computerized Tomography (SPECT) of two frontotemporal dementia patients who show hypoperfusion of the frontal lobes (patient on the left), and frontal and anterior temporal lobes (patient on the right). Both patients show increased pain threshold and pain tolerance. See p.245.

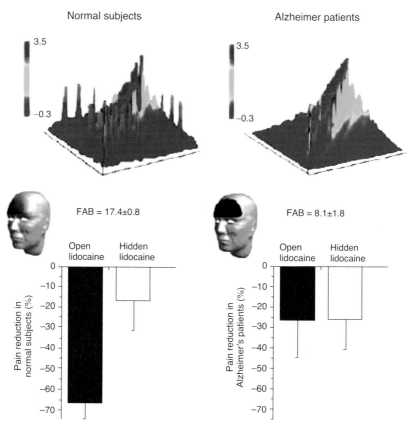

Plate 20 Correlation between electroencephalographic connectivity analysis (assessed by means of 'mutual information analysis': top panel), cognitive status (assessed by means of Frontal Assessment Battery or FAB) and the placebo component of open (black bars) and hidden (white bars) application of the local analgesic lidocaine. Note the differences between normal subjects (on the left) and Alzheimer patients (on the right). Alzheimer patients show reduced electroencephalographic connectivity, as shown by the disappearance of the orange peaks (top panel), reduced FAB scores, and reduced effects of open lidocaine. See p.250.

Source: From Benedetti et al. 2006 and Colloca et al. 2008 with permission from Springer, Copyright 2008.

produces a reduction of proencephalic dopamine as large as about 90%, along with a reduction in electrical self-stmulation (Fibiger et al. 1987). Likewise, a lesion of the nucleus accumbens reduces drug reward (Kelsey et al. 1989).

The mesolimbic dopaminergic system is activated in many reward-seeking behaviours (Schultz et al. 2000; Schultz 2002), as we have seen for hunger, sex, electrical self-stimulation, and drug self-administration. All these behaviours are present in both animals and humans. It is worth noting that there are reward-seeking behaviours that are typical of human beings, in which the very same reward network is activated. For example, monetary reward typically activates the mesolimbic dopaminergic system. Figure 4.3A shows the Monetary Incentive Delay task used in the studies by Knutson et al. (2001) and Scott et al. (2007). A trial consisted of a cue, followed by a variable delay interval, followed by a button-press response to a target. Subjects were then informed of their success on the preceding trial, as well as their monetary gain or loss. The cue could be one of seven types, representing three different levels of monetary gain ($0.20, $1, and $5), a null condition ($0), or three levels of monetary loss (−$0.20, −$1, −$5). In monetary gain trials, subjects would win the cued amount of money if they successfully responded during the target presentation. In monetary loss trials, subjects had to successfully respond to the target to avoid losing the cued monetary amount. In the null trials, subjects experienced no monetary gain or loss but were still instructed to respond to the target. Figure 4.3B shows the activation of the nucleus accumbens, as measured with functional magnetic resonance imaging. Figure 4.3C depicts the percent change in the nucleus accumbens magnetic resonance signal from low ($0.20) to intermediate ($1) to high ($5) monetary reward trials. It can be seen that the brain responses are proportional to the reward value.

There is thus experimental evidence that in gamble the nucleus accumbens increases its activity. In another study, neural responses accompanying anticipation and experience of monetary gains and losses were recorded by using functional magnetic resonance imaging. Trials comprised an initial expectancy phase, whereby a set of three monetary amounts was displayed, and a subsequent outcome phase, whereby one of these amounts was awarded. Responses were consistent with the activation of the mesolimbic dopaminergic network and increased monotonically with monetary value in the nucleus accumbens, sublenticular extended amygdala, and hypothalamus (Breiter et al. 2001). In a different study, pathological gamblers showed a reduction of nucleus accumbens and ventromedial prefrontal activation that was negatively correlated with gambling severity, linking hypoactivation of these areas to disease severity (Reuter et al. 2005).

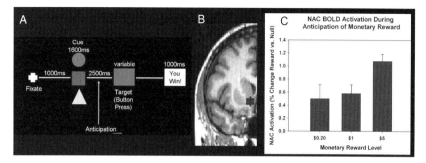

Fig 4.3 Activation of the nucleus accumbens by monetary reward. (A) Experimental design showing the Monetary Incentive Delay task. A cue representing a monetary value is followed by an anticipation phase and a neutral target requiring button press. The cue could be one of seven types, representing three different levels of monetary gain ($0.20, $1, and $5), a null condition ($0), or three levels of monetary loss (−$0.20, −$1, −$5). (B) Functional magnetic resonance image showing nucleus accumbens activation. (C) Percent change in the nucleus accumbens magnetic resonance signal from low ($0.20) to intermediate ($1) to high ($5) monetary reward trials. Note that the brain responses are proportional to the reward value. NAC, nucleus accumbens. See colour plate 6.
Source: From Scott et al. 2007 with permission from Elsevier and Cell Press, Copyright 2007.

The overlap of the observed activations of the mesolimbic dopamine system in response to a variety of motivated behaviours and rewards, such as alimentary stimuli and food intake, sexual arousal and sexual activity, drugs of abuse and euphoria-inducing drugs, and monetary incentives and gamble, is consistent with a contribution of common circuitry to the processing of diverse rewards as well as to the initiation of different motivation-induced behavioural repertoires. Therefore, motivated behaviour that aims to suppress discomfort from sickness and to seek the reward of clinical amelioration can be approached within the context of motivation/reward mechanisms.

4.2 **Suppressing discomfort from sickness**

4.2.1 **Seeking relief from sickness is a motivated behaviour**

The general model of Fig 4.1A can be reframed as shown in Fig 4.4. Pathological processes, e.g. tissue damage, represent the variable to be controlled, whereas the afferent pathway originates from receptors in the impaired tissue. This is a sensory pathway that gives rise to a symptom, e.g. pain, through interoceptive and/or nociceptive afferents, and to negative emotions such as anxiety. It turns out that negative emotions trigger the motivational system, with increased motivation to suppress the discomfort. Finally, a specific behavioural repertoire

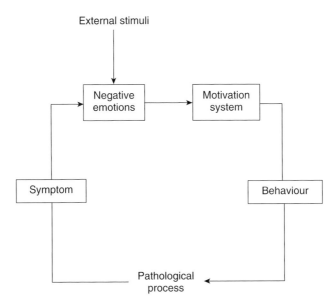

Fig 4.4 Motivated behaviour that aims to suppress sickness. This schema is reframed from the more general model of Fig 4.1. A pathological process, e.g. tissue damage, is the variable to be controlled. Thence, a symptom, e.g. pain, travels along the afferent pathway and gives rise to negative emotions, e.g. anxiety. The motivational system is activated, with increased motivation to suppress the discomfort. Finally, a specific behavioural repertoire is started that is aimed at seeking relief by suppressing the pathological process. External stimuli, e.g. a negative diagnosis, may induce negative emotions directly, without the presence of any symptom.

is started that is aimed at seeking relief. It should be noted that a symptom is not always necessary to evoke negative emotions and to trigger the motivational system. External stimuli, for example the negative diagnosis by a doctor, may induce negative emotions directly, without the presence of any symptom.

From an evolutionary perspective, it is interesting to note that motivated behaviour that is triggered by sickness is present in animals, with more or less simple behavioural repertoires, as well as in humans, with much more complex behavioural acts, such as going to a doctor's office (see section 4.2.2). In animals, behaviour that aims to fight sickness is adaptive in nature, that is, animals may adopt the most appropriate behavioural repertoires that can reduce the severity and shorten the duration of illness (Weary et al. 2009). Many of the behaviours shown by ill animals are part of a coordinated strategy to fight disease (Hart 1988; Dantzer 2004). For example, heat conservation during infection is achieved through both physiological responses, like vasoconstriction, and behavioural responses, such as postural changes. These strategies allow energy to be preserved, particularly by considering that sick animals may reduce food intake. In this regard, reduction in appetite helps promote recovery (Johnson 2002; Weary et al. 2009). In a study, experimentally infected mice were allowed to consume food ad libitum, whereas others were force-fed to the level of uninfected controls. Infected mice that regulated their own intake ate only 58% as much as the controls, and showed longer survival compared to mice that were force-fed (Murray and Murray 1979).

Animal behaviour that aims to fight sickness may have even more complex meanings. It may signal vigour and/or need (Weary et al. 2009). Where and when possible, sick animals can mask any signs of vulnerability, especially if the illness makes them an easier target for predation. This may be true in early and mild stages of a disease, for it is more difficult to mask signs of vulnerability when the illness is more severe. In Figure 4.4, the external stimuli may be represented in this case by the presence of a predator, which inhibits sickness-related negative emotions and motivated behaviour. By contrast, animals may benefit from signalling their infirmity, for example, for soliciting parental care. Therefore, different forms of motivated behaviour may take place in different situations. Preys that are continuously exposed to predators are likely to mask their sickness, while domestic animals are more likely to signal their infirmity. As occurs in animals, different motivated behaviours are also present in humans, and these depend mainly on cultural differences.

4.2.2 Motivated behaviour varies according to cultural differences

In the schema of Fig 4.4, the behaviour that is adopted varies from individual to individual. Of course, the purpose is always the same, i.e. seeking someone or something that can provide some form of relief, but the way this is accomplished is based on personal beliefs, expectancies, cultural differences, or, in other words, on the memories about how discomfort and pathological processes can be suppressed. Mainstream medicine and the conventional doctor is the most common means through which this motivated behaviour is accomplished in Western societies, but alternative medicines are also common. Conversely, in non-Western societies, traditional practices and shamanism are more usual. As described in section 2.2.2, there are plenty of medical practices all over the world, from traditional Chinese medicine to Ayurvedic medicine of India, and from Muti in Southern Africa to Ifà in Western Africa. Individual beliefs, e.g. distrust in doctors, may even lead to self-healing behaviours, whereby the individual tries to suppress his own discomfort in himself through a number of procedures learned within the context of his family and/or social group. Even within the context of Western societies, there are rural areas, for example in Europe and North America, where people have never seen a conventional modern doctor, and whose motivated behaviour to suppress sickness is based on irrational procedures.

According to these cultural differences, it is clear that what the sick does first is to rely on the healer who, he believes, is capable of suppressing the pathological process. The following step, which will be the topic of Chapter 5, is to interact with the healer. For the sake of this chapter, it is important to realize that the ability, competence, and skills of the healer do not matter at all. What counts is the patient's behaviour, regardless of the healer whom he refers to. It is like a thirsty man who wants to placate his discomfort. In the study of motivation, what matters is his water-seeking behaviour, regardless of the place where he goes. He can choose either the right or the wrong place, according to his beliefs and expectations. Therefore, it must be clear that, when studying motivation to suppress sickness, the behavioural repertoire that is adopted (Fig 4.4) does not have to be necessarily the correct choice.

4.2.3 The motivation/reward system is activated when seeking and expecting relief

There is compelling experimental evidence that the mesolimbic dopaminergic system may be activated when a subject expects clinical improvement. Most, if not all, of this evidence comes from the placebo literature, whereby an inert medical treatment is administered along with verbal suggestions of improvement. When a patient seeks relief, he eventually expects the reward of the positive therapeutic outcome, irrespective of whether or not a therapy has been started. In other words, the patient expects that his own seeking behaviour will probably lead to a successful outcome. In this regard, there is no clear-cut distinction between a doctor and a positive therapeutic outcome as rewards: both are the objective of the motivated behaviour. It should also be noted that, from a strict experimental point of view, it is not easy to investigate brain processes during the reward-seeking behaviour, thus some manipulations are necessary in an experimental setting, for example, the administration of a placebo procedure. The arguments of this section will also be treated in Chapter 6, when the therapeutic act itself will represent the main topic.

In 2001, de la Fuente-Fernandez et al. (2001) assessed the release of endogenous dopamine by using positron emission tomography with raclopride, a radiotracer which binds to dopamine D2 and D3 receptors and competes with endogenous dopamine. In this study, Parkinson patients were aware that they would be receiving an injection of either active drug (apomorphine, a dopamine receptor agonist) or placebo, according to classical clinical trial methodology. After placebo administration, that is, an inert substance that the patient believed to be apomorphine, it was found that dopamine was released in the striatum, corresponding to a change of 200% or more in extracellular dopamine concentration and comparable to the response to amphetamine in subjects with an intact dopamine system. The release of dopamine in the motor striatum (putamen and dorsal caudate) was greater in those patients who reported clinical improvement. Although in the studies by de la Fuente-Fernandez et al. (2001, 2002) all patients showed dopamine placebo responses, only half of the patients reported motor improvement. These patients also released larger amounts of dopamine in the dorsal motor striatum, suggesting a relationship between the amount of dorsal striatal dopamine release and clinical benefit. This relationship was not present in the ventral striatum, i.e. in the nucleus accumbens, in which all patients showed increased dopamine release, irrespective of whether they perceived any improvement. Accordingly, the investigators proposed that the dopamine released in the nucleus accumbens was associated with the patients' expectation of improvement in their symptoms, which could in turn be considered a form of reward.

In 2002, another brain imaging study was carried out (Mayberg et al. 2002). Changes in brain glucose metabolism were measured by means of positron emission tomography in male patients with unipolar depression who were treated with either placebo or fluoxetine for six weeks. Common and unique responses were described. In fact, both placebo and fluoxetine treatment induced regional metabolic increases in the prefrontal, anterior cingulate, premotor, parietal, posterior insula, and posterior cingulate, and metabolic decreases in the subgenual, para-hippocampus, and thalamus. The magnitude of regional fluoxetine changes was generally greater than placebo. However, fluoxetine responses were associated with additional subcortical and limbic changes in the brainstem, striatum, anterior insula, and hippocampus. There were no regional changes unique to placebo at six weeks. Interestingly, there were unique ventral striatal (nucleus accumbens) and orbital frontal changes in both placebo and drug responders at one week of treatment, that is, well before clinical benefit. Thus these changes are not associated to the clinical response, but rather to expectation and anticipation of the clinical benefit. Such changes were seen neither in the eventual drug non-responders nor at six weeks when the antidepressant response was well established, consistent with an expectation pattern of response (Mayberg et al. 2002; Benedetti et al. 2005). This pattern of activation of the nucleus accumbens is in agreement with an involvement of reward mechanisms in antidepressant placebo responses.

In another brain imaging study in which both positron emission tomography and functional magnetic resonance imaging were used, Scott et al. (2007) tested the correlation between the responsiveness to placebo and that to monetary reward. By using a model of experimental pain in healthy subjects, they found that placebo responsiveness was related to the activation of dopamine in the nucleus accumbens, as assessed by using *in vivo* receptor binding positron emission tomography with raclopride. The very same subjects were then tested with functional magnetic resonance imaging for monetary responses in the nucleus accumbens. A correlation between the placebo responses and the monetary responses was found: the larger the nucleus accumbens responses to monetary reward, the stronger the nucleus accumbens responses to placebos (Fig 4.5A). In addition, subjects who found the placebo either more or equally effective than anticipated demonstrated increasing right nucleus accumbens responses to increasing levels of expected reward value. Individuals who rated the placebo as less effective than anticipated did not demonstrate increasing nucleus accumbens responses as a function of reward values (Fig 4.5B). This study indicates common reward mechanisms for placebo responsiveness and monetary responses.

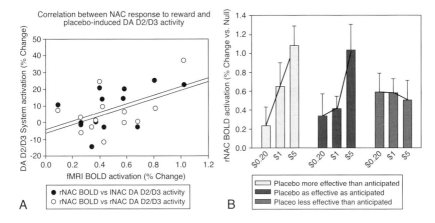

Fig 4.5 Nucleus accumbens responses to both monetary rewards and placebo-induced expectation of pain relief. (A) Correlation between the magnitude of right nucleus accumbens activity during the monetary reward task (x axis) and the placebo induced dopamine activation in the right (white circles) and left (black circles) nucleus accumbens (y axis). Note that the larger the nucleus accumbens responses to monetary reward are, the stronger the nucleus accumbens responses to placebos. (B) Subjects that found the placebo either more or equally effective than anticipated demonstrated increasing right nucleus accumbens responses to increasing levels of expected reward value. Individuals who rated the placebo as less effective than anticipated did not demonstrate increasing nucleus accumbens responses as a function of reward values (mean ± S.E.M.). Monetary reward was assessed with the method shown in Fig 4.3. NAC, nucleus accumbens; rNAC, right nucleus accumbens; lNAC, left nucleus accumbens; DA, dopamine.
Source: From Scott et al. 2007 with permission from Elsevier and Cell Press, Copyright 2007.

The same group (Scott et al. 2008) studied the endogenous opioid and the dopaminergic systems in different brain regions, including the nucleus accumbens. Subjects underwent a pain challenge, in the absence and presence of a placebo with expected analgesic properties. By using positron emission tomography with ^{11}C-labeled raclopride for the analysis of dopamine and ^{11}C-carfentanil for the study of opioids, it was found that placebo induced activation of opioid neurotransmission in the anterior cingulate, orbitofrontal and insular cortices, nucleus accumbens, amygdala, and periaqueductal grey matter. Dopaminergic activation was observed in the ventral basal ganglia, including the nucleus accumbens. Both dopaminergic and opioid activity were associated with both anticipation and perceived effectiveness of the placebo, as shown by the reduction in pain ratings. Large placebo responses were associated with greater dopamine and opioid activity in the nucleus accumbens. Interestingly, nocebo responses, which are opposite to placebo responses, were associated with a deactivation of dopamine and opioids. The release of dopamine in the nucleus accumbens accounted for 25% of the variance in placebo analgesic effects. Therefore, placebo and nocebo effects seem to be associated with opposite responses of dopamine and endogenous opioids in a distributed network of regions that form part of the reward and motivation circuit.

References

Benedetti F, Colloca L, Lanotte M, Bergamasco B, Torre E and Lopiano L (2004). Autonomic and emotional responses to open and hidden stimulation of the human subthalamic region. *Brain Research Bulletin*, **63**, 203–11.

Benedetti F, Mayberg HS, Wager TD, Stohler CS and Zubieta JK (2005). Neurobiological mechanisms of the placebo effect. *Journal of Neuroscience*, **25**, 10390–402.

Bloch GJ, Butler PC and Kohlert JG (1996). Galanin microinjected into the medial preoptic nucleus facilitates female- and male-typical sexual behaviors in the female rat. *Physiology and Behavior*, **59**, 1147–54.

Bloch GJ, Butler PC, Kohlert JG and Bloch DA (1993). Microinjection of galanin into the medial preoptic nucleus facilitates copulatory behaviour in the male rat. *Physiology and Behavior*, **54**, 615–24.

Bolles RC (1975). *Theory of motivation*. Harper & Row, New York, NY.

Bozarth MA and Wise RA (1984). Anatomically distinct opiate receptor fields mediate reward and physical dependence. *Science*, **224**, 516–7.

Breiter HC, Aharon I, Kahneman D, Dale A and Shizgal P (2001). Functional imaging of neural responses to expectancy and experience of monetary gains and losses. *Neuron*, **30**, 619–39.

Considine RV, Sinha MK, Heiman ML, Kriauciunas A, Stephens TW, Nyce MR et al. (1996). Serum immunoreactive-leptin concentrations in normal-weight and obese humans. *New England Journal of Medicine*, **334**, 292–5.

Corbett D and Wise RA (1980). Intracranial self-stimulation in relation to the ascending dopaminergic systems of the midbrain: a moveable electrode mapping study. *Brain Research*, **185**, 1–15.

Dantzer R (2004). Cytokine-induced sickness behaviour: a neuroimmune response to activation of innate immunity. *European Journal of Pharmacology*, **500**, 399–411.

de Jonge FH, Louwerse AL, Ooms MP, Evers P, Endert E and Van de Poll NE (1989). Lesions of the SDN-POA inhibit sexual behaviour of male Wistar rats. *Brain Research Bulletin*, **23**, 483–92.

de la Fuente-Fernandez R, Ruth TJ, Sossi V, Schulzer M, Calne DB and Stoessl AJ (2001). Expectation and dopamine release: mechanism of the placebo effect in Parkinson's disease. *Science,* **293**, 1164–6.

de la Fuente-Fernández R, Phillips AG, Zamburlini M, Sossi V, Calne DB, Ruth TJ et al. (2002). Dopamine release in human ventral striatum and expectation of reward. *Behavioural. Brain Research*, **136**, 359–63.

Dominguez JM and Hull EM (2001). Stimulation of the medial amygdala enhances medial preoptic dopamine release; implications for male rat sexual behaviour. *Brain Research*, **917**, 225–9.

Fibiger HC, LePiane FG, Jakubovic A and Phillips AG (1987). The role of dopamine in intracranial self-stimulation of the ventral tegmental area. *Journal of Neuroscience*, **7**, 3888–96.

Fiorino DF, Coury A and Phillips AG (1997). Dynamic changes in nucleus accumbens dopamine efflux during the Coolidge effect in male rats. *Journal of Neuroscience*, **17**, 4849–55.

Fitzsimons JT and Moore-Gillon MJ (1980). Drinking and anti-diuresis in response to reductions in venous return in the dog: neural and endocrine mechanisms. *Journal of Physiology*, **308**, 403–16.

Flood JF and Morley JE (1991). Increased food intake by neuropeptide Y is due to an increased motivation to eat. *Peptides*, **12**, 1329–32.

Hart BL (1988). Biological basis of the behaviour of sick animals. *Neuroscience and Biobehavioral Reviews*, **12**, 123–37.

Heath RG (1963). Electrical self-stimulation of the brain in man. *American Journal of Psychiatry*, **120**, 571–7.

Hoebel BG, Monaco A, Hernandes L, Aulisi E, Stanley BG and Lenard L (1983). Self injection of amphetamine directly into the brain. *Psychopharmacology*, **81**, 158–63.

Hull CL (1951). *Essentials of behavior*. Yale University Press, New Haven, CT.

Ingelfinger FJ (1944). The late effects of total and subtotal gastrectomy. *New England Journal of Medicine*, **231**, 321–7.

Johnson R W (2002). The concept of sickness behaviour: a brief chronological account of four key discoveries. *Veterinary Immunology and Immunopathology*, **87**, 443–50.

Kelsey JE, Carlezon WA Jr and Falls WA (1989). Lesions of the nucleus accumbens in rats reduce opiate reward but do not alter context-specific opiate tolerance. *Behavioral Neuroscience*, **103**, 1327–34.

Knutson B, Adams CM, Fong GW and Hommer D (2001). Anticipation of increasing monetary reward selectively recruits nucleus accumbens. *Journal of Neuroscience*, **21**, RC159, 1–5.

Mas M, Fumero B and Gonzalez-Mora JL (1995). Voltammetric and microdialysis monitoring of brain monoamine neurotransmitter release during sociosexual interactions. *Behavioural Brain Research*, **71**, 69–79.

Masters W and Johnson V (1966). *The human sexual response*. Little Brown, Boston, MA.

Matuszewich L, Lorrain DS and Hull EM (2000). Dopamine release in the medial preoptic area of female rats in response to hormonal manipulation and sexual activity. *Behavioral Neuroscience*, **114**, 772–82.

Mayberg HS, Silva JA, Brannan SK, Tekell JL, Mahurin RK, McGinnis S et al. (2002). The functional neuroanatomy of the placebo effect. *American Journal of Psychiatry*, **159**, 728–37.

Meston CM and Frohlich PF (2000). The neurobiology of sexual function. *Archives of General Psychiatry*, **57**, 1012–30.

Murray MJ and Murray AB (1979). Anorexia of infection as a mechanism of host defence. *American Journal of Clinical Nutrition*, **32**, 593–6.

Nakahara D, Ozaki N, Miura Y, Miura H and Nagatsu T (1989). Increased dopamine and serotonin metabolism in rat nucleus accumbens produced by intracranial self-stimulation of medial forebrain bundle as measured by in vivo microdialysis. *Brain Research*, **495**, 178–81.

Nakashima T, Pierau FK, Simon E and Hori T (1987). Comparison between hypothalamic thermoresponsive neurons from duck and rat slices. *Pfluegers Archive: European Journal of Physiology*, **409**, 236–43.

Novin D, VanderWeele DA and Rezek M (1973). Infusion of 2-deoxy D-glucose into the hepatic portal system causes eating: evidence for peripheral glucoreceptors. *Science*, **181**, 858–60.

Olds J and Milner P (1954). Positive reinforcement produced by electrical stimulation of the septal area and other regions of the rat brain. *Journal of Comparative Physiological Psychology*, **47**, 419–27.

Olson BR, Freilino M, Hoffman GE, Stricker EM, Sved AF and Verbalis JG (1993). C-fos expression in rat brain and brainstem nuclei in response to treatments that alter food intake and gastric motility. *Molecular and Cellular Neuroscience*, **4**, 93–106.

Palmiter RD (2007). Is dopamine a physiologically relevant mediator of feeding behavior? *Trends in Neurosciences*, **30**, 375–81.

Pfaff DW and Sakuma Y (1979). Deficit in the lordosis reflex of female rats caused by lesions in the ventromedial nucleus of the hypothalamus. *Journal of Physiology*, **288**, 203–10.

Pfaus JG, Kleopoulos SP, Mobbs CV, Gibbs RB and Pfaff DW (1993). Sexual stimulation activates c-fos within estrogen-concentrating regions of the female rat forebrain. *Brain Research*, **624**, 253–67.

Pi-Sunyer X, Kissilef HR, Thornton J and Smith GP (1982). C terminal octapeptide of cholecystokinin decreases food intake in obese men. *Physiology and Behavior*, **29**, 627–30.

Reuter J, Raedler T, Rose M, Hand I, Gläscher J and Büchel C (2005). Pathological gambling is linked to reduced activation of the mesolimbic reward system. *Nature Neuroscience*, **8**, 147–8.

Ritter S and Taylor JS (1990). Vagal sensory neurons are required for lipoprivic but not glucoprivic feeding in rats. *American Journal of Physiology*, **258**, R1395–401.

Schultz W (2002). Getting formal with dopamine and reward. *Neuron*, **36**, 241–63.

Schultz W, Tremblay L and Hollerman JR (2000). Reward processing in primate orbitofrontal cortex and basal ganglia. *Cerebral Cortex*, **10**, 272–8.

Schwartz MW and Seeley RJ (1997). The new biology of body weight regulation. *Journal of the American Dietetic Association*, **97**, 54–8.

Scott DJ, Stohler CS, Egnatuk CM, Wang H, Koeppe RA and Zubieta JK (2007). Individual differences in reward responding explain placebo-induced expectations and effects. *Neuron*, **55**, 325–36.

—— (2008). Placebo and nocebo effects are defined by opposite opioid and dopaminergic responses. *Archives of General Psychiatry*, **65**, 220–31.

Simpson JB, Epstein AN and Camardo JS Jr (1978). Localization of receptors for the dipsogenic action of angiotensin II in the subfornical organ of rat. *Journal of Comparative and Physiological Psychology*, **92**, 581–601.

Smith GP, Jerome C and Norgren R (1985). Afferent axons in abdominal vagus mediate satiety effect of cholecystokinin in rats. *American Journal of Physiology*, **249**, R638–41.

Stanley BG, Kyrkouli SE, Lampert S and Leibowitz SF (1986). Neuropeptide Y chronically injected into the hypothalamus: a powerful neurochemical inducer of hyperphagia and obesity. *Peptides*, **7**, 1189–92.

Stellar JR and Stellar E (1985). *The neurobiology of motivation and reward*. Springer-Verlag, New York, NY.

Thrasher TN and Keil LC (1987). Regulation of drinking and vasopressin secretion: role of organum vasculosum laminae terminalis. *American Journal of Physiology*, **253**, R108–20.

Warner RK, Thompson JT, Markowski VP, Loucks JA, Bazzett TJ, Eaton RC et al. (1991). Microinjection of the dopamine antagonist cis-flupenthixol into the MPOA impairs copulation, penile reflexes and sexual motivation in male rats. *Brain Research*, **540**, 177–82.

Weary DM, Huzzey JM and von Keyserlingk MAG (2009). Using behaviour to predict and identify ill health in animals. *Journal of Animal Sciences*, **87**, 770–7.

Wise RA (1996). Neurobiology of addiction. *Current Opinion in Neurobiology*, **6**, 243–51.

Wise RA and Rompre P. -P. (1989). Brain dopamine and reward. *Annual Review of Psychology*, **40**, 191–225.

Woods SC, Schwartz MW, Baskin DG and Seeley RJ (2000). Food intake and the regulation of body weight. *Annual Review of Psychology*, **51**, 255–77.

Chapter 5

Meeting the therapist: a look into trust, hope, empathy, and compassion mechanisms

Summary and relevance to the clinician

1) In this chapter, several aspects of the doctor–patient interaction are considered, from the patient's trust and admiration towards the therapist to the doctor's empathic and compassionate behaviour. All these highly complex brain functions have been described from a neuroscientific perspective, and represent what is called social neuroscience, a branch of the neurosciences which investigates complex social behaviours.

2) Trustworthiness decisions are based on several environmental stimuli, first and foremost, facial expressions. The decision on whether a face is trustworthy or untrustworthy depends on the amygdala. This region increases its activity as the facial expression is judged to be untrustworthy, and vice versa.

3) Oxytocin is a hormone that has been found to stimulate pro-social behaviour. In particular, it is produced in the hypothalamus and then secreted by the pituitary gland, and is capable of increasing trust. This effect is likely to be due to the presence of oxytocin receptors with inhibitory action in the amygdala. As amygdala hyperactivity is associated to untrustworthiness, oxytocin may inhibit this effect when binding to amygdala neurons.

4) Although admiration differs from trust, these two emotions are related to each other. If one admires a person, he is likely to trust him. The opposite often holds true. Admiration and trust may represent a very important aspect of the therapist–patient encounter. There is experimental evidence that admiration engages two different neural systems, depending on the type of admiration. If it is related to someone else's psychological state, e.g. admiration for moral virtue, it recruits a network involving the inferior/posterior posteromedial cortices and the anterior middle cingulate, which are affiliated with interoceptive information. If it is related to someone else's physical state, e.g. admiration for virtuosic skill, it recruits the superior/anterior part of the posterolateral cortices most connected with lateral parietal cortices, which deal with exteroception and musculoskeletal information.

5) Sensory stimuli are particularly important during the doctor–patient interaction. For example, subtle differences in verbal communication may lead to different outcomes. Likewise, visual stimuli are crucial for nonverbal communication, whereby gestures and postures can communicate plenty of meaningful information. The mirror neuron system plays a crucial role in these functions. Finally, the somatosensory input, e.g. tactile, may contain important emotional information. For example, being touched by a beloved one while in pain may reduce the unpleasantness of the pain itself.

6) Hope is also a basic aspect of the therapist–patient interaction. It can be defined as a positive motivational state that is based on a sense of successful goal-directed energy and planning to meet goals. Two key elements take part in hope: expectation and motivation. With the former, the patient expects the future to be better than the present. With the latter, the patient adopts the adequate behavioural repertoire to do so. Hope and hopelessness may influence the course of a disease, and even mortality. Therefore, high levels of hope should always be induced in the patient.

7) The study of hopelessness, and related helplessness, has shown that both the serotoninergic and noradrenergic systems are involved. For example, there is a negative correlation between the activation of serotonin receptors in the dorsolateral prefrontal cortex and the degree of hopelessness.

8) One of the main characteristics of health professionals should be their empathic behaviour. Empathy is distinguished from sympathy or empathic concern or compassion. An emotion produced by empathy is isomorphic with the other's emotion. This is not necessarily true for sympathy or compassion. Nor is empathy necessarily linked to pro-social motivation, namely, the concern about the others' well being. By contrast, pro-social motivation is involved in both sympathy and compassion.

9) There is evidence suggesting that at least two mechanisms mediate empathy: emotional contagion on the one hand and cognitive perspective-taking on the other. Whereas emotional contagion is thought to support our ability to empathize emotionally, that is, to share the other person's emotional feelings, empathic perspective-taking involves complex cognitive components, whereby one infers the state of the other person. This distinction is particularly important from a neuroscientific point of view. In fact, whereas cognitive perspective taking activates the medial prefrontal regions, the superior temporal sulcus, the temporal pole, and the temporo-parietal junction, empathizing with another person has been found to activate somatosensory and insular cortices as well as the anterior cingulate cortex.

10) As for admiration, there are two different neural networks for compassion. Compassion for social pain is associated with strong activation in the inferior/posterior portion of the posteromedial cortices, whereas compassion for physical pain produces a larger activation in the superior/ anterior portion of the posteromedial cortices.

11) In order to suppress distress in everyday medical practice, health professionals, particularly those involved in invasive and painful procedures, have developed mechanisms of self-control that are aimed at reducing negative emotions while watching the suffering of their patients. For example, the somatosensory cortex of physicians who practice acupuncture shows less activation compared to naive subjects when observing animated visual stimuli depicting needles being inserted into different body parts.

12) A good interaction between doctors and patients may lead to positive therapeutic outcomes and this represents the basis of different placebo effects, which will be discussed in Chapter 6. Therefore, health professionals must always adopt empathic and compassionate behaviours, which are aimed at modulating the patient's brain through the activation of the neural mechanisms of trust and hope. Even a mere diagnostic procedure may produce positive effects if performed in the appropriate context.

13) On the other hand, a bad interaction between health professionals and their patients may lead to negative outcomes. For example, anxiety may be induced, and we have seen in section 3.3.3 that negative emotions amplify the perception of pain. Although anxiety-induced hyperalgesia is the best-known model to understand the link between negative emotions and the perception of a symptom (see section 3.3.3), symptoms other than pain can be amplified by anxiety and other negative emotions.

14) This chapter is of particular relevance to psychotherapy. In fact, in psychotherapy the therapist–patient interaction is at the very heart of the therapeutic outcome. Several authors suggest that psychotherapy works only through a benign positive interaction, and several studies support this notion. There are common elements in any form of psychotherapy, such as trust, belief, hope, motivation, expectations, and these may represent the key to successful outcomes.

5.1 Trusting the therapist

5.1.1 Trust in doctors can be measured

Trust can be conceptualized as a set of beliefs that the therapist will behave in a certain way (Thom and Campbell 1997). The therapist's behaviours on which patients usually base their trust are competence, compassion, confidentiality, reliability, and communication (Pearson and Raeke 2000). As emphasized by Mechanic and Schlesinger (1996) and by Pearson and Raeke (2000), there are at least two types of trust. Interpersonal trust refers to the trust that derives from the repeated interactions with a person, whose trustworthy behaviour can be tested over time. Conversely, social trust is a more general concept, whereby the trust is in society and collective institutions. By analogy with state and trait anxiety, interpersonal trust can be conceptualized as state trust, whereby we trust a specific person in a specific circumstance, while social trust can be viewed as trait trust, whereby we trust the society as a whole.

Treating trust as a psychological, cognitive, and affective parameter to be measured with rigorous scientific methodology is not an easy task. The multi-dimensional nature of trust, which is constituted of complex cognitive and emotional components, makes it difficult to pursue rigorous research. The first study that was aimed at measuring the patient's trust was performed by Anderson and Dedrick (1990), who created an 11-item Trust in Physician Scale. To better understand the complex nature of the psychological variables that are at work here, it is useful to list the 11 items as follows:

1) I doubt that my doctor really cares about me as a person.

2) My doctor is usually considerate of my needs and puts them first.

3) I trust my doctor so much that I always try to follow his/her advice.

4) If my doctor tells me something is so, then it must be true.

5) I sometimes distrust my doctor's opinion and would like a second one.

6) I trust my doctor's judgement about my medical care.

7) I feel my doctor does not do everything he/she should for my medical care.

8) I trust my doctor to put my medical needs above all other considerations when treating my medical problems.

9) My doctor is a real expert in taking care of medical problems like mine.

10) I trust my doctor to tell me if a mistake was made about my treatment.

11) I sometimes worry that my doctor may not keep the information we discuss totally private.

Many variants of this Trust in Physician Scale as well as new scales have been developed over the last years (e.g. Kao et al. 1998a, b; Safran et al. 1998). For example, the Patient Trust Scale by Kao et al. (1998a, b) reveals once again the complex nature of the psychological variables that come into play in the measurement of patients' trust. In this psychometric evaluation, patients are asked how much they trust their physician:

1) to put their health and well-being above keeping down health plan's costs,

2) to keep personally sensitive medical information private,

3) to provide them with information on all potential medical options and not just options covered by the health plan,

4) to refer them to a specialist when necessary,

5) to admit them to the hospital when needed,

6) to make appropriate medical decisions regardless of health plan rules and guidelines,

7) to judge about their medical care,

8) to perform necessary medical tests and procedures regardless of costs,

9) to offer them high-quality medical care,

10) to perform only medically necessary tests and procedures.

It is interesting to note how much the concerns about health costs are represented in this psychometric evaluation and, in particular, the concerns about the priority of health and well-being over health plan rules, guidelines and costs. Not surprisingly, this reflects the patient's concerns about receiving appropriate medical care, regardless of health plan rules and costs.

Overall, these scales reveal the complex nature of the cognitive/affective factors that constitute trust as a whole, ranging from the balance between patient's and doctor's needs to the doctor's competence and the patient's privacy. Interestingly, the payment method and system has also been found to be correlated to trust, along with trust in health plan, length of patient–physician relationship, whether there had been choice of physician, race of the doctor, and self-reported health status (Kao et al. 1998a, b). Patients' trust in their physicians has always been considered as an important element that per se may have beneficial effects on the overall health status. This may occur through a better adherence to treatments as well as the reinforcement of clinical relationship and patient satisfaction (Pearson and Raeke 2000).

5.1.2 The amygdala is a key region in trustworthiness decisions

During social interactions, deciding if an unfamiliar person is trustworthy represents one of the most important decisions in everyday life. Either a good or a bad interaction very much depends on this decision. The brain is capable of making such decisions very quickly. One hundred milliseconds of exposure to a neutral face is sufficient for this complex task. Willis and Todorov (2006) investigated the minimal conditions under which people make such inferences. To do this, these authors manipulated the exposure time of unfamiliar faces, and found that judgments made after a 100-ms exposure were highly correlated with judgments made in the absence of time constraints, thereby suggesting that this exposure time was enough for subjects to form an impression. Five judgments were tested: trustworthiness, attractiveness, likeability, competence, and aggressiveness. When the exposure time was increased from 100 ms to 500 ms, subjects' judgments became more negative, response times for judgments decreased, and confidence in judgments increased. When the exposure time was increased from 500 ms to 1000 ms, overall trait judgments and response times did not change significantly, but confidence increased for some of the judgments. Therefore, additional time may simply boost confidence in judgments. Interestingly, trustworthiness judgments showed the highest correlation, supporting the notion that people can be especially efficient in making inferences of trustworthiness because, from an evolutionary perspective, the detection of trustworthiness is essential for survival (Cosmides and Tooby 1992). This very short period of time, i.e. one tenth of a second, for trustworthiness judgments shows that face exploration is not necessary, and the first impression of whether or not an individual is deemed to be trustworthy does not require eye exploratory movements. In fact, a time lag of 100 ms is not sufficient for saccadic eye movements (Todorov 2008).

Trustworthiness is correlated with other judgement traits. In fact, a positive correlation is present between trustworthiness, attractiveness (Fig 5.1A), and intelligence (Fig 5.1B), whereas a negative correlation is present between trustworthiness and aggressiveness (Fig 5.1C). According to Todorov (2008), in situations where no context is provided, trustworthiness judgments from faces reflect inferences about positivity/negativity of the face. Judgments of trustworthiness may serve the function of automatic approach/avoidance in social interactions, determining whether to approach or avoid a stranger. Therefore, trustworthiness judgments are an attempt to infer emotional expressions signalling either approach or avoidance behaviours. For the positive ratings of trustworthiness, these are expressions of happiness, whereas for the negative ratings (i.e. untrustworthiness), these are expressions of anger. In other words, expressions of anger communicate that the person should be avoided, and expressions of happiness communicate that the person can be approached. Indeed, some studies showed that angry faces trigger automatic avoidance responses (Marsh et al. 2005; Adams et al. 2006).

Examples of faces with trustworthiness features that range from negative (i.e. untrustworthiness) to positive (total trustworthiness) are shown in Fig 5.2A. Whereas the faces in the centre column were randomly generated, the left three columns show the exaggerated features to decrease their perceived trustworthiness, and the right three columns to increase their perceived trustworthiness. In Fig 5.2B, the categorization of faces as angry, happy, and neutral as a function of their trustworthiness is shown. As the facial features become more

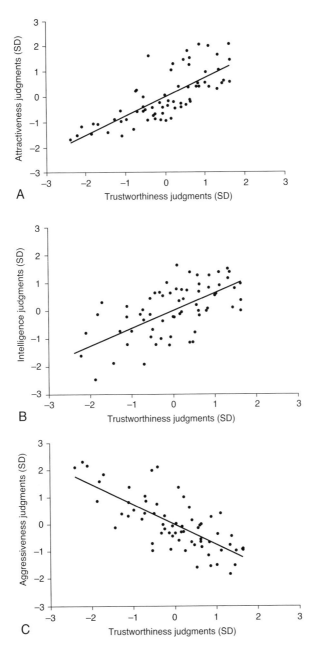

Fig 5.1 Correlation between judgments of trustworthiness from emotionally neutral faces with judgments of attractiveness (A), judgments of intelligence (B), and judgments of aggressiveness (C). Each point represents a face. Note the positive correlation between trustworthiness, attractiveness, and intelligence judgments, and the negative correlation between trustworthiness and aggressiveness.
Source: From Todorov 2008 with permission from John Wiley & Sons and the New York Academy of Sciences, Copyright 2008.

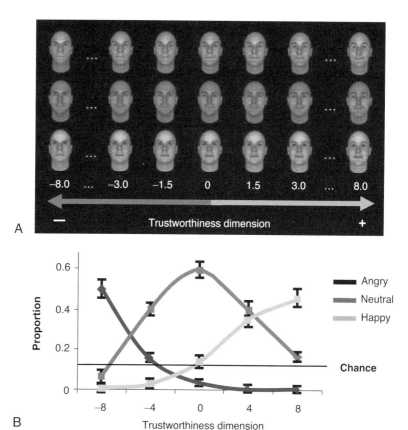

Fig 5.2 (A) Examples of faces with trustworthiness features that range from negative (i.e. untrustworthiness) to positive (total trustworthiness). The faces in the centre column were randomly generated and then their features were exaggerated to decrease (left three columns) and increase (right three columns) their perceived trustworthiness. (B) Categorization of faces as angry, happy, and neutral as a function of their trustworthiness. The x-axis represents the extent of exaggeration of facial features in standard deviation units. As the facial features become more exaggerated, the neutral categorization approaches chance, and this is particularly clear on the negative end of the continuum. As the facial features become more exaggerated in the negative direction (−8), the faces are mostly classified as angry, whereas when the trustworthy facial features become more exaggerated in the positive direction (+8), the faces are mostly classified as happy. See colour plate 8. Source: From Todorov 2008 with permission from John Wiley & Sons and the New York Academy of Sciences, Copyright 2008.

exaggerated, the neutral categorization approaches chance, and this is particularly clear on the negative end of the continuum. As the facial features become more exaggerated in the negative direction, the faces are mostly classified as angry, whereas when the trustworthy facial features become more exaggerated in the positive direction, the faces are mostly classified as happy.

Patients with amygdala damage show an impairment in recognizing emotional facial expressions (Adolphs et al. 1994, 1998; Young et al. 1995; Broks et al. 1998). In particular, patients with bilateral amygdala lesion show a bias to perceive untrustworthy faces as trustworthy. Adolphs et al. (1998) asked three subjects with complete bilateral amygdala damage to judge faces of unfamiliar people with respect to two attributes important in real-life social encounters: approachability and trustworthiness. These two judgments were analysed for the 50 faces to which normal subjects assign the most negative ratings, and for the 50 most positive faces. Whereas bilateral damage of the amygdala produced significantly more positive ratings for the most negative faces compared to normal controls, unilateral lesions did not differ from the controls. These findings lead to at least two conclusions. First, the human amygdala triggers socially and emotionally relevant information in response to visual stimuli. Second, its role appears to be of special importance for social judgment of faces that are normally classified as unapproachable and untrustworthy. This latter conclusion is consistent with the role of amygdala in processing threatening and aversive stimuli (Amaral 2003; Phelps and LeDoux 2005). For example, damage to the amygdala results in an impairment in interpreting the intensity of fear expressions in others (Adolphs et al. 1999).

Since face evaluation can be subserved by the mechanisms underlying perception of emotional expressions, it is possible that a dissociation between processing of face evaluation and facial identity may be present. Indeed, there are prosopagnosic patients who can recognize emotional expressions but not identity (Tranel et al. 1988; Damasio et al. 1990; Duchaine et al. 2003; Bentin et al. 2007). Likewise, there is some evidence that individuals with developmental prosopagnosia can make normal trustworthiness judgments but show impaired perception of face identity (Todorov 2008).

Besides the lesion studies mentioned above, there is compelling evidence on the role of the amygdala in trustworthiness judgements that comes from imaging studies. Winston et al. (2002) used functional magnetic resonance imaging to unravel the neural underpinnings of trustworthiness judgments. In this study, subjects were asked to make explicit trustworthiness judgments and implicit (with respect to trustworthiness) age judgments of unfamiliar faces. It was found that, independent of the task, the amygdala activity increased in relation to subjective untrustworthiness. In fact, trustworthiness judgments ratings were correlated with magnetic resonance signal change to reveal task-independent increased activity in bilateral amygdala and right insula in response to faces judged untrustworthy. Conversely, the right superior temporal sulcus showed enhanced signal change during explicit trustworthiness judgments alone. Thus, a functional dissociation between automatic engagement of amygdala versus intentional engagement of the superior temporal sulcus in social judgment is present. Figure 5.3 shows the activation of the superior temporal sulcus during the explicit social judgments (A), and the activation of the left and right amygdala as well as of the right insula during the more automatic implicit task (B). Overall, social judgments about faces reflect a combination of brain responses that are stimulus driven, in the case of the amygdala, and driven by processes relating to inferences concerning the intentionality of others, in the case of superior temporal sulcus (Winston et al. 2002).

In a subsequent study, Engell et al. (2007) used a different implicit task, whereby the subjects were engaged in a memory task. They were presented with blocks of faces and asked to indicate whether a test face was presented in the preceding block or not. Judgments of trustworthiness or person evaluation were never mentioned during the course of the experiment. Although the task did not demand face evaluation, the amygdala response to faces increased as the untrustworthiness of the faces increased (Fig 5.4). Again, as in the above-described study by Winston et al. (2002), these findings suggest that the amygdala automatically categorizes faces according to face properties commonly perceived to signal untrustworthiness.

5.1.3 Oxytocin enhances trust

Trust behaviour has been found to undergo hormonal modulation by oxytocin. In general, this hormone is known to have pro-social effects in mammals, such as to stimulate the ability to form social attachments and affiliations, including parental care, pair bonding, and social memory (Carter 1998, 2003; Insel and Young 2001; Ferguson et al. 2002; Young and Wang 2004; Lim and Young 2006). Oxytocin also has pro-social effects in humans, like the modulation of social interaction behaviour and social cognition (Bartz and Hollander 2006; Heinrichs and Domes 2008) and the influence on a person's ability to infer another's mental state, an ability that is referred to as 'mind-reading' (Domes et al. 2007). It should be noted that these pro-social effects were not the first to be discovered. In fact, the functions of oxytocin that were first described were its uterine-contracting properties (Dale 1906) and, shortly thereafter, the milk ejection property (Ott and Scott 1910; Schafer and Mackenzie 1911). Thus oxytocin was first considered to be a hormone important for parturition and lactation.

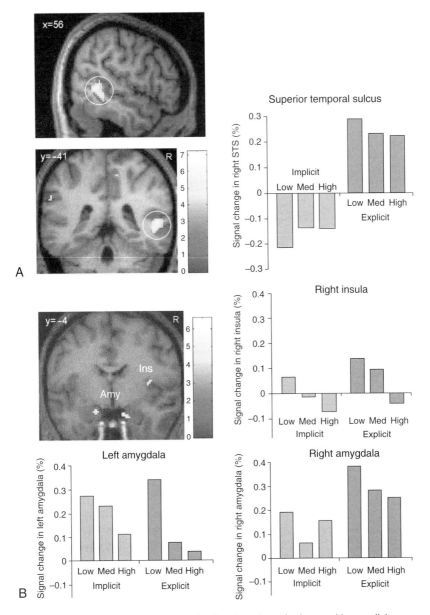

Fig 5.3 (A) The right superior temporal sulcus is activated when making explicit judgments about trustworthiness compared to age. On the right, magnetic resonance signal measure categorized by task and trustworthiness of faces. 'Low', 'med', and 'high' refer to trustworthiness. The y-axis represents mean percentage signal change. Note that there is no clear pattern of response to the faces according to trustworthiness. (B) Bilateral amygdala and right insula are activated by untrustworthy faces. The graphs indicate the responses to faces as a function of degree of individually rated trustworthiness for right insula, left amygdala, and right amygdala. Note greater responses to less trustworthy faces across all these regions. Source: Partially modified from Winston et al. 2002 with permission from the Nature Publishing Group, Copyright 2002.

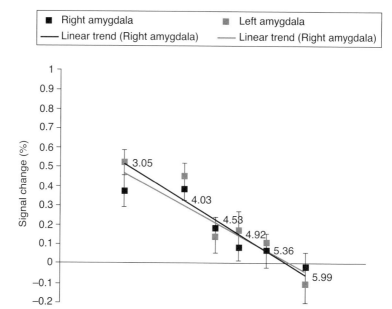

Fig 5.4 Functional magnetic resonance imaging response (% signal change) in the amygdala showing a significant linear trend as a function of trustworthiness ratings of novel faces. It can be seen that the smaller the trustworthiness ratings, the larger the magnetic resonance signal change in both the right and left amygdala.
Source: From Engell et al. 2007 with permission from the Massachusetts Institute of Technology, Copyright 2007.

Oxytocin was the first peptide to have its structure chemically identified and synthesized in the laboratory (du Vigneaud et al. 1953a, b, 1954; Tuppy 1953), and its receptor was then cloned by Kimura et al. (1992). It is composed of nine amino acids (Cys–Tyr–Ile–Gln–Asn–Cys–Pro–Leu–GlyNH2) and its structure is very similar to another nonapeptide, vasopressin, which differs from oxytocin by two amino acids (Cys–Tyr–Phe–Gln–Asn–Cys–Pro–Arg–GlyNH2). It is primarily synthesized in magnocellular neurons of the paraventricular and supraoptic nuclei of the hypothalamus, and the bulk of it is transported to the posterior pituitary where it is released into the blood stream (Fig 5.5). The distribution of oxytocin receptors, Oxtr, varies across species but, overall, they can be found throughout the nervous system (Lee et al. 2009) (Fig 5.5). Whereas in rodents they are expressed particularly in the olfactory bulb, hippocampus, amygdala, nucleus accumbens, neocortex, and hypothalamus (Insel et al. 1991; Veinante and Freund-Mercier 1997), in humans they can be found in the basal nucleus of Meynert,

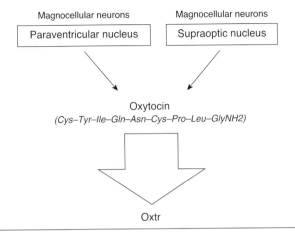

Fig 5.5 The oxytocin system. The nonapeptide oxytocin is produced in the magnocellular neurons of the paraventricular nucleus and supraoptic nucleus of the hypothalamus, transported to the pituitary gland and here released into the blood stream. Oxytocin binds to its receptors, Oxtr, which can be found in a variety of tissues throughout the body, including the uterus and the central nervous system. Here only the Oxtr distribution in the main regions of the brain is shown.

lateral septal nucleus, hypothalamus, substantia nigra pars compacta, substantia gelatinosa of the trigeminal nucleus and spinal cord (Loup et al. 1989, 1991).

Although a large amount of research on the pro-social effects of oxytocin has been performed in animals, human social behaviour has been found to be affected by oxytocin as well (Lee et al. 2009; Ross and Young 2009). For example, couples receiving intranasal oxytocin prior to a videotaped 'conflict discussion' show an increase in positive communication behaviours, e.g. eye contact and positive body language (Ditzen et al. 2009). Oxytocin has also been found to strengthen the anxiolytic effect of the presence of a friend during public speaking (Heinrichs et al. 2003). Women viewing pictures of loved ones have high brain activity in dopamine-associated reward regions, which contain high levels of oxytocin and vasopressin receptors (Bartels and Zeki 2004). This also occurs in people self-describing as being 'intensely in love' (Fisher et al. 2005, 2006). It is also interesting to note that dog owners who receive a 'long' duration of gaze from their dogs, and report a high degree of attachment to their dogs, show an increase in urinary oxytocin levels (Nagasawa et al. 2008).

Genetic variants of the serotonin transporter (5-HTT SLC6A4 polymorphism) and the oxytocin receptor (OXTR rs53576 polymorphism), have been studied in different populations. For example, mothers with these two polymorphisms present lower levels of sensitive responsiveness to their children, like the aid given to their children on cognitively difficult tasks (Bakermans-Kranenburg and van Ijzendoorn 2008), which suggests systems involved in production and bonding of oxytocin in maternal responsiveness.

It has also been found that the intranasal administration of oxytocin increases the time spent gazing at the eyes of human faces (Guastella et al. 2008a), the likelihood of recalling happy faces (Guastella et al. 2008b), and the ability to infer the mental state of others from social cues in the eye region (Domes et al. 2007). Petrovic et al. (2008) also found that oxytocin attenuates the negative evaluations of conditioned faces. These findings point at the important role of oxytocin in many complex social behaviours, including those derived from the exploration of human facial expressions.

One of the pro-social behaviours that are affected by oxytocin is trustworthy behaviour. Zak et al. (2004) found an increase in plasma oxytocin in subjects who participated in a trust game whereby cooperative behaviour can benefit both parties. In the experimental paradigm, one participant must make a monetary sacrifice to signal the degree of trust in the other before the other's behavioural response is known. Indeed, the receipt of a signal of trust of this kind is associated with an increase in plasma oxytocin. In a different study, Kosfeld et al. (2005) found that in a trust game the intranasal administration of oxytocin was associated to a larger amount of money given by an investor to a trustee. It is worth noting that intranasal oxytocin was not effective if the investor gave the money to a 'project' instead of a trustee, thus indicating specific effects on trustworthiness.

We have seen in section 5.1.2 that the amygdala plays a crucial role in trustworthy behaviour. Interestingly, oxytocin receptors are abundant in the amygdala (Huber et al. 2005), thus the amygdala should be expected to be affected by oxytocin administration. Indeed, Baumgartner et al. (2008) examined the neural circuitry of trustworthy behaviour by combining the intranasal administration of oxytocin with functional magnetic resonance imaging. It was found that oxytocin induced no change in trusting behaviour after the subjects learned that their trust had been breached several times, while the control subjects who had not received oxytocin decreased their trust. This difference in trust adaptation was associated with a specific reduction in activation in the amygdala, the midbrain regions, and the dorsal striatum in subjects receiving oxytocin, which suggests that neural systems mediating fear processing (amygdala and midbrain regions) and behavioural adaptations to feedback information (dorsal striatum) modulate the effects of oxytocin on trust (Fig 5.6).

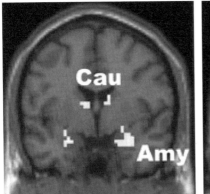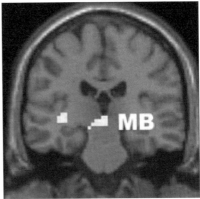

Fig 5.6 Subjects who receive oxytocin show no change in their trusting behaviour after they learned that their trust had been breached several times while control subjects (who did not receive oxytocin) decrease their trust. This difference in trust adaptation is associated with a specific reduction in activation in the amygdala, the midbrain regions, and the caudate nucleus in subjects receiving oxytocin. Amy, amygdala; Cau, caudate nucleus; MB, midbrain. See colour plate 7.
Source: From Baumgartner et al. 2008 with permission from Elsevier and Cell Press, Copyright 2008.

Taken together, the findings on the amygdala and oxytocin reveal a specific neuronal circuitry which is involved in trustworthy behaviour. Oxytocin receptors are abundant in the amygdala, thus they can modulate its activity in a number of ways. In general, the functioning of this circuitry can be summarized as follows. The higher the activity in the amygdala, the higher an emotion of untrustworthiness is generated. Oxytocin acts on its own receptors in the amygdala by reducing neural activity, thereby restoring an emotion of trustworthiness.

5.1.4 Admiration for virtue and skills involves two separate neural systems

Although admiration differs from trust, these two emotional aspects are certainly related to each other. If one admires a person, he is likely to trust him. Of course, the opposite is often true: if one trusts a person, this is because he may have an emotional feeling of admiration towards him. Therefore, admiration may represent a very important aspect of the therapist–patient encounter. For example, admiration can be evoked by witnessing virtuous behaviour aimed at reducing the suffering of others, known also as elevation, or by displays of virtuosic skill. In the first case, admiration has to do with social/psychological circumstances, i.e. virtue, whereas in the second case it pertains to another person's immediate physical circumstances, i.e. skilful abilities (Immordino-Yang et al. 2009).

In a study by Immordino-Yang et al. (2009), admiration was found to engage a territory encompassing three contiguous cortical areas, the posterior cingulate cortex, the retrosplenial area, and the precuneus, which together comprise the posteromedial cortices. Interestingly, admiration for virtue was associated with strong activation in the inferior/posterior portion of the posteromedial cortices, whereas admiration for skills produced a larger activation in the superior/anterior portion of the posteromedial cortices. It is worth noting that the superior/anterior portion of the posteromedial cortices is strongly interconnected with lateral parietal cortices, while the inferior/posterior portion is closely associated with the anterior middle cingulate cortex (Parvizi et al. 2006). Therefore, the study by Immordino-Yang et al. (2009) suggests that those emotions related to someone else's psychological state, e.g. virtue, may preferentially recruit a network involving the inferior/posterior posteromedial cortices and the anterior middle cingulate, which are affiliated with interoceptive information (see section 3.1). Conversely, those emotional states that are related to someone else's physical state, e.g. virtuosic skill, may recruit the superior/anterior part of the posterolateral cortices most connected with lateral parietal cortices, which deal with exteroception and musculoskeletal information.

Interestingly, a similar organization is found for compassionate behaviour, whereby these two neural systems are also involved (Immordino-Yang et al. 2009). In section 5.4.4, these two networks will be described again for compassion.

5.2 Sensory inputs can make the difference

5.2.1 Subtle differences in verbal communication may lead to different outcomes

The auditory/language systems play a critical role in the doctor–patient relationship. This is not surprising, of course, for verbal communication represents one of the most important social interaction between therapists and their patients. Indeed, some subtle differences in verbal communication may produce different effects. For example, the uncertainty of the doctor's words and attitudes may affect the outcome of a medical treatment, and different sentences such as 'This painkiller may work' or 'Rest assured, this painkiller does work' may lead to different therapeutic outcomes (Benedetti 2002, 2008).

In this regard, Thomas (1987) conducted either positive or negative general practice consultations in patients with different kinds of pain, cough, giddiness, nasal congestion, and tiredness. In the positive consultations, the patients were given a firm diagnosis and therapeutic assurance. If no prescription was to be given, they were told that they required none, and if a prescription was to be given, that the therapy would certainly make them better. In the negative consultations, no firm assurance was given. For example, if no prescription was to be given, the following statement was made: 'I cannot be certain what your problem is, therefore I will give you no treatment.' Conversely, if a prescription was to be given, the patients were told: 'I am not sure that the treatment I am going to give you will have an effect'. The treatment was a placebo in all cases. Two weeks after consultation there was a significant difference in recovery between the positive and negative groups but not between the treated and untreated groups, and the therapeutic outcome went in the same direction of the verbal suggestions that were delivered: certain suggestions led to positive outcomes, while uncertain suggestions led to negative outcomes. Therefore, the words the doctor use may be crucial for recovery.

The importance of verbal communication is also shown by the emotional impact that the anaesthetist may have upon his patient (Egbert et al. 1963, 1964). Egbert et al. (1964) found a reduction in postoperative pain in patients who had been informed about the course of their postoperative pain and encouraged to overcome it. Moreover, the requirement of narcotics of these patients was much lower compared with a control group.

Another study by Kirsch and Weixel (1988), albeit outside the clinical setting, showed that different verbal contexts produce different outcomes. In this study, coffee and decaffeinated coffee were administered following different verbal instructions. In one case they were given according to the usual double-blind design (i.e. subjects knew either the active substance or a placebo was being administered), in the other case decaffeinated coffee was deceptively presented as real coffee. It was found that the placebo response was stronger following the deceptive administration than the double-blind paradigm. The authors concluded that this was attributable to the fact that the double-blind administration induces less certain expectations about the outcome.

In the light of the importance of these subtle differences in verbal communication between doctors and patients, Pollo et al. (2001) carried out a similar study in the clinical setting in order to investigate the differences between the double-blind and the deceptive paradigm. Post-operative patients were treated with buprenorphine on request for three consecutive days, and with a basal infusion of saline solution. However, the symbolic meaning of this saline basal infusion varied in three different groups of patients. The first group was told nothing (natural history or no-treatment group), the second was told that the infusion could be either a potent analgesic or a placebo (classic double-blind administration), and the third group was told that the infusion was a potent painkiller (deceptive administration). The placebo effect of the saline basal infusion was measured by recording the doses of buprenorphine requested over the three-day treatment. It is important to stress once again that the double-blind group received uncertain verbal instructions ('It can be either a placebo or a painkiller. Thus we are not certain that the pain will subside'), whereas the deceptive administration group received certain instructions ('It is a painkiller. Thus pain will subside soon'). A decrease in buprenorphine intake was found with the double-blind administration and even more with the deceptive administration of the saline basal infusion. The reduction of buprenorphine requests in the double-blind group was as large as 20.8% compared with the natural history group, and the reduction in the deceptive administration group was even larger, reaching 33.8%. It is important to point out that the time-course of pain was the same in the three groups over the three-day period of treatment. Thus the same analgesic effect was obtained with different doses of buprenorphine.

The above studies teach us that the uncertainty of verbal instructions and attitudes indeed leads to different results. Thus, as Thomas (1987) says, there is a point in being positive. Subtle differences in verbal communication may have a significant impact on the therapeutic outcome. In section 6.2.1, we will see that even more dramatic effects can be found when verbal communication about the therapy that is being administered is totally lacking, for example when the therapy is given unbeknownst to the patient.

Another important example of the powerful effects of verbal communication is represented by hypnosis. Through hypnotic verbal suggestions it is possible to obtain impressive effects, such as reduced colour-naming conflict in a Stroop task with an associated decrease in functional magnetic resonance imaging signal in the anterior cingulate cortex and visual areas (Raz et al. 2005, 2007), and activation of colour-processing regions following the verbal suggestions to see black-and-white pictures in colour (Kosslyn et al. 2000). In addition, in highly hypnotizable subjects, verbal suggestions to perceive pain in a hand that was not touched by any means activates part of the pain-processing circuitry (Raij et al. 2005). Placebo and nocebo verbal suggestions represent another example of the powerful effects of the doctor's words, and these effects are described in different parts of this volume such as section 3.3.3 and Chapter 6.

5.2.2 Visual stimuli are the basis for nonverbal communication

Among the great variety of visual information that reaches the patient's brain when he meets a therapist, we have seen in section 5.1.2 that facial expressions play a key role in complex cognitive functions such as trustworthiness decisions. The face is an excellent source of information and plays a fundamental role in signalling social intentions from which people infer meaning, such as personality traits and complex social characteristics (Frith and Frith 1999). Generally, people form reliable and strong impressions on the basis of facial appearance. Figure 5.2 shows that when judgements are aimed at detecting either trustworthy or untrustworthy faces, they are also entangled with other features of the facial expressions, such happiness and anger. Indeed, several brain regions are involved in detecting subtle differences in facial expressions, and these regions make up a complex network which is specifically aimed at processing facial emotions, whereas facial identity is processed by a different network (Todorov 2008; see also section 5.1.2).

Face perception is in many ways a microcosm of object recognition. The specialness of face processing is shown by the fact that even a split-second glimpse of a person's face tells us his/her identity, sex, mood, age, race, and direction of attention (Tsao and Livingstone 2008). Even monkeys have been found to respond selectively to faces, and neurons in the inferotemporal cortex and superior temporal sulcus have been found to be driven by complex biologically relevant stimuli, such as hands or faces (Gross et al. 1969, 1972; Foldiak et al. 2004). Face cells are not just selective for individual features but rather they require an intact face. For example, Kobatake and Tanaka (1994) recorded from the inferotemporal cortex of monkeys and found that neurons only responded when the stimulus looked like a face, no matter how simplified. Figure 5.7 shows a cell that responds best to the face of a toy monkey (a), as well as to a configuration of two black dots over a horizontal line within a disk (b), but not in the absence of either the line (c) or the spots (d) or the circular outline (e). The circular outline alone does not produce any response either (f). The contrast between the inside and the outside of the circle is not critical, as the cell still responds (g). White spots and white horizontal line do not elicit any response (h). Therefore, face-responsive neurons detect a particular spatial configuration that looks like a face as a whole.

In human brain imaging studies, although face-specific activation can be seen in the superior temporal sulcus and in part of the occipital lobe, a number of studies support the idea that the lateral side of the right mid-fusiform gyrus, the 'fusiform face area' or FFA, is activated robustly and specifically by faces (Kanwisher et al. 1997; Tsao and Livingstone 2008). It should be noted, however that the FFA does not respond only to face stimuli but also to non-face objects, albeit less robustly. This might indicate that the FFA may have more general functions, for example the processing of any sets of stimuli that share a common shape and for which the subject has gained some expertise (Tarr and Gauthier 2000; Tsao and Livingstone 2008).

The detection of faces, together with their emotional content, is crucial in non-verbal communication. The information that is gained from faces is fundamental

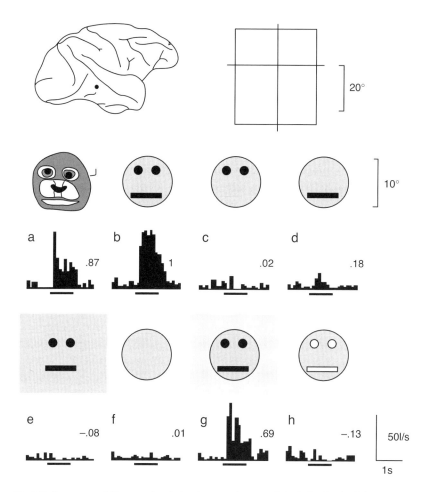

Fig 5.7 A neuron of the monkey inferotemporal cortex (black dot in the left top panel) responding to visual stimuli that look like a face. This neuron responds to the face of a toy monkey (a), to a configuration of two black dots over a horizontal line within a disk (b, g), but not in the absence of either the line (c) or the spots (d) or the circular outline (e). Nor does it respond to the circular outline alone (f), or to white spots and white horizontal line (h). The visual angle of the stimuli is shown. Source: From Kobatake and Tanaka 1994 with permission from the American Physiological Society, Copyright 1994.

for social interaction, including the doctor–patient encounter. Although recognition of face identities, along with spatial features and configuration, by regions such the FFA, and perception of face emotions by regions such as the amygdala (section 5.1.2) are at the very heart of social relationships, they are not the only ones. Nonverbal cues such as gestures, postures, and eye contact contribute substantially to social interactions. Therefore, beyond verbal communication, social relationships are supported and boosted by visual stimuli (facial emotions, gestures, postures, eye contact, and the like) that convey important pieces of information (Hari and Kujala 2009).

For example, eye contact, i.e. the mutual eye gaze that connects people together, represents an important aspect of social interaction and solicits attention and interest of the interacting persons (Senju and Johnson 2009). In contrast to many species, whereby eye contact induces aversive responses and represents a potential threat (Emery 2000), human social interactions rely on eye contact and, indeed, mutual eye gaze triggers attention and interest. At least five regions have been found to be activated more by direct gaze than by averted gaze, as shown in Fig 5.8: the fusiform gyrus (or FFA), the anterior part of the right superior temporal sulcus, the posterior part of right superior temporal sulcus, the medial prefrontal cortex and orbitofrontal cortex, and the amygdala (Senju and Johnson 2009). There are several explanations of how these regions may be activated by direct gaze. First, eye contact may activate directly the arousal system and may elicit strong emotional responses (Kawashima et al. 1999), which in turn affect subsequent perceptual and cognitive processing. Second, eye contact may activate a communicative intention detector, which is subserved by specific cortical structures such as medial prefrontal cortex and superior temporal sulcus (Frith and Frith 2006). Third, an alternative 'fast-track modulator' model has been proposed, whereby the eye contact effect is mediated by the subcortical face detection pathway, hypothesized to include the superior colliculus, pulvinar, and amygdala (Senju and Johnson 2009). Interestingly, damage to the amygdala has been found to impair eye contact during conversation and to enhance focus on the mouth of the speaker (Spezio et al. 2007).

Gestures and postures represent another important aspect of social interactions. During social encounters, related social knowledge arises automatically from memory and unconsciously affects the persons' judgments and appreciation of other people (Ferguson and Bargh 2004). Likewise, the perceived behaviour of others affects one's own behaviour unconsciously. For example, people are likely to rub their face if their conversation partner does so (Chartrand and Bargh 1999). When observing the gestures of and interacting with others, one can also infer his intentions and, accordingly, adapt his own behaviour. Mirror neurons are at the very heart of this social behaviour and play a critical role whenever the behaviour of others is observed (Rizzolatti and Craighero 2004).

The mirror neuron system was first discovered in area F5 of the monkey premotor cortex. This type of neurons fire both when the monkey does a

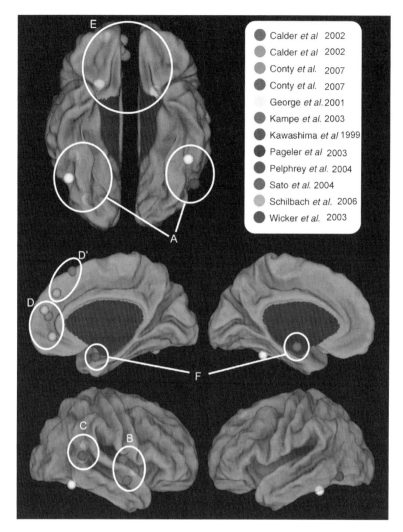

Fig 5.8 Cortical and subcortical regions that are activated by eye contact (mutual eye gaze that connects people together) in different studies. (A) Fusiform gyrus, particularly in the right hemisphere. (B) Anterior part of the right superior temporal sulcus. (C) Posterior part of right superior temporal sulcus. (D) Right medial prefrontal cortex (in two studies averted gaze was more effective than direct gaze (D')). (E) Orbitofrontal cortex. (F) Right and left amygdala. See colour plate 9.
Source: From Senju and Johnson 2009 with permission from Elsevier and Cell Press, Copyright 2009.

particular action and when it observes another individual, be it monkey or human, doing a similar action (Di Pellegrino et al. 1992; Gallese et al. 1996; Rizzolatti et al. 1996). They are visuomotor neurons that encode an object-directed action. Presenting widely different visual stimuli, but which all represent the same action, is equally effective for their activation. For example, they can respond equally to a human hand grasping as well as when the grasping hand is that of a monkey. The response is not affected by the size of the observed grasping hand, thereby a near or far action is equally effective. Likewise, mirror neurons fire with the same intensity if the experimenter grasps the food and gives it to the recorded monkey or to another monkey in the room, which indicates that reward is not crucial. All these neurons have been found in the monkey brain in at least three regions: the frontal premotor area F5, the superior temporal sulcus, and the inferior parietal lobule. There are several differences among these areas, for example, the superior temporal sulcus appears to code a much larger number of movements than F5, and does not appear to be endowed with motor properties (Rizzolatti and Craighero 2004).

There is compelling experimental evidence that mirror neurons mediate action understanding, that is, the meaning of the observed action and not its visual features. For example, in a study by Umiltà et al. (2001), a monkey either was shown a fully visible action directed towards an object ('full vision' condition) or saw the same action but with its final, critical part hidden ('hidden' condition). Before each trial, a piece of food was placed behind the screen so that the monkey knew there was an object there. As shown in Fig 5.9, the neuron responded to the observation of grasping and holding (A, full vision) as well as when the hand approaching the stimulus and subsequently holding it was hidden from monkey's vision (B, hidden condition). Conversely, the observation of a mimed action did not activate the neuron (C, full vision, and D, hidden condition). It is important to point out that visual stimulation in B and D is identical, thereby demonstrating that it was the understanding of the meaning of the observed actions that determined the discharge in the hidden condition.

That a mirror neuron system is also present in humans is shown by at least two experimental approaches. First, several studies with electroencephalography and magnetoencephalography techniques have shown that neurophysiological responses occur not only during active movements but also during the observation of others performing the same movements (Hari et al. 1998; Cochin et al. 1999; Caetano et al. 2007). Likewise, motor potentials evoked by transcranial magnetic stimulation of the motor cortex have been found to be modulated selectively during the observation of others' movements (Fadiga et al. 1995). Second, there are a number of brain imaging studies suggesting

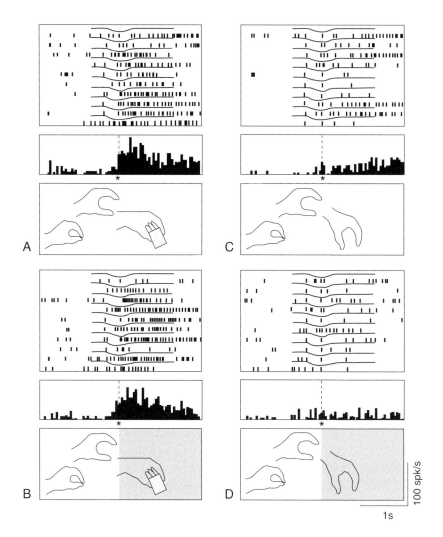

Fig 5.9 Response of a mirror neuron to action observation in full vision (A and C) and in hidden condition (B and D). The lower part of each panel shows the experimenter's action as observed from the monkey's vantage point. In hidden conditions the experimenter's hand started to disappear from the monkey's vision when crossing the asterisk. In each panel above the illustration of the experimenter's hand, raster displays and histograms of ten consecutive trials recorded are shown. Above each raster, the line represents the kinematics of the experimenter's hand movements.

Source: From Umiltà et al. 2001 with permission from Elsevier and Cell Press, Copyright 2001.

mirror properties of several brain regions. In general, a complex network encompassing occipital, temporal, and parietal visual areas, as well as cortical regions involved in motor control, has been described (Rizzolatti and Craighero 2004; Iacoboni and Dapretto 2006). Figure 5.10 shows that an anterior area with mirror neuron properties is located in the inferior frontal cortex. This includes the posterior inferior frontal gyrus and the ventral premotor cortex. A posterior area with mirror neuron properties is also present and is located in the rostral part of the inferior parietal lobule. The main visual input to the mirror neuron system originates from the posterior portion of the superior temporal sulcus.

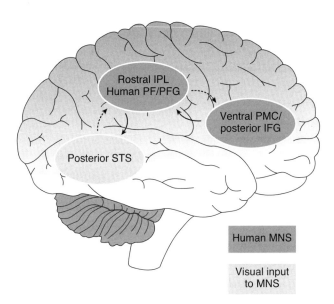

Fig 5.10 The mirror neuron system (MNS, dark grey) with its main visual input (light grey) in the human brain. An anterior area with mirror neuron properties is located in the inferior frontal cortex, encompassing the posterior inferior frontal gyrus (IFG) and adjacent ventral premotor cortex (PMC). A posterior area with mirror neuron properties is located in the rostral part of the inferior parietal lobule (IPL) and prefrontal gyrus (PFG). The main visual input to the MNS originates from the posterior part of the superior temporal sulcus (STS). The visual input from the STS to the MNS is represented by a broken arrow. The other broken arrow represents the information flow from the parietal MNS, which is mostly concerned with the motoric description of the action, to the frontal MNS, which is more concerned with the goal of the action. The solid arrows represent efference copies of motor imitative commands that are sent back to the STS to allow matching between the sensory predictions of imitative motor plans and the visual description of the observed action.
Source: Modified from Iacoboni and Dapretto 2006, with permission from Nature Publishing Group, Copyright 2006.

Besides eye-contact and mirror neural mechanisms, there are other regions that are involved in social interaction and, overall, cortical midline structures have been proposed to play a key role in social cognition (Northoff and Bermpohl 2004). For example, the anterior cingulate cortex has been proposed to be related to monitoring, the dorsomedial prefrontal cortex to evaluation, the orbitomedial prefrontal cortex to representation, and the posterior cingulate cortex to integration of self-referential stimuli. Interestingly, the dorsomedial prefrontal cortex and medial parietal areas are activated when subjects watch social interaction between other people (Iacoboni et al. 2004), and the anterior paracingulate cortex is engaged when subjects watch other interacting subjects and try to understand their intentions (Walter et al. 2004).

Overall, nonverbal communication relies on all these mechanisms, from facial expressions to eye contact and directed gaze, and from the observation of others' gestures to guessing the others' intentions. Nonverbal communication is critical in any social encounter, including the special situation of doctor–patient interaction. Nonverbal messages and intentions can be communicated either consciously or unconsciously to the other, and indeed gestural communication may have represented a primitive form of language. Some authors suggest that this visually mediated gestural language may have then evolved into speech, thus substituting visual stimuli with auditory ones (Rizzolatti and Arbib 1998).

5.2.3 Being touched by a beloved makes the pain more bearable

After auditory input and verbal communication and visual stimuli, touch is the third modality that is considered in this section. Touch and somatosensory inputs are signals that convey strong emotional information in many circumstances. For example, we have seen in section 1.3 that social grooming, or allogrooming, is an important mediator of social relationships in nonhuman primates. It promotes social interaction and boosts social bonding. The very act of grooming, scratching, rubbing, and licking is a complex concertation of neural, hormonal, and genetic events, which take place in both cortical and subcortical areas. A powerful somatosensory emotional stimulus is represented by hand-holding, which can be considered a nonverbal supportive social behaviour in all respects. It expresses social support and affection, and it has even been observed in nonhuman primates during periods of dyadic reconciliation and soothing (de Waal 2000). It has also been found to reduce autonomic arousal and anxiety under stressful conditions, for example in cataract surgery patients under local anaesthesia (Jung-Soon and Kyung-Sook 2001).

A study investigating the biological effects of hand-holding was performed on married women who were subjected to the threat of electric shock in three different conditions: while holding their husband's hand, while holding the hand of an anonymous male experimenter, or holding no hand at all (Coan et al. 2006). Whereas holding the spouse's hand produced a decrease in unpleasantness ratings compared to no hand-holding, holding the stranger's hand did not decrease unpleasantness (Fig 5.11A). By using functional magnetic resonance imaging, these investigators also found attenuation of activation in the neural systems supporting emotional and behavioural threat responses when the women held their husband's hand, for example in right dorsolateral prefrontal cortex, left caudate–nucleus accumbens, and superior colliculus (Fig 5.11B). A more limited attenuation of activation in these systems occurred when they held the hand of a stranger, for example in the ventral anterior cingulate cortex, posterior cingulate, right postcentral gyrus, and left supramarginal gyrus. Interestingly, the effects of spousal hand-holding on these neural threat responses varied as a function of marital quality, with higher marital quality predicting less threat-related neural activation in the right anterior insula, superior frontal gyrus, and hypothalamus during spousal, but not stranger, hand-holding. This suggests that individuals in higher quality relationships benefit from greater regulatory effects on the neural systems involved in negative emotions, e.g. the affective component of pain.

It should be noted that hand-holding by a close relative or friend is not always necessary to induce these effect. Sometimes the presence of a beloved one in the room is enough. For example, fibromyalgia patients were tested for thermal pain thresholds and somatosensory magnetoencephalographic responses under two experimental conditions of social support: patient alone and patient's significant other present (Montoya et al. 2004). Thermal pain thresholds indicated greater sensitivity in fibromyalgia patients than in controls. This pain sensitivity as well as subjective pain ratings were reduced in the presence of their significant others as compared with the ratings when the patients were alone. Brain activity elicited by elbow stimulation was also significantly reduced when a significant other was present as compared with the activity when the patient was alone. These findings indicate that social support through the presence of a significant other can influence pain processing at the subjective-behavioural level as well as at the central nervous system level.

5.3 The patient wants the future to be better than the present

5.3.1 Hope and hopelessness may impact on health

Defining hope is not an easy task. It can be defined as a positive motivational state that is based on a sense of successful goal-directed energy and planning to

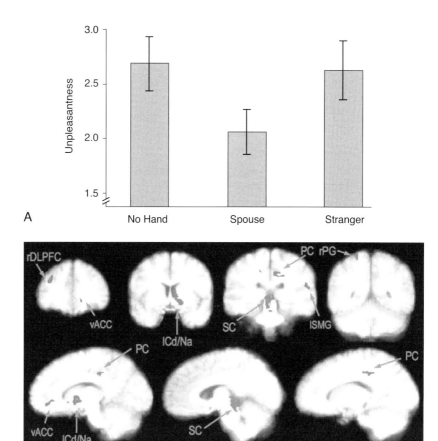

Fig 5.11 (A) Effect of hand-holding on unpleasantness about threat of an electric shock. Whereas there is no difference between the no-hand condition and holding a stranger's hand, a significant reduction in unpleasantness is present when holding the spouse's hand. (B) Threat-responsive regions affected by hand-holding condition. Green clusters indicate attenuation in the right dorsolateral prefrontal cortex (rDLPFC), left caudate–nucleus accumbens (lCd/Na), and superior colliculus (SC) when hoding the spouse's hand. Blue clusters indicate attenuation in the ventral anterior cingulate cortex (vACC), posterior cingulate (PC), right postcentral gyrus (rPG), and left supramarginal gyrus (lSMG) associated with both spouse and stranger hand-holding. See colour plate 10.

Source: Adapted from Coan et al. 2006 with permission from
John Wiley & Sons and the Association for Psychological Science, Copyright 2006.

meet goals (Snyder et al. 1991b; Snyder 2002). A fundamental condition of hope seems to be the current unsatisfactory conditions of life, which may involve deprivation, damage, or threat (Lazarus 1999), although this definition precludes hopeful thoughts about building on what already is satisfactory, the so-called enhancement goals (Snyder 2002). In any case, motivational behaviour is central to hope, and actually it interacts with goal-directed behaviour. In other words, once an individual has planned his own pathway to reach a goal, a strong motivational state is necessary to reach the desired goal. In this sense, high-hope individuals are capable of using alternative pathways if an impediment of any sort occurs in the planned pathways, so that the same goal can be reached in a different way (Snyder 2002). Although motivation and emotions have often been considered central to hope, and indeed hope itself has often been conceptualized as an emotion (Farina et al. 1995), according to Snyder (2002), what really matters in dispositional hope is not so much enduring emotions but rather an interaction between emotions and goal-directed thinking. The unsatisfactory and stressful current circumstances of life can be made less stressful through the appropriate thoughts and actions, a set of regulatory thought processes that, as a whole, have been called 'coping' (Lazarus 1999, 2000).

That hope is not easy to define is also shown by several similarities with other constructs, such as optimism, self-efficacy, self-esteem, and problem-solving. For example, in optimism, outcome expectancies, that is, the perception as being able to move towards desirable goals and away from undesirable goals, can play a critical role (Scheier and Carver 1985), and these are very similar to the motivational state in hope theory (Snyder 2002). Likewise, as occurs in the hope construct by Snyder (2002), in self-efficacy thinking, an important goal-related outcome must be involved (Bandura 1977), and in problem-solving a desired goal (e.g. a problem solution) is assumed to be involved (Heppner and Hillerbrand 1991).

In order to understand the complexity of the psychological factors that are at work in hope, it is worth considering at least two scales that have been developed over the past years. The first scale assesses trait hope, i.e. hope as a trait of personality (Snyder et al. 1991a). Its items are the following:

1) I can think of many ways to get out of a jam.

2) I energetically pursue my goals.

3) I feel tired most of the time.

4) There are lots of ways around any problem.

5) I am easily downed in an argument.

6) I can think of many ways to get the things in life that are important to me.

7) I worry about my health.

8) Even when others get discouraged, I know I can find a way to solve the problem.

9) My past experiences have prepared me well for my future.

10) I've been pretty successful in life.

11) I usually find myself worrying about something.

12) I meet the goals that I set for myself.

It is clear that all the key elements in Snyder's theory of hope (Snyder 2002) are tested, namely, goals, pathways, and planning to meet goals, as well as the motivational components. For example, in items 6 and 8, it is explicitly asked whether individuals are capable of using alternative pathways in order to reach the goals they had set for themselves.

The second scale is about state hope and is not very different from the first one. However, in this case the main emphasis is on how respondents describe themselves as they are 'right now' (Snyder et al. 1996). The items are as follows:

1) If I should find myself in a jam, I could think of many ways to get out of it.

2) At the present time, I am energetically pursuing my goals.

3) There are lots of ways around any problem that I am facing now.

4) Right now, I see myself as being pretty successful.

5) I can think of many ways to reach my current goals.

6) At this time, I am meeting the goals that I have set for myself.

Thus, although many elements take part in hope, at least two key factors can be identified: expectation and motivation. The subject expects the future to be better than the present and is strongly motivated to adopt the necessary behavioural repertoire in order to get the goals that he had set for himself.

Several studies indicate that hope has beneficial effects on health, thus the therapist should strive to induce hope in his patients. For example, researchers have found that higher hope is related to better adjustment in coping with severe arthritis (Snyder 2002), burn injuries (Barnum et al. 1998), spinal cord injuries (Elliott et al. 1991), fibromyalgia (Affleck and Tennen 1996; Tennen and Affleck 1999), blindness (Jackson et al. 1998), and cancer (Stanton et al. 2000). Likewise, high-hope individuals have been found to tolerate pain better than low-hope individuals. This has also been tested experimentally in the laboratory setting by using the cold pressor test as an experimental pain (Snyder 1998, 2002). These authors found that the high-hope persons tolerate pain about twice as long as the low-hope people.

In a similar study on experimental pain, Breznitz (1999) manipulated expectations about how long the pain might last, in order to see whether hope for a relatively early end would indeed allow subjects to tolerate pain better. Subjects were required to keep one of their hands in ice-cold water until they could no longer stand the pain. Subjects in one group were told that the test would be over in four minutes, while those in another group were not told anything. Actually, the test lasted a maximum of four minutes in both cases. The researchers found that 60% of those who knew when the test would end were able to endure the full four minutes, whereas only 30% of those who were kept in the dark were.

Some studies have found that high hopers show higher adherence to prescribed medications, and high Hope Scale scores predict staying in a drug treatment programme (Snyder 2002). Hopelessness and pessimism have been found to be associated with illness and mortality (Engel 1968; Schmale and Iker 1971; Peterson et al. 1988; Stein et al. 1989). For example, hopelessness is associated with a major risk of developing fatal ischemic heart disease (Anda et al. 1993) an to increased risk of dying from both cardiovascular and noncardiovascular causes in subjects with a history of cardiovascular disease, diabetes, cancer, or respiratory disease (Everson et al. 1996; Stern et al. 2001). In addition, Frank (1961, 1971, 1981), by analysing the healing process in psychotherapy within the context of patient's expectations, proposed that hope is the primary mechanism of change in folk tradition of healing and in psychotherapy.

Although the association between hope/hopeless and illness/mortality have been found in many studies, these findings should be taken with some caution for at least two reasons. First, some other studies have not found such correlation. For example, Schulz et al. (1996) observed that pessimism may not affect mortality in the elderly population, and explained this finding with the possibility that pessimism or hopelessness may be more normative in older persons. Second, helplessness and hopelessness are typical symptoms of depressive disorders among others such as anhedonia, feelings of guilt, loss of energy, or sleep disturbances, thus it is often hard to disentangle hopelessness and depression. Therefore, the specificity of hopelessness is not very clear in many circumstances, and some effects can sometime be attributed to depressive symptoms.

Despite the fact that hopelessness belong to a set of symptoms which characterize depression, there are some specific aspects that are worthy of analysis. Hopelessness has been considered as the key variable linking depression to suicidal behaviour by Minkoff et al. (1973) and by Beck et al. (1975) and, indeed, in the next section we will see that part of the neurobiological mechanisms that are known overlap with those involved in suicidal behaviour. Hopelessness and helplessness are often considered together, e.g. in some animal models of depression, however it should be remembered that whereas hopelessness can be considered as a negative expectation with respect to the future, helplessness can be viewed as unrealistically low concepts of the own capabilities (e.g. see Henkel et al. 2002). The association of hopelessness with helplessness is likely to derive from Beck's theory of depression, whereby three elements are at the very heart of depressive symptoms. This triad consists of negative attitudes to the self, to the future, and to the environment (Beck et al. 1985). Helplessness may be viewed as a negative attitude to the self (low concepts of the own capabilities) and hopelessness as a negative attitude to the future (negative expectations).

5.3.2 Hopelessness/helplessness involve serotoninergic and noradrenergic systems

In 1967 it was reported that dogs undergoing electric shocks not contingent on their behaviour showed a subsequent difficulty to escape and avoid the shocks (Overmier and Seligman 1967). In other words, the experience of uncontrollable events and the expectation that no action can control outcomes led to symptoms of passivity, emotional deficits, anxiety, and hostility. This occurred because the dogs learned that the shocks were independent of any responses. Indeed, they showed a motivational deficit, whereby only a few attempts to escape the shocks were conducted, as well as an emotional deficit, with no overt emotional responses (Overmier and Seligman 1967). This phenomenon, which was called 'learned helplessness', has been used as an animal model of depression, despite many criticisms and a reformulation in more cognitive terms by Abramson et al. (1978, 1989). In such reformulation, a hopelessness theory of depression was proposed, whereby hopelessness was viewed as a subset of helplessness, which means that if hopelessness occurs then helplessness also occurs, but not vice versa.

Despite this confusion in terminology and overlapping between hopelessness on the one hand and helplessness on the other, the animal models of learned helplessness have provided some interesting insights into the neurobiological mechanisms of these phenomena. First of all, serotonin has been found to be involved in learned helplessness (Amat et al. 1998; Edwards et al. 1991, 1992). For example, in some experiments rats could be separated into two different groups after exposure to uncontrollable shocks. Whereas one group of rats did not learn to escape a controllable shock after the previous experience of uncontrollable shocks (learned helpless rats), another group learned an adequate response (non-learned helpless rats). The learned helpless rats showed an up-regulation of serotonin receptors in the cortex, hippocampus, septum, and hypothalamus and a down-regulation in the hypothalamus. In addition, changes of presynaptic serotoninergic activity caused by uncontrollable shocks has been described in

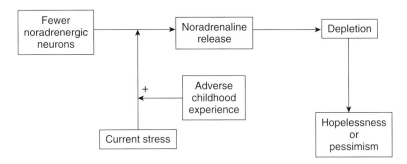

Fig 5.12 Relationship between stress sensitivity and hopelessness. Different stressful situations, such as adverse childhood experiences, might lead to stress sensitivity that is manifested in excessive noradrenaline release from fewer noradrenergic neurons. This, in turn, would lead to depletion of noradrenaline that might underlie hopelessness. Source: From Mann 2003 with permission from the Nature Publishing Group, Copyright 2003.

the hippocampus and hypothalamus of learned helpless rats (Edwards et al. 1991, 1992; Amat et al. 1998).

In another study by van Heeringen et al. (2003), a negative correlation between prefrontal (mainly dorsolateral) binding to serotonin 5-HT2A receptors and levels of hopelessness was found; in other words, the lower the binding to serotonin receptors, the higher the degree of hopelessness. In the same study, both prefrontal 5-HT2A binding and levels of hopelessness correlated with scores on the temperamental dimension 'harm avoidance', which is a trait-dependent measure of behavioural inhibition or regulation of anxiety.

Not surprisingly, together with the involvement of serotoninergic mechanisms, an activation of the hypothalamus-pituitary-adrenal axis has been found in a number of studies that used inescapable shocks as a model (Henkel et al. 2002). Indeed, adverse experiences might lead to stress sensitivity that is manifested in excessive noradrenaline release and its possible subsequent depletion (Fig 5.12). This, in turn, might be a mechanism which leads to hopelessness (Mann 2003). Interestingly, hopelessness and pessimistic traits, together with other psychological factors such as aggressive/impulsive traits and history of physical or sexual abuse during childhood, is one of the clinical features that increase the risk for suicidal behaviour (Mann 2003; van Heeringen 2003). Therefore, the same neurochemical changes that are present in hopelessness, like a dysfunction of serotoninergic and noradrenergic systems, have also been found in suicide victims (Mann 2003; van Heeringen 2003).

5.4 **A look into the doctor's brain**

5.4.1 Face expressions of pain are likely to have evolved for eliciting medical attention from others

Facial expressions are an important means of communicating emotions to others. Expressions such as happiness, fear, anger, sadness, and disgust are universally recognized (Ekman and Friesen 1986; Ekman 1992). Although pain per se is often not considered as an emotion, specific facial movements associated with pain have been identified, such as lowering the brow, narrowing the eyes by tightening the lids and raising the cheeks or even fully closing the eyes, raising the upper lip, deepening the nasolabial fold and wrinkling the nose as well as opening the lips and mouth in varying degrees (LeResche and Dworkin 1984, 1988; Craig and Patrick 1985; Prkachin 1992; Kappesser and Williams 2002). Complex associations have also been described, such as expressions of disgust, anger, fear, and sadness during pain. For example, Hale and Hadjistavropoulos (1997) found that the intensity of disgust expression increased on venipuncture with pain expression, while happiness expression decreased in anticipation of it. Interestingly, there are strong consistencies in the morphology of facial pain expression from birth through old age, but sensitive to cultural differences and to social context (Williams 2002).

According to Williams (2002), facial expressions are likely to have evolved for eliciting medical attention from others. According to this evolutionary perspective, a greater facial expression of pain in the presence of potential caregivers than in their absence is of primary importance, so that the presence of potential caregivers would prompt the release of suppression of pain facial expression. According to Williams (2002), a propensity characterized as 'Don't hide pain in the presence of a potential caregiver', would encourage free expression of pain in the presence of solicitous others and of those whose professional duty is to attend and minister to pain. Conversely, in the presence of others not expected to provide support of any sort, or alone, facial expression of pain would tend to be suppressed. Indeed, in the presence of their parents, children may disinhibit some pain expressions and rate pain lower when their parents are absent (Craig et al. 1996). Interestingly, in adulthood grief is expressed among kin and friends rather than among strangers or alone (Parkes 1972), which supports the powerful social meaning of the facial expression of negative emotions.

5.4.2 Empathy and compassion have different meanings and mechanisms

The patient's face expressions of pain, fear, grief, and negative emotions are the critical factor, albeit not the only one, triggering the doctor's empathic behaviour.

Besides technical skills, empathic behaviour should represent the main characteristic of any health professional. We have seen in section 1.3.2 that social grooming is likely to have evolved to empathy first and then to altruism. Empathic behaviour is an important step in evolution of mankind and its social interactions, for it allows to share the emotional state of another and to adopt his perspective. In this regard, the social connection between the suffering patient, who expresses his discomfort, and the empathic doctor is at the very heart of the doctor–patient relationship. Empathy thus refers to an inter-subjective process through which the cognitive and emotional experiences of another come to be shared, without losing sight of the original source of the experience (Decety and Jackson 2004). Empathy can be approached from different perspectives, for example through social psychology or cognitive neuroscience, and clearly involves both bottom-up and top-down information processing components (Decety and Moriguchi 2007; Goubert et al. 2009). Whereas the bottom-up processes involve an automatic and covert mimicry component, which drives emotional contagion during inter-individual interactions, top-down processes modulate and self-regulate both this automatic system and subsequent pro-social behaviours (Decety et al. 2010). Therefore, emotional and cognitive components are both involved in empathic behaviour, but whereas the former supports our ability to empathize emotionally ('I feel what you feel'), the latter includes complex cognitive components such as empathic perspective-taking and mentalizing ('I understand what you feel') (Shamay-Tsoory et al. 2009).

There are powerful cultural influences upon empathic behaviour. In a study by Decety et al. (2010), participants were exposed to a series of short video clips featuring individuals experiencing pain who were (i) similar to the participant (i.e. healthy), (ii) stigmatized but not responsible for their stigmatized condition (infected with AIDS as a result of an infected blood transfusion), or (iii) stigmatized and responsible for their stigmatized condition (infected with AIDS as a result of intravenous drug use). It was found that the participants were significantly more sensitive to the pain of AIDS transfusion targets as compared with healthy and AIDS drug targets, together with greater hemodynamic activity in areas associated with pain processing, such as the right anterior insula, anterior midcingulate cortex, and periaqueductal grey. Conversely, lower activity was observed in the anterior midcingulate cortex for AIDS drug targets as compared with healthy controls. Interestingly, the more the participants blamed these targets, the less pain they attributed to them as compared with healthy controls. In another study by Xu et al. (2009), empathic neural responses of the pain matrix were recorded to see whether differences were present between racial groups. Whereas painful stimulations applied to racial in-group faces induced increased activations in the anterior cingulate cortex and inferior frontal/insula cortex in both Caucasians and Chinese, the empathic neural response in the anterior cingulate cortex decreased significantly when participants viewed faces of other races. Thus empathy is modulated by a priori attitudes towards the target group.

As emphasized by Hein and Singer (2008), it is important to note that empathy is distinguished from sympathy or empathic concern or compassion (see also Batson et al. 2007; Eisenberg 2007). An emotion produced by empathy is isomorphic with the other's emotion. This is not necessarily true for sympathy or compassion (Eisenberg 2007). Nor is empathy necessarily linked to pro-social motivation, namely, the concern about the others' well-being. By contrast, pro-social motivation is involved in both sympathy and compassion. In fact, compassion enable individuals to enter into and maintain relationships of caring and tends to motivate us to help people who are emotionally suffering, thus it represents an important aspect of pro-social behaviour. Furthermore, it has also been known that a positive intrinsic reward feeling may occur as a result of experiencing compassion for others (Sprecher and Fehr 2006). Therefore, having compassion towards a sad person goes beyond the simple sharing of the person's sadness, involving motivational and reward components that lead to pro-social behaviours.

In the next sections, empathy and compassion will be treated separately. This separation is not only necessary from a behavioural standpoint, but also from a neuroscientific perspective. In fact, different neural systems are involved in the many aspects of empathic behaviour, e.g. emotional contagion and empathic perspective-taking, and in compassion, which emphasizes once again the different meanings of these words.

5.4.3 There are two different neural systems for empathy

Accumulating evidence suggests that there are at least two mechanisms mediating empathy: emotional contagion on the one hand and cognitive perspective-taking on the other (De Waal 2007; see also section 1.3.2). Whereas emotional contagion is thought to support our ability to empathize emotionally, that is, to share the other person's emotional feelings, empathic perspective-taking involves complex cognitive components, whereby one infers the state of the other person, also known as theory of mind (Premack and Woodruff 1978), or mentalizing (Frith and Frith 2003), or mindreading (Baron-Cohen 1995).

The distinction between the emotional and the cognitive component is particularly important from a neuroscientific point of view, for findings from brain imaging studies suggest that understanding others on the basis of cognitive perspective taking and empathy recruit different neural networks (Hein and Singer 2008). Figure 5.13 shows the two main systems that mediate

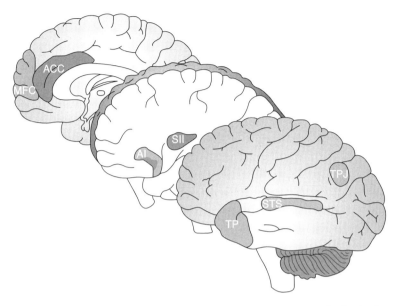

Fig 5.13 Brain regions typically involved in understanding others on the basis of cognitive perspective taking (green) and empathic emotional abilities (orange). MFC, medial prefrontal cortex; ACC, anterior cingulate cortex; AI, anterior insula; SII, secondary somatosensory cortex; TP, temporal poles; STS, superior temporal sulcus; TPF, temporo-parietal junction. See color plate 11.
Source: From Hein and Singer 2008 with permission from Elsevier, Copyright 2008.

empathic emotional behaviour on the one hand (orange) and cognitive perspective taking on the other (green). Whereas cognitive perspective taking, in which subjects are typically asked to take the perspective of a person shown on a cartoon, activates the medial prefrontal regions, the superior temporal sulcus, the temporal pole, and the temporo-parietal junction (Frith and Frith 2006; Saxe 2006), empathizing with another person has been found to activate somatosensory and insular cortices as well as the anterior cingulate cortex (Hein and Singer 2008). For example, in a study by Singer et al. (2004), the bilateral anterior insula and the rostral anterior cingulate cortex were activated when a female experienced pain herself as well as when she saw that her husband had experienced pain. As these areas are involved in the processing of the affective component of pain (see section 3.2), both the experience of pain to oneself and the knowledge that the other person is experiencing pain activates the same affective pain circuits. In a different study by the same group (Singer et al. 2006), the empathic brain responses in the anterior insula and anterior cingulate cortex were not restricted to a beloved partner, but also occurred when an unknown but likable person was in pain. Therefore, the neural simulation of the pain of another person occurs independently of the affective link between the empathizer and the person in pain (Hein and Singer 2008), which has obvious implications for the therapist–patient encounter.

That there are two independent systems for empathic emotional abilities and cognitive empathy is also shown by lesion studies, although some differences are present compared to the organization of Fig 5.13. Shamay-Tsoory et al. (2009) investigated subjects with lesions either in the ventromedial prefrontal cortex or in the inferior frontal gyrus, whose measures of empathy that incorporate both cognitive and affective dimensions were assessed. A remarkable behavioural and anatomic double dissociation between deficits in cognitive empathy (ventromedial prefrontal lesion) and emotional empathy (inferior frontal gyrus lesion) was found. In addition, precise anatomical mapping of lesions revealed Brodmann area 44 to be critical for emotional empathy while areas 11 and 10 were found necessary for cognitive empathy. Figure 5.14 shows the double dissociation between the emotional and cognitive indices. Patients with ventromedial prefrontal lesions are significantly impaired in the cognitive index as compared to patients with the inferior frontal gyrus lesions, non-frontal

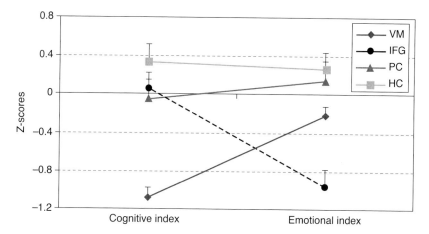

Fig 5.14 Double dissociation between emotional index (emotional empathy, emotion recognition) and cognitive index (cognitive empathy, mentalizing). Patients with ventromedial prefrontal lesions (VM) are significantly impaired in the cognitive index as compared to patients with the inferior frontal gyrus lesions (IFG), with non-frontal lesions (PC) and to healthy controls (HC). Patients with IFG lesions are impaired in the emotional index as compared to the VM patients, PC and HC groups.
Source: From Shamay-Tsoory et al. 2009 with permission from Oxford University Press, Copyright 2009.

lesions, and healthy controls, whereas patients with inferior frontal gyrus lesions are impaired in the emotional index as compared to the ventromedial prefrontal patients, non-frontal lesion, and healthy control groups.

The inclusion of the inferior frontal gyrus in empathic emotional abilities but not in cognitive perspective taking, as suggested by the study of Shamay-Tsoory et al. (2009), is particularly interesting. In fact, some studies have found the activation of the mirror neuron system of the inferior frontal gyrus not only with respect to motor actions but to emotion recognition or evaluation (Carr et al. 2003; Seitz et al. 2008) and emotional empathy (Jabbi et al. 2007; Schulte-Ruther et al. 2007) as well.

Empathic responses have been found to depend on a variety of factors, such as the intensity of the stimulation or the displayed emotion. For example, Saarela et al. (2007) presented faces of patients being in chronic or acute pain and showing different degrees of emotional expression. Stronger activations were found in the anterior insula and anterior cingulate cortex when the subjects empathized with people in acute pain as compared with chronic pain. Likewise, in the study by Avenanti et al. (2006), participants were shown a needle piercing body parts of a human model (high-intensity pain) or just scratching the surface of the skin (low-intensity pain). Muscle evoked potentials following trans-cranial magnetic stimulation, which are known to be affected by empathy (Avenanti et al. 2005), were found to be inhibited in the high-intensity condition, but not in the low-intensity condition. As we have seen in the previous section 5.4.2, other factors can modulate empathic responses, like cultural and racial differences and a priori attitudes. For example, painful stimulations applied to racial in-group faces induce increased activations in the anterior cingulate cortex and inferior frontal/insula cortex in both Caucasians and Chinese, yet the empathic neural response in the anterior cingulate cortex decreases significantly when participants view faces of other races (Xu et al. 2009). Similarly, individuals are more sensitive to the pain of targets who are not responsible for their stigmatized condition (AIDS as the result of a blood transfusion) than targets who are held responsible for their condition (AIDS through illegal drug use), and this is associated to different brain responses in regions of pain processing (Decety et al. 2010).

While pain is surely the modality that has been investigated in more detail, it should be emphasized that similar empathic responses have also been described in other modalities, like touch and taste, as well as in emotions such as disgust. For example, both observation of touch and first-hand experience of touch activate the secondary somatosensory cortex (Keysers et al. 2004), and video clips showing people sampling pleasant and unpleasant tastes make observers experience the same tastes, along with activation in anterior insula cortex when both observing and experiencing disgust (Jabbi et al. 2007).

5.4.4 **Compassion for social and physical pain engages two separate neural systems**

There are similarities in the neural mechanisms of admiration and compassion. We have seen in section 5.1.4 that admiration can be evoked by witnessing virtuous behaviour aimed at reducing the suffering of others or by displays of virtuosic skill. Whereas the former has to do with social/psychological circumstances, i.e. virtue, the latter pertains to another person's immediate physical circumstances, i.e. skilful abilities. The same distinction can be adopted for compassion. In fact, compassion can be evoked by witnessing situations of personal loss and social deprivation, i.e. social pain, or by witnessing bodily injury, i.e. physical pain. As for admiration, whereas the former pertains to social/psychological circumstances, the latter has to do with immediate physical circumstances (Immordino-Yang et al. 2009).

Interestingly, in the study by Immordino-Yang et al. (2009) already described in section 5.1.4 for admiration, compassion for social and physical pain was found to engage two different neural circuits. Compassion for social pain was associated with strong activation in the inferior/posterior portion of the posteromedial cortices, whereas compassion for physical pain produced a larger activation in the superior/anterior portion of the posteromedial cortices (Fig 5.15). Since the superior/anterior portion of the posteromedial cortices is strongly interconnected with lateral parietal cortices and the inferior/posterior portion is closely associated with the anterior middle cingulate cortex (Parvizi et al. 2006), the study by Immordino-Yang et al. (2009) suggests that those emotions related to someone else's psychological state, e.g. social pain, may preferentially recruit a network involving the inferior/posterior posteromedial cortices and the anterior middle cingulate, which are affiliated with interoceptive information. By contrast, those emotions that are related to someone else's physical state, e.g. physical pain, may recruit the superior/anterior part of the posterolateral cortices most connected with lateral parietal cortices, which deal with exteroception and musculoskeletal information. These neural networks, one for the emotions related to someone else's psychological state and the other for the emotions related to someone else's physical state, are engaged by both admiration and compassion, as shown in Fig 5.15. Therefore, the crucial point here is the distinction between recognizing another's social or physical situation and emotionally reacting to it, which represents two complex social functions subserved by two discrete neural systems.

It should be noted that compassionate concern towards a suffering person is related to the motivation to approach, help, comfort, and alleviate his suffering, and, accordingly, a positive intrinsic reward feeling may occur as a result of experiencing compassion for others (Sprecher and Fehr 2006). Therefore, having

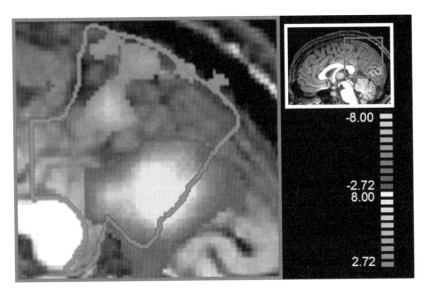

Fig 5.15 Activation in the posteromedial cortices (outlined in pink) for admiration for virtue and compassion for social pain (blue/green) versus admiration for skill and compassion for physical pain (orange/yellow). The red box frames the location of the magnified view. Note the clear separation between the anterosuperior sector activated by admiration for skill and compassion for physical pain, and the posteroinferior activated by admiration for virtue and compassion for social pain. See colour plate 12. Source: From Immordino-Yang et al. 2009 with permission from the National Academy of Sciences USA, Copyright 2009.

compassion towards a person should be expected to activate the reward system (see Chapter 4). Indeed, Kim et al. (2009) found that compassionate attitude activated a neural network encompassing the medial frontal cortex, the subgenual frontal cortex, the inferior frontal cortex, and the midbrain regions. In particular, a test of the interaction between a compassionate attitude and sad facial affect revealed significant activations in the midbrain/ventral striatum/septal network region, a key region involved in pro-social/social approach motivation and reward mechanisms (see Chapter 4). These findings emphasize the differences between empathic behaviour, which does not necessarily involve motivational systems, and compassionate behaviour, whereby the motivation to alleviate others' suffering represents the central element.

5.4.5 Doctors can regulate their emotional responses to others' suffering

In order to suppress distress in everyday medical practice, health professionals, particularly those involved in invasive and painful procedures, may have developed mechanisms of self-control that is aimed at reducing negative emotions while watching the suffering of their patients. In other words, nurses and clinicians have to develop a defensive shield towards the negative emotions or seen pain in order to prevent strenuous coping and maintain their own health. The danger of this habituation to others' suffering is represented by the possible underestimation of patients' pain by health professionals (Kappesser and Williams 2002).

There is some experimental evidence that, indeed, habituation to others' suffering occurs in clinical practice. Cheng et al. (2007) conducted a functional magnetic resonance imaging study, whereby physicians who practice acupuncture were compared to naive participants while observing animated visual stimuli depicting needles being inserted into different body parts, such as the mouth region, the hands, and the feet. It was found that the anterior insula, the somatosensory cortex, the periaqueducal grey, and the anterior cingulate cortex were significantly activated in the naive group, but not in the expert group. The latter showed activation of the medial and superior prefrontal cortices and the temporoparietal junction, which are known to be involved in emotion regulation and theory of mind. Figure 5.16 shows the regions within the somatosensory cortex when watching different body parts being pricked by a needle or touched by a Q-tip in experienced acupuncturists and in naive subjects. It can be seen that the somatosensory activations are modulated by the expertise of the participants and the level of pain inferred. In fact, whereas in naive subjects (controls), watching the body parts pricked by a needle (red columns) was associated with stronger signal than was watching a Q-tip (orange columns), in experienced acupuncturists (experts), the Q-tip and needle resulted in similar signal changes in the somatosensory cortex.

The difference in activation of the somatosensory cortex between the two groups of naive and expert subjects is likely to reflect top-down processes induced by one's degree of knowledge about acupuncture. Therefore, health professionals are capable of regulating their emotions by relying on higher cognitive processes involving knowledge in working memory and long-term memory.

5.5 The doctor–patient interaction may have both positive and negative effects

5.5.1 A positive interaction may lead to positive outcomes

There is compelling experimental and clinical evidence that a positive doctor–patient relationship and the very act of meeting a therapist may lead to positive outcomes. Indeed, these effects are described throughout this volume, for example in section 5.2.1. In particular, they represent a critical factor for the

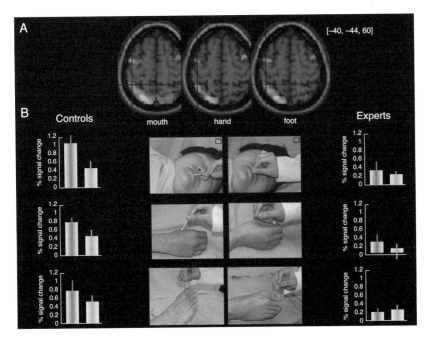

Fig 5.16 Regions within the somatosensory cortex when watching different body parts being pricked by a needle or touched by a Q-tip in experienced acupuncturists (experts) and in naive subjects (controls). (A) Watching different body parts (from left to right: mouth region, hand, foot) elicits differential activations around the somatosensory cortex. (B) The somatosensory activations are modulated by the expertise of the participants and the level of pain inferred. In controls, watching the body parts pricked by a needle (red columns) was associated with stronger signal than was watching a Q-tip (orange columns). In experts, the Q-tip and needle resulted in similar signal changes in the somatosensory cortex. See colour plate 13. Source: From Cheng et al. 2007 with permission by Elsevier, Copyright 2007.

occurrence of placebo effects and, accordingly, a detailed description will be given in Chapter 6. Therefore, this section is only a brief anticipation of the positive effects that have been described when a patient starts interacting with his therapist. The reader has to refer to Chapter 6 for a more detailed and thorough discussion on how the patient's expectations of therapeutic benefit and the subsequent clinical improvement may lead to real amelioration of his illness.

In general, physicians have long known the powerful effect of their relationship with their patients and, accordingly, have used the appropriate words and attitudes with their patients. Apart from the clinical observations and experiments described in section 5.2.1, other examples can be considered to illustrate the positive outcomes resulting from a good doctor–patient interaction. Kaplan et al. (1989) found that blood pressure, blood sugar, functional status, and overall health status were consistently related to specific aspects of the physician–patient communication. There are also a number of studies in which the doctor–patient relationship has been found to be correlated to the outcome of illness (Stewart et al. 1979; Starfield et al. 1981; Gracely et al. 1985; Greenfield et al. 1985; Bass et al. 1986; Stewart 1995). Even diagnostic tests, which have nothing to do with therapy, have been found to induce clinical improvement (Sox et al. 1981).

Although the underlying mechanisms are not always understood, many factors could be at work here. For example, besides expectations of improvement, it is possible that a better interaction between the doctor and the patient might lead to a better compliance with the drug regimens (Inui et al. 1976). In this regard, it is worth mentioning the Coronary Drug Project (1980), a randomized double-blind placebo-controlled trial evaluating the efficacy of lipid lowering drugs in the long-term treatment of coronary heart disease. The five years mortality in 1103 men treated with clofibrate was 20%. Similarly, the 2789 treated with placebo showed a mortality of 20.9%. Those patients who were found to take at least 80% of their prescribed medication (good adherers) had significantly lower mortality (15%) than poor adherers (24.6%). Virtually identical findings occurred in those assigned to the placebo group, in which good adherers had 15.1% mortality and poor adherers 28.3% mortality. This suggests that placebo may be quite powerful, and its effects may be intertwined with other phenomena, such as compliance and adherence.

In some conditions, the number of the doctor's visits have been found to be a good predictor of clinical improvement. For example, three or less visits were found to be less likely to induce large remissions in those patients who received a placebo than four or more visits (Ilnyckyj et al. 1997). Similarly, the number of study visits during a clinical trial, as well as the duration of the study and the severity of disease at entry, were good predictors of remission in the placebo groups of clinical trials of Crohn's disease (Su et al. 2004).

The positive effects of a good relationship is of particular relevance in psychotherapy. Indeed, several authors claim that psychotherapy works only through a benign human relationship. For example, it is worth noting that there are more than 400 types of psychotherapy, each with its theory and working hypothesis and, surprisingly, all of them effective (Parloff 1986; Moerman 2002). In a widely known and influential review of about 40 studies that used different psychotherapeutic approaches, Luborsky et al. (1975) found that all the psychotherapies were effective, even those in which minimal treatment was carried out. In a different analysis of 375 studies of different kinds of psychotherapy by Smith and

Glass (1977), negligible differences were found in the effects produced by different therapy types. In 1982, Landman and Dawes (1982) went through these 375 studies and found that many of them did not have random allocation of patients to the different groups. Therefore, they re-analysed the 375 studies plus 60 they added, and were able to extract 42 studies that used true random assignment. Surprisingly, Landman and Dawes (1982) found that the results were similar to those of the 375 studies analysed by Smith and Glass (1977), which indicates that it did not matter whether the studies had a true random assignment: psychotherapy was effective regardless of its theories. Therefore, all psychotherapies work more or less pretty well and there are little differences across the different therapeutic approaches. In other words, psychotherapy might be nothing more than good human interaction between patient and therapist, so that trust, belief, expectation, motivation, and hope, that are common in all types of psychotherapy, would be the factors responsible for the successful therapeutic outcomes.

Another study is worthy mentioning. In 1979, Strupp and Hadley (1979) conducted an interesting experiment whereby disturbed college students were allocated to either psychotherapy carried out by practiced psychotherapists with an average experience of more than 20 years, or interaction with professors of English, philosophy, history, or mathemathics with renowned reputation for warmth and trustworthiness but with no previous experience as therapists. Both groups improved and there was no significant difference between the improvement of those who interacted with psychotherapists or with the professors. In addition, two control groups, one receiving minimal treatment and one only receiving diagnostic testing, also showed improvement, although significantly smaller than the experimental groups. Strupp and Hadley (1979) concluded that the positive changes experienced by the patients of both experimental groups was attributable to the healing effects of a benign human relationship.

All these studies suggest that factors other than specific elements of each psychotherapy are at work. This concept was expressed by Frank (1961, 1971, 1981), who proposed that all forms of psychotherapy work because they contain similar elements, such as a ritual to reinforce the therapist–patient relationship and the presence of a thoughtful listener. He analysed the healing process within the context of patient's expectations, and proposed that hope is the primary mechanism of change in folk tradition of healing and in psychotherapy.

5.5.2 A negative interaction may lead to negative outcomes

As for the positive effects, the negative effects following a negative interaction are described in other parts of this volume. For example, the nocebo effect and anxiety-induced hyperalgesia are discussed in section 3.3.3. Indeed, words and attitudes by the provider may induce negative expectations in the patient and may lead to clinical worsening. Interestingly, the primary reason for lawsuits in the United States is not medical injury itself, but the failure of communication between doctors and their patients (Beckman et al. 1994; Levinson 1994), thereby pointing out the key role of a good patient–provider interaction. Unfortunately, empathic and compassionate behaviour is not always included in the doctor's background and armamentarium, and bad communication is sometimes the rule in routine medical practice. One good example is represented by the way in communicating negative diagnoses, a task that requires powerful empathic and compassionate abilities. The impact of a negative diagnosis on the patient's brain and body can be substantial and can induce real worsening, for example of pain (see section 3.3.3). Anxiety plays a key role in these situations and a bad interaction may indeed increase the patient's anxiety state and negative emotions. In this regard, the mechanisms underlying anxiety-induced hyperalgesia have been investigated in some detail, such as the involvement of some brain regions and of the neurotransmitter/hormone cholecystokinin, and are described in section 3.3.3.

As for a positive interaction, in this case also, the issue is relevant to psychotherapy. In fact, it is worth noting that in psychotherapy the therapist–patient relationship does not necessarily go always in the positive direction. Bootzin and Bailey (2005) emphasized how negative iatrogenic (literally, therapist-caused) effects may also occur during a psychotherapy. These negative effects have been described in different types of psychotherapy, such as critical incident stress debriefing for the treatment of post-traumatic stress disorder, group therapy for conduct disorder adolescents, and psychotherapy for dissociative identity disorder (Bootzin and Bailey 2005). For example, in group therapy for conduct disorder adolescents, the interaction between juvenile delinquents during group treatments may strengthen antisocial behaviour through the lack of positive expectancies (Bootzin and Bailey 2005). Therefore, not only may negative effects derive from a bad therapist–patient interaction, but also from uncontrolled variables during the psychotherapeutic procedure, like the negative interaction with other members of the therapeutic group.

References

Abramson LY, Metalsky GI and Alloy LB (1989). Hopelessness depression: a theory-based subtype of depression. *Psychological Reviews*, **96**, 358–72.

Abramson LY, Seligman MEP and Teasdale J (1978). Learned helplessness in humans: critique and reformulation. *Journal of Abnormal Psychology*, **87**, 49–74.

Adams RB, Ambady N, Macrae N and Kleck RE (2006). Emotional expressions forecast approach-avoidance behavior. *Motivation & Emotion*, **30**, 179–88.

Adolphs R, Tranel D, Damasio H and Damasio A (1994). Impaired recognition of emotion in facial expressions following bilateral damage to the human amygdala. *Nature*, **372**, 669–72.

Adolphs R, Tranel D and Damasio AR (1998). The human amygdala in social judgment. *Nature*, **393**, 470–4.

Adolphs R, Tranel D, Hamann S, Young AW, Calder AJ, Phelps EA et al. (1999). Recognition of facial emotion in nine individuals with bilateral amygdala damage. *Neuropsychologia*, **37**, 1111–7.

Affleck G and Tennen H (1996). Construing benefits from adversity: adaptational significance and dispositional underpinnings. *Journal of Personality*, **64**, 899–922.

Amaral DG (2003). The amygdala, social behavior, and danger detection. *Annals of the New York Academy of Sciences*, **1000**, 337–47.

Amat J, Matus-Amat P, Watkins LR and Maier SF (1998). Escapable and inescapable stress differentially and selectively alter extracellular levels of 5-HT in the ventral hippocampus and dorsal periaqueductal gray of the brain. *Brain Research*, **797**, 12–22.

Anda R, Williamson D, Jones D, Macera C, Eaker E, Glassman A et al. (1993). Depressed affect, hopelessness, and the risk of ischemic heart disease in a cohort of U.S. adults. *Epidemiology*, **4**, 285–94.

Anderson LA and Dedrick RF (1990). Development of the trust in physician scale: a measure to assess interpersonal trust in patient-physician relationships. *Psychological Reports*, **67**, 1091–100.

Avenanti A, Bueti D, Galati G and Aglioti S (2005). Transcranial magnetic stimulation highlights the sensorimotor side of empathy for pain. *Nature Neuroscience*, **8**, 955–60.

Avenanti A, Paluello IM, Bufalari I and Aglioti SM (2006). Stimulus-driven modulation of motor-evoked potentials during observation of others' pain. *Neuroimage*, **32**, 316–24.

Bakermans-Kranenburg MJ and van Ijzendoorn MH (2008). Oxytocin receptor (OXTR) and serotonin transporter (5-HTT) genes associated with observed parenting. *Social Cognitive and Affective Neuroscience*, **3**, 128–34.

Bandura A (1977). Self-efficacy: toward a unifying theory of behavior change. *Psychological Review*, **84**, 191–215.

Barnum DD, Snyder CR, Rapoff MA, Mani MM and Thompson R (1998). Hope and social support in the psychological adjustment of pediatric burn survivors and matched controls. *Children's Health Care*, **27**, 15–30.

Baron-Cohen S (1995). *Mindblindness: an essay on autism and theory of mind*. MIT Press, Cambridge, MA.

Bartz JA and Hollander E (2006). The neuroscience of affiliation: forging links between basic and clinical research on neuropeptides and social behavior. *Hormones and Behavior*, **50**, 518–28.

Bartels A and Zeki S (2004). The neural correlates of maternal and romantic love. *Neuroimage*, **21**, 1155–66.

Bass MJ, Buck C, Turner L, Dickie G, Pratt G and Campbell Robinson H (1986). The physician's actions and the outcome of illness in family practice. *Journal of Family Practice*, **23**, 43–7.

Batson CD, Eklund JH, Chermok VL, Hoyt JL and Ortiz BG (2007). An additional antecedent of empathic concern: valuing the welfare of the person in need. *Journal of Personality and Social Psychology*, **93**, 65–74.

Baumgartner T, Heinrichs M, Vonlanthen A, Fischbacher U and Fehr E (2008). Oxytocin shapes the neural circuitry of trust and trust adaptation in humans. *Neuron*, **58**, 639–50.

Beck AT, Kovacs M and Weissman A (1975). Hopelessness and suicidal behavior: an overview. *Journal of the American Medical Association*, **234**, 1146–9.

Beck AT, Steer RA, Kovacs M and Garrison B (1985). Hopelessness and eventual suicide: a 10 year prospective study of patients hospitalized with suicidal ideation. *American Journal of Psychiatry*, **142**, 559–63.

Beckman HB, Markakis KM, Suchman AL and Frankel RM (1994). The doctor–patient relationship and malpractice: lessons from plaintiff depositions. *Archives of Internal Medicine*, **154**, 1365–70.

Benedetti F (2002). How the doctor's words affect the patient's brain. *Evaluation and the Health Professions*, **25**, 369–86.

—— (2008). *Placebo effects: understanding the mechanisms in health and disease.* Oxford University Press, Oxford.

Bentin S, Degutis JM, D'Esposito M and Robertson LC (2007). Too many trees to see the forest: performance, event-related potential, and functional magnetic resonance imaging manifestations of integrative congenital prosopagnosia. *Journal of Cognitive Neuroscience*, **19**, 132–46.

Bootzin RR and Bailey E (2005). Understanding placebo, nocebo, and iatrogenic treatment effects. *Journal of Clinical Psychology*, **61**, 871–80.

Breznitz S (1999). The effect of hope on pain tolerance. *Social Research*, **66**, 629–52.

Broks P, Young AW, Maratos EJ, Coffey PJ, Calder AJ, Isaac CL et al. (1998). Face processing impairments after encephalitis: amygdala damage and recognition of fear. *Neuropsychologia*, **36**, 59–70.

Caetano G, Jousmaki V and Hari R (2007). Actor's and viewer's primary motor cortices stabilize similarly after seen or heard motor actions. *Proceedings National Academy of Sciences USA*, **104**, 9058–62.

Calder AJ, Lawrence AD, Keane J, Scott SK, Owen AM, Christoffels I et al. (2002). Reading the mind from eye gaze. *Neuropsychologia*, **40**, 1129–38.

Carr L, Iacoboni M, Dubeau MC, Mazziotta JC and Lenzi GL (2003). Neural mechanisms of empathy in humans: a relay from neural systems for imitation to limbic areas. *Proceedings of the National Academy of Sciences USA*, **100**, 5497–502.

Carter CS (1998). Neuroendocrine perspectives on social attachment and love. *Psychoneuroendocrinology*, **23**, 779–818.

—— (2003). Developmental consequences of oxytocin. *Physiology and Behavior*, **79**, 383–97.

Chartrand TL and Bargh JA (1999). The chameleon effect: the perception behavior link and social interaction. *Journal of Personality and Social Psychology*, **76**, 893–910.

Cheng Y, Lin CP, Liu HL, Hsu YY, Lim KE, Hung D et al. (2007). Expertise modulates the perception of pain in others. *Current Biology*, **17**, 1708–13.

Coan JA, Schaefer HS and Davidson RJ (2006). Lending a hand. Social regulation of the neural response to theat. *Psychological Science*, **17**, 1032–9.

Cochin S, Barthelemy C, Roux S and Martineau J (1999). Observation and execution of movement: similarities demonstrated by quantified electroencephalography. *European Journal of Neuroscience*, **11**, 1839–42.

Conty L, N'Diaye K, Tijus C and George N (2007). When eye creates the contact! ERP evidence for early dissociation between direct and averted gaze motion processing. *Neuropsychologia*, **45**, 3024–37.

Coronary Drug Project (1980). Influence of adherence to treatment and response of cholesterol on mortality in the coronary drug project. *New England Journal of Medicine*, **303**, 1038–41.

Cosmides L and Tooby J (1992). Cognitive adaptations for social exchange. In: JH Barkow, L Cosmides and J Tooby, eds. *The adapted mind: evolutionary psychology and the generation of culture*, pp. 163–228. Oxford University Press, London.

Craig KD and Patrick CJ (1985). Facial expression during induced pain. *Journal of Personality and Social Psychology*, **48**, 1080–91.

Craig KD, Lilley CM and Gilbert CA (1996). Social barriers to optimal pain management in infants and children. *Clinical Journal of Pain*, **12**, 232–42.

Dale HH (1906). On some physiological actions of ergot. *Journal of Physiology*, **34**, 163–206.

Damasio AR, Tranel D and Damasio H (1990). Face agnosiaand the neural substrates of memory. *Annual Review of Neuroscience*, **13**, 89–109.

Decety J and Jackson PL (2004). The functional architecture of human empathy. *Behavioral and Cognitive Neuroscience Reviews*, **3**, 71–100.

Decety J and Moriguchi Y (2007). The empathic brain and its dysfunction in psychiatric populations: implications for intervention across different clinical conditions. *Biopsychosocial Medicine*, **1**, 22–65.

Decety J, Echols S and Correll J (2010). The blame game: the effect of responsibility and social stigma on empathy for pain. *Journal of Cognitive Neuroscience*, **22**, 985–97 10.1162/jocn.2009.21266.

De Waal FB (2000). Primates – a natural heritage of conflict resolution. *Science*, **289**, 586–90.

—— (2007). Putting the altruism back into altruism: the evolution of empathy. *Annual Review Psychology*, **59**, 1–22.

Di Pellegrino G, Fadiga L, Fogassi L, Gallese V and Rizzolatti G (1992). Understanding motor events: a neurophysiological study. *Experimental Brain Research*, **91**, 176–80.

Ditzen B, Schaer M, Gabriel B, Bodenmann G, Ehlert U and Heinrichs M (2009). Intranasal oxytocin increases positive communication and reduces cortisol levels during couple conflict. *Biological Psychiatry*, **65**, 728–31.

Domes G, Heinrichs M, Michel A, Berger C and Herpertz SC (2007). Oxytocin improves 'mind-reading' in humans. *Biological Psychiatry*, **61**, 731–3.

Duchaine BC, Parker H and Nakayama K (2003). Normal emotion recognition in a developmental prosopagnosic. *Perception*, **32**, 827–38.

du Vigneaud V, Ressler C, Swan JM, Roberts CW and Katsoyannis PG (1954). The synthesis of oxytocin. *Journal of the American Chemical Society*, **76**, 3115–21.

du Vigneaud V, Ressler C, Swan JM, Roberts CW, Katsoyannis, PG and Gordon S (1953a). The synthesis of an octapeptide amide with the hormonal activity of oxytocin. *Journal of the American Chemical Society*, **75**, 4879–80.

du Vigneaud V, Ressler C and Trippett S (1953b). The sequence of amino acids in oxytocin, with a proposal for the structure of oxytocin. *Journal of Biological Chemistry*, **205**, 949–57.

Edwards E, Harkins K, Wright G and Henn FA (1991). 5-HT1b receptors in an animal model of depression. *Neuropharmacology*, **30**, 101–5.

Edwards E, Kornich W, Houtten PV and Henn FA (1992). Presynaptic serotonin mechanisms in rats subjected to inescapable shock. *Neuropharmacology*, **31**, 323–30.

Egbert LD, Battit GE, Turndorf H and Beecher HK (1963). The value of the preoperative visit by an anesthetist. *Journal of American Medical Association,* **185**, 553–5.

Egbert LD, Battit GE, Welch CE and Bartlett MK (1964). Reduction of postoperative pain by encouragement and instruction of patients. *New England Journal of Medicine,* **270**, 825–7.

Eisenberg N (2007). Empathy-related responding and prosocial behaviour. *Novartis Foundation Symposia,* **278**, 71–80.

Ekman P (1992). An argument for basic emotions. *Cognition & Emotion*, **6**, 169–200.

Ekman P and Friesen WV (1986). A new pan cultural expression of emotion. *Motivation & Emotion,* **10**, 159–68.

Elliott TR, Witty TE, Herrick S and Hoffman JT (1991). Negotiating reality after physical loss: hope, depression, and disability. *Journal of Personality and Social Psychology,* **61**, 608–13.

Emery NJ (2000). The eyes have it: the neuroethology, function and evolution of social gaze. *Neuroscience and Biobehavioral Reviews*, **24**, 581–604.

Engel GL (1968). A life setting conducive to illness: the givingup–given-up complex. *Annals of Internal Medicine*, **69**, 293–9.

Engell AD, Haxby JV and Todorov A (2007). Implicit trustworthiness decisions: automatic coding of face properties in human amygdala. *Journal of Cognitive Neuroscience*, **19**, 1508–19.

Everson SA, Goldberg DE, Kaplan GA, Cohen RD, Pukkala E, Tuomilehto J et al. (1996). Hopelessness and risk of mortality and incidence of myocardial infarction and cancer. *Psychosomatic Medicine*, **58**, 113–21.

Fadiga L, Fogassi L, Pavesi G and Rizzolatti G (1995). Motor facilitation during action observation: a magnetic stimulation study. *Journal of Neurophysiology,* **73**, 2608–11.

Farina CJ, Hearth AK and Popovich JM (1995). *Hope and hopelessness: critical clinical constructs.* Sage, Thousand Oaks, CA.

Ferguson MJ and Bargh JA (2004). How social perception can automatically influence behavior. *Trends in Cognitive Sciences,* **8**, 33–9.

Ferguson JN, Young LJ and Insel TR (2002). The neuroendocrine basis of social recognition. *Frontiers in Neuroendocrinology*, **23**, 200–24.

Fisher H, Aron A and Brown LL (2005). Romantic love: an fMRI study of a neural mechanism for mate choice. *Journal of Comparative Neurology*, **493**, 58–62.

—— (2006). Romantic love: a mammalian brain system for mate choice. *Philosophical Transactions of the Royal Society of London B, Biological Sciences*, **361**, 2173–86.

Foldiak P, Xiao D, Keysers C, Edwards R and Perrett DI (2004). Rapid serial visual presentation for the determination of neural selectivity in area STSa. *Progress in Brain Research*, **144**, 107–16.

Frank JD (1961). *Persuasion and healing: a comparative study of psychotherapy.* Schocken Books, New York. Johns Hopkins University Press, Baltimore.

—— (1971). Therapeutic factors in psychotherapy. *American Journal of Psychotherapy,* **25**, 350–61.

—— (1981). Therapeutic components shared by all psychotherapies. In: JH Hawey and MM Parks, eds. *Psychotherapy research and behavior change.* American Psychological Association, Washington, DC.

Frith CD and Frith U (1999). Interacting minds – a biological basis. *Science*, **286**, 1692–5.

—— (2003). Development and neurophysiology of mentalizing. *Philosophical Transactions of the Royal Society of London B Biological Sciences*, **358**, 459–73.

— (2006). The neural basis of mentalizing. *Neuron*, **50**, 531–4.

Gallese V, Fadiga L, Fogassi L and Rizzolatti G (1996). Action recognition in the premotor cortex. *Brain*, **119**, 593–609.

George N, Driver J and Dolan RJ (2001). Seen gaze-direction modulates fusiform activity and its coupling with other brain areas during face processing. *Neuroimage*, **13**, 1102–12.

Goubert L, Craig KD and Buysse A (2009). Perceiving others in pain: Experimental and clinical evidence on the role of empathy. In: J Decety and W Ickes, eds. *The social neuroscience of empathy*, pp. 153–65. MIT Press, Cambridge, MA.

Gracely RH, Dubner R, Deeter WR and Wolskee PJ (1985). Clinicians' expectations influence placebo analgesia. *Lancet*, **1**, 43.

Greenfield S, Kaplan S and Ware JE (1985). Expanding patient involvement in care. *Annals of Internal Medicine*, **102**, 520–8.

Gross CG, Bender DB and Rocha-Miranda CE (1969). Visual receptive fields of neurons in inferotemporal cortex of the monkey. *Science*, **166**, 1303–6.

Gross CG, Rocha-Miranda CE and Bender DB (1972). Visual properties of neurons in inferotemporal cortex of the Macaque. *Journal of Neurophysiology*, **35**, 96–111.

Guastella AJ, Mitchell PB and Dadds MR (2008a). Oxytocin increases gaze to the eye region of human faces. *Biological Psychiatry*, **63**, 3–5.

Guastella AJ, Mitchell PB and Mathews F (2008b). Oxytocin enhances the encoding of positive social memories in humans. *Biological Psychiatry*, **64**, 256–8.

Hale CJ and Hadjistavropoulos T (1997). Emotional components of pain. *Pain Research and Management*, **2**, 217–25.

Hari R and Kujala MV (2009). Brain basis of human social interaction: from concepts to brain imaging. *Physiological Reviews*, **89**, 453–79.

Hari R, Forss N, Avikainen S, Kirveskari S, Salenius S and Rizzolatti G (1998). Activation of human primary motor cortex during action observation: a neuromagnetic study. *Proceedings of the National Academy of Sciences USA*, **95**, 15061–5.

Hein G and Singer T (2008). I feel how you feel but not always: the empathic brain and its modulation. *Current Opinion in Neurobiology*, **18**, 153–8.

Heinrichs M and Domes G (2008). Neuropeptides and social behavior: effects of oxytocin and vasopressin in humans. *Progress in Brain Research*, **170**, 337–50.

Heinrichs M, Baumgartner T, Kirschbaum C and Ehlert U (2003). Social support and oxytocin interact to suppress cortisol and subjective responses to psychosocial stress. *Biological Psychiatry*, **54**, 1389–98.

Henkel V, Bussfeld P, Moller H-J and Hegerl U (2002). Cognitive-behavioural theories of helplessness/hopelessness: valid models for depression? *European Archives of Psychiatry and Clinical Neuroscience*, **252**, 240–9.

Heppner PP and Hillerbrand ET (1991). Problem-solving training implications for remedial and preventive training. In: CR Snyder and DR Forsyth, eds. *Handbook of social and clinical psychology: the health perspective*, pp. 681–98. Pergamon, Elmsford, NY.

Huber D, Veinante P and Stoop R (2005). Vasopressin and oxytocin excite distinct neuronal populations in the central amygdala. *Science*, **308**, 245–8.

Iacoboni M and Dapretto M (2006). The mirror neuron system and the consequences of its dysfunction. *Nature Reviews Neuroscience*, **7**, 942–51.

Iacoboni M, Lieberman MD, Knowlton BJ, Molnar-Szakacs I, Moritz M, Throop CJ et al. (2004). Watching social interactions produces dorsomedial prefrontal and medial parietal BOLD fMRI signal increases compared to a resting baseline. *Neuroimage*, **21**, 1167–73.

Ilnyckyj A, Shanahan F, Anton PA, Cheang M and Bernstein CN (1997). Quantification of the placebo response in ulcerative colitis. *Gastroenterology*, **112**, 1854–8.

Immordino-Yang MH, McColl A, Damasio H and Damasio A (2009). Neural correlates of admiration and compassion. *Proceedings of the National Academy of Sciences USA*, **106**, 8021–6.

Insel TR and Young LJ (2001). The neurobiology of attachment. *Nature Reviews Neuroscience*, **2**, 129–36.

Insel TR, Gelhard R and Shapiro LE (1991). The comparative distribution of forebrain receptors for neurohypophyseal peptides in monogamous and polygamous mice. *Neuroscience*, **43**, 623–30.

Inui TS, Yourtee EL and Williamson JW (1976). Improved outcomes in hypertension after physician tutorials. *Annals of Internal Medicine*, **84**, 646–51.

Jabbi M, Swart M and Keysers C (2007). Empathy for positive and negative emotions in the gustatory cortex. *Neuroimage*, **34**, 1744–53.

Jackson WT, Taylor RE, Palmatier AD, Elliott TR and Elliott JL (1998). Negotiating the reality of visual impairment: hope, coping, and functional ability. *Journal of Clinical Psychology in Medical Settings*, **5**, 173–85.

Jung-Soon M and Kyung-Sook C (2001). The effects of hand holding on anxiety in cataract surgery patients under local anaesthesia. *Journal of Advanced Nursing*, **35**, 407–15.

Kampe KK, Frith CD and Frith U (2003). Hey John': signals conveying communicative intention toward the self activate brain regions associated with 'mentalizing' regardless of modality. *Journal of Neuroscience*, **23**, 5258–63.

Kanwisher NG, McDermott J and Chun MM (1997). The fusiform face area: a module in human extrastriate cortex specialized for face perception. *Journal of Neuroscience*, **17**, 4302–11.

Kao AC, Green DC, Davis NA, Koplan JP and Cleary PD (1998a). Patients' trust in their physicians: effects of choice, continuity, and payment method. *Journal of General Internal Medicine*, **13**, 681–6.

Kao AC, Green DC, Zaslavsky AM, Koplan JP and Cleary PD (1998b). The relationship between method of physician payment and patient trust. *Journal of American Medical Association*, **280**, 1708–14.

Kaplan SH, Greenfield S and Ware JE Jr. (1989). Assessing the effects of physician-patient interactions on the outcomes of chronic disease. *Medical Care*, **27**(Suppl 3), S110–27.

Kappesser J and Williams AC de C (2002). Pain and negative emotions in the face: judgements by health care professionals. *Pain*, **99**, 197–206.

Kawashima R, Sugiura M, Kato T, Nakamura A, Hatano K, Ito K et al. (1999). The human amygdala plays an important role in gaze monitoring. A PET study. *Brain*, **122**, 779–83.

Keysers C, Wicker B, Gazzola V, Anton JL, Forgassi L and Gallese V (2004). A touching sight: SII/PV activation during the observation and experience of touch. *Neuron*, **42**, 335–46.

Kim JW, Kim SE, Kim JJ, Jeong B, Park CH, Son AR et al. (2009). Compassionate attitude towards others' suffering activates the mesolimbic neural system. *Neuropsychologia*, **47**, 2073–81.

Kimura T, Tanizawa O, Mori K, Brownstein MJ and Okayama H (1992). Structure and expression of a human oxytocin receptor. *Nature*, **356**, 526–9.

Kirsch I and Weixel LJ (1988). Double-blind versus deceptive administration of a placebo. *Behavioral Neuroscience*, **102**, 319–23.

Kobatake E and Tanaka K (1994). Neuronal selectivities to complex object features in the ventral visual pathway of the macaque cerebral cortex. *Journal of Neurophysiology*, **71**, 856–67.

Kosfeld M, Heinrichs M, Zak PJ, Fischbacher U and Fehr E (2005). Oxytocin increases trust in humans. *Nature*, **435**, 673–6.

Kosslyn SM, Thompson WL, Costantini-Ferrando MF, Alpert NM and Spiegel D (2000). Hypnotic visual illusion alters color processing in the brain. *American Journal of Psychiatry*, **157**, 1279–84.

Landman JT and Dawes RM (1982). Psychotherapy outcome. Smith and Glass' conclusions stand up under scrutiny. *American Psychologist*, **37**, 504–16.

Lazarus RS (1999). Hope: an emotion and a vital coping resource against despair. *Social Research*, **66**, 665–9.

—— (2000). Toward better research on stress and coping. *American Psychologist*, **55**, 653–78.

Lee H-J, Macbeth AH, Pagani JH and Young WS 3rd (2009). Oxytocin: the great facilitator of life. *Progress in Neurobiology*, **88**, 127–51.

LeResche L and Dworkin SF (1984). Facial expression accompanying pain. *Social Science and Medicine*, **19**, 1325–30.

—— (1988). Facial expressions of pain and emotions in chronic TMD patients. *Pain*, **35**, 71–8.

Levinson W (1994). Physician–patient communication: a key to malpractice prevention. *Journal of American Medical Association*, **272**, 1619–20.

Lim MM and Young LJ (2006). Neuropeptidergic regulation of affiliative behavior and social bonding in animals. *Hormones and Behavior*, **50**, 506–17.

Loup F, Tribollet E, Dubois-Dauphin M, Pizzolato G and Dreifuss JJ (1989). Localization of oxytocin binding sites in the human brainstem and upper spinal cord: an autoradiographic study. *Brain Research*, **500**, 223–30.

Loup F, Tribollet E, Dubois-Dauphin M and Dreifuss JJ (1991). Localization of high affinity binding sites for oxytocin and vasopressin in the human brain. An autoradiographic study. *Brain Research*, **555**, 220–32.

Luborsky L, Singer B and Luborsky L (1975). Comparative studies of psychotherapies. Is it true that 'everyone has won and all must have prizes'? *Archives of General Psychiatry*, **32**, 995–1008.

Mann JJ (2003). Neurobiology of suicidal behaviour. *Nature Reviews Neuroscience*, **4**, 819–28.

Marsh AA, Ambady N and Kleck RE (2005). The effects of fear and anger facial expressions on approach- and avoidance-related behaviors. *Emotion*, **5**, 119–24.

Mechanic D and Schlesinger M (1996). The impact of managed care on patients' trust in medical care and their physicians. *Journal of American Medical Association*, **275**, 1693–7.

Minkoff K, Bergmann E, Beck AT and Beck R (1973). Hopelessness, depression and attempted suicide. *American Journal of Psychiatry*, **130**, 455–9.

Moerman DE (2002). *Meaning, medicine and the placebo effect.* Cambridge University Press, Cambridge, MA.

Montoya P, Larbig W, Braun C, Preissl H and Birbaumer N (2004). Influence of social support and emotional context on pain processing and magnetic brain responses in fibromyalgia. *Arthritis & Rheumatism*, **50**, 4035–44.

Nagasawa M, Kikusui T, Onaka T and Ohta M (2008). Dog's gaze at its owner increases owner's urinary oxytocin during social interaction. *Hormones and Behavior*, **55**, 434–41.

Northoff G and Bermpohl F (2004). Cortical midline structures and the self. *Trends in Cognitive Sciences,* **8**, 102–7.

Ott I and Scott JC (1910). The action of infundibulum upon mammary secretion. *Proceedings of the Society of Experimental Biology*, **8**, 48–9.

Overmier JB and Seligman MEP (1967). Effects of inescapable shock upon subsequent escape and avoidance learning. *Journal of Comparative Physiology and Psychology*, **63**, 23–33.

Pageler NM, Menon V, Merin NM, Eliez S, Brown WE and Reiss AL (2003). Effect of head orientation on gaze processing in fusiform gyrus and superior temporal sulcus. *Neuroimage*, **20**, 318–29.

Parkes CM (1972). *Bereavement: studies of grief in adult life.* Tavistock, London.

Parloff MB (1986). Frank's 'common elements' in psychotherapy: non-specific factors and placebos. *American Journal of Orthopsychiatry,* **56**, 521–30.

Parvizi J, Van Hoesen GW, Buckwalter J and Damasio AR (2006). Neural connections of the posteromedial cortex in the macaque. *Proceedings of the National Academy of Sciences USA,* **103**, 1563–8.

Pearson SD and Raeke LH (2000). Patients' trust in physicians: many theories, few measures, and little data. *Journal of General Internal Medicine*, **15**, 509–13.

Pelphrey KA, Viola RJ and McCarthy G (2004). When strangers pass: processing of mutual and averted social gaze in the superior temporal sulcus. *Psychological Sciences*, **15**, 598–603.

Peterson C, Seligman MEP and Vaillant G (1988). Pessimistic explanatory style is a risk factor for physical illness: a thirty-five year longitudinal follow-up. *Journal of Personality and Social Psychology*, **55**, 23–7.

Petrovic P, Kalisch R, Singer T and Dolan RJ (2008). Oxytocin attenuates affective evaluations of conditioned faces and amygdala activity. *Journal of Neuroscience*, **28**, 6607–15.

Phelps EA and LeDoux JE (2005). Contributions of the amygdale to emotion processing: from animal models to human behavior. *Neuron*, **48**, 175–87.

Pollo A, Amanzio M, Arslanian A, Casadio C, Maggi G and Benedetti F (2001). Response expectancies in placebo analgesia and their clinical relevance. *Pain*, **93**, 77–84.

Premack D and Woodruff G (1978). Does the chimpanzee have a theory of mind? *Behavioral and Brain Sciences*, **1**, 515–26.

Prkachin KM (1992). The consistency of facial expressions of pain. A comparison across modalities. *Pain*, **51**, 297–306.

Raij TT, Numminen J, Narvanen S, Hiltunen J and Hari R (2005). Brain correlates of subjective reality of physically and psychologically induced pain. *Proceedings of the National Academy of Sciences USA,* **102**, 2147–51.

Raz A, Fan J and Posner MI (2005). Hypnotic suggestion reduces conflict in the human brain. *Proceedings of the National Academy of Sciences USA*, **102**, 9978–83.

Raz A, Moreno-Iniguez M, Martin L and Zhu H (2007). Suggestion overrides the Stroop effect in highly hypnotizable individuals. *Consciousness and Cognition*, **16**, 331–8.

Rizzolatti G and Arbib MA (1998). Language within our grasp. *Trends in Neuroscience*, **21**, 188–94.

Rizzolatti G and Craighero L (2004). The mirro-neuron system. *Annual Review of Neuroscience*, **27**, 169–92.

Rizzolatti G, Fadiga L, Fogassi L and Gallese V (1996). Premotor cortex and the recognition of motor actions. *Cognitive Brain Research*, **3**, 131–41.

Ross EH and Young LJ (2009). Oxytocin and the mechanisms regulating social cognition and affiliative behavior. *Frontiers in Neuroendocrinology*, **30**, 534–47.

Saarela MV, Hlushchuk Y, Williams AC, Schurmann M, Kalso E and Hari R (2007). The compassionate brain: humans detect intensity of pain from another…s face. *Cerebral Cortex*, **17**, 230–7.

Safran DG, Kosinski M, Tarlov AR, Rogers WH, Taira DH, Lieberman N et al. (1998). The Primary Care Assessment Survey: tests of data quality and measurement performance. *Medical Care*, **36**, 728–39.

Sato W, Yoshikawa S, Kochiyama T and Matsumura M (2004). The amygdala processes the emotional significance of facial expressions: an fMRI investigation using the interaction between expression and face direction. *Neuroimage*, **22**, 1006–13.

Saxe R (2006). Uniquely human social cognition. *Current Opinion in Neurobiology*, **16**, 235–9.

Schafer EA and Mackenzie K (1911). The action of animal extracts on milk secretion. *Proceedings of the Royal Society of London Series B*, **84**, 16–22.

Scheier MF and Carver CS (1985). Optimism, coping, and health: assessment and implications of generalized outcome expectancies. *Health Psychology*, **4**, 219–47.

Schilbach L, Wohlschlaeger AM, Kraemer NC, Newen A, Shah NJ, Fink GR et al. (2006). Being with virtual others: neural correlates of social interaction. *Neuropsychologia*, **44**, 718–30.

Schmale AH Jr and Iker HP (1971). Hopelessness as a predictor of cervical cancer. *Social Science & Medicine*, **5**, 95–100.

Schulte-Ruther M, Markowitsch HJ, Fink GR and Piefke M (2007). Mirror neuron and theory of mind mechanisms involved in face-to-face interactions: a functional magnetic resonance imaging approach to empathy. *Journal of Cognitive Neuroscience*, **19**, 1354–72.

Schulz R, Bookwala J, Knapp JE, Scheier M and Williamson GM (1996). Pessimism, age, and cancer mortality. *Psychology & Aging*, **11**, 304–9.

Seitz RJ, Schafer R, Scherfeld D et al. (2008). Valuating other people's emotional face expression: a combined functional magnetic resonance imaging and electroencephalography study. *Neuroscience*, **152**, 713–22.

Senju A and Johnson MH (2009). The eye contact effect: mechanisms and development. *Trends in Cognitive Sciences*, **13**, 127–34.

Shamay-Tsoory SG, Aharon-Peretz J and Perry D (2009). Two systems for empathy: a double dissociation between emotional and cognitive empathy in inferior frontal gyrus versus ventromedial prefrontal lesions. *Brain*, **132**, 617–27.

Singer T, Seymour B, O'Doherty J, Kaube H, Dolan RJ and Frith CD (2004). Empathy for pain involves the affective but not sensory components of pain. *Science*, **303**, 1157–62.

Singer T, Seymour B, O'Doherty JP, Stephan KE, Dolan RJ and Frith CD (2006). Empathic neural responses are modulated by the perceived fairness of others. *Nature*, **439**, 466–9.

Smith ML and Glass GV (1977). Meta-analysis of psychotherapy outcome studies. *American Psychologist*, **32**, 752–60.

Snyder CR (1998). A case for hope in pain, loss, and suffering. In: JH Harvey, J Omarzu and E Miller, eds. *Perspectives on loss: a sourcebook*, pp. 63–79. Taylor & Francis, Washington DC.

Snyder CR (2002). Hope theory: rainbows in the mind. *Psychological Inquiry*, **13**, 249–75.

Snyder CR, Harris C, Anderson JR, Holleran SA, Irving LM, Sigmon ST et al. (1991a). The will and the ways: development and validation of an individual-differences measure of hope. *Journal of Personality and Social Psychology*, **60**, 570–85.

Snyder CR, Irving L and Anderson JR (1991b). Hope and health: measuring the will and the ways. In: CR Snyder and DR Forsyth, eds. *Handbook of social and clinical psychology: the health perspective*, pp. 285–305. Pergamon, Elmsford, NY.

Snyder CR, Sympson SC, Ybasco FC, Borders TF, Babyak MA and Higgins RL (1996). Development and validation of the State Hope Scale. *Journal of Personality and Social Psychology*, **70**, 321–35.

Sox HC, Margulies I and Sox CH (1981). Psychologically mediated effects of diagnostic tests. *Annals of Internal Medicine*, **95**, 680–5.

Spezio ML, Huang PY, Castelli F and Adolphs R (2007). Amygdala damage impairs eye contact during conversations with real people. *Journal of Neuroscience*, **27**, 3994–7.

Sprecher S and Fehr B (2006). Enhancement of mood and self-esteem as a result of giving and receiving compassionate love. *Current Research in Social Psychology*, **11**, 227–42.

Stanton AL, Danoff-Burg S, Cameron CL, Bishop M, Collins CA, Kirk SB et al. (2000). Emotionally expressive coping predicts psychological and physical adjustment to breast cancer. *Journal of Consulting and Clinical Psychology*, **68**, 875–82.

Starfield B, Wray C, Hess K, Gross R, Birk PS and D'Lugoff BC (1981). The influence of patient–practitioner agreement on outcome of care. *American Journal of Public Health*, **71**, 127–32.

Stein S, Linn MW and Stein EM (1989). Psychological correlates of survival in nursing home cancer patients. *Gerontologist*, **29**, 224–8.

Stern SL, Dhanda R and Hazuda HP (2001). Hopelessness predicts mortality in older Mexican and European Americans. *Psychosomatic Medicine*, **63**, 344–51.

Stewart MA (1995). Effective physician–patient communication and health outcomes: a review. *Canadian Medical Association Journal*, **152**, 1423–33.

Stewart MA, McWhinney IR and Buck CW (1979). The doctor–patient relationship and its effect upon outcome. *Journal of Royal College of General Practice*, **29**, 77–82.

Strupp HH and Hadley SW (1979). Specific vs non-specific factors in psychotherapy. A controlled study of outcome. *Archives of General Psychiatry*, **36**, 1125–36.

Su C, Lichtenstein GR, Krok K, Brensinger CM and Lewis JD (2004). A meta-analysis of the placebo response rates of remission and response in clinical trials of active Crohn's disease. *Gastroenterology*, **126**, 1257–69.

Tarr MJ and Gauthier I (2000). FFA: a flexible fusiform area for subordinate-level visual processing automatized by expertise. *Nature Neuroscience*, **3**, 764–9.

Tennen H and Affleck G (1999). Finding benefits in adversity. In: CR Snyder, ed. *Coping: the psychology of what works*, pp. 279–304. Oxford University Press, New York, NY.

Thom DH and Campbell B (1997). Patient–physician trust: an exploratory study. *Journal of Family Practice*, **44**, 169–76.

Thomas KB (1987). General practice consultations: is there any point in being positive? *British Medical Journal*, **294**, 1200–2.

Todorov A (2008). Evaluating faces from trustworthiness. An extension of systems for recognition of emotion signaling approach/avoidance behaviours. *Annals of the New York Academy of Sciences*, **1124**, 208–24.

Tranel D, Damasio AR and Damasio H (1988). Intact recognition of facial expression, gender, and age in patients with impaired recognition of face identity. *Neurology*, **38**, 690–6.

Tsao DY and Livingstone MS (2008). Mechanisms of face perception. *Annual Review of Neuroscience*, **31**, 411–37.

Tuppy H (1953). The amino-acid sequence in oxytocin. *Biochimica and Biophysica Acta*, **11**, 449–50.

Umiltà MA, Kohler E, Gallese V, Fogassi L, Fadiga L, Keysers C et al. (2001). 'I know what you are doing': a neurophysiological study. *Neuron*, **31**, 155–65.

van Heeringen K (2003). The neurobiology of suicide and suicidality. *Canadian Journal of Psychiatry*, **48**, 292–300.

van Heeringen C, Audenaert K, Van Laere K, Dumont F, Slegers G, Mertens J et al. (2003). Prefrontal 5-HT2a receptor binding potential, hopelessness and personality characteristics in attempted suicide. *Journal of Affective Disorders*, **74**, 149–58.

Veinante P and Freund-Mercier MJ (1997). Distribution of oxytocin- and vasopressin binding sites in the rat extended amygdala: a histoautoradiographic study. *Journal of Comparative Neurology*, **383**, 305–25.

Walter H, Adenzato M, Ciaramidaro A, Enrici I, Pia L and Bara BG (2004). Understanding intentions in social interaction: the role of the anterior paracingulate cortex. *Journal of Cognitive Neuroscience*, **16**, 1854–63.

Wicker B, Perrett DI, Baron-Cohen S and Decety J (2003). Being the target of another's emotion: a PET study. *Neuropsychologia*, **41**, 139–46.

Williams AC de C (2002). Facial expression of pain: an evolutionary account. *Behavioral and Brain Sciences*, **25**, 439–55.

Willis J and Todorov A (2006). First impressions: making up your mind after 100 ms exposure to a face. *Psychological Science*, **17**, 592–8.

Winston J, Strange B, O'Doherty J and Dolan R (2002). Automatic and intentional brain responses during evaluation of trustworthiness of face. *Nature Neuroscience*, **5**, 277–83.

Xu X, Zuo X, Wang X and Han S (2009). Do you feel my pain? Racial group membership modulates empathic neural responses. *Journal of Neuroscience*, **29**, 8525–9.

Young AW, Aggleton JP, Hellawell DJ, Johnson M, Broks P and Hanley JR (1995). Face processing impairments after amygdalotomy. *Brain*, **118**, 15–24.

Young LJ and Wang Z (2004). The neurobiology of pair bonding. *Nature Neuroscience*, **7**, 1048–54.

Zak PJ, Kurzban R and Matzner WT (2004). The neurobiology of trust. *Annals of the New York Academy of Sciences*, **1032**, 224–7.

Chapter 6

Receiving the therapy: the activation of expectation and placebo mechanisms

Summary and relevance to the clinician

1) This chapter aims to elucidate the effects of the ritual of the therapeutic act on the patient's brain. The term 'therapeutic act' is meant to include all sensory and social stimuli that surround a therapy and that let the patient know that a treatment is being administered. In addition, all the patient's internal psychological states, such as expectations and beliefs, contribute to these effects. Therefore, the therapeutic act itself is not the specific effect of a medical treatment but rather the context that is around it.

2) The study of different placebo effects across a variety of medical conditions has been crucial in understanding the role of the psychosocial context in the therapeutic outcome. There are many placebo effects, and many mechanisms can be involved. For example, when the patient expects a benefit from a therapy, his anxiety can decrease or, otherwise, reward mechanisms can be activated, whereby the reward is represented by the benefit itself. Learning and previous experience is crucial, and this may occur through both conscious expectation mechanisms and unconscious Pavlovian conditioning.

3) Understanding the biological mechanisms of placebo effects means to understand how the psychosocial context affects the patient's brain. Different social stimuli, such as the verbal suggestions of amelioration, have been found to activate a number of neurotransmitters, e.g. opioid neuropeptides, dopamine, cholecystokinin. By using neuroimaging techniques and single-cell recordings from awake patients, different regions and neuronal circuits in the patient's brain have been found to be affected by placebos, i.e. by the ritual of the therapeutic act.

4) One need not trust his doctor or believe in the treatment in order for a placebo response to occur. Totally unconscious placebo responses may

take place in the immune and endocrine systems, and these are attributable to Pavlovian conditioning. Genetic subgroups of patients have also been found to respond to placebo differently, e.g. in social anxiety and major depressive disorder.

5) Knowledge about a therapy affects the therapeutic outcome. If a treatment is administered covertly (unexpectedly), with the patient unaware that a therapy is being administered, its efficacy is reduced. This indicates that expectations about the outcome are critical. Therefore, in clinical practice, all efforts should be made in order to make the patient aware of what is going on, why a procedure is being carried out and what kind of outcome should be expected. The higher efficacy of open administrations (in full view of the patient, according to routine medical practice) compared to hidden administrations of therapies (unbeknownst to the patient) should induce all health professionals to further increase their interaction with patients. Even when a treatment has to be stopped, what the therapist tells his patient is essential. The way in which treatments are delivered or interrupted plays an important role in the therapeutic outcome.

6) The concept that is emerging today is that psychosocially activated brain mechanisms are similar to those activated by drugs. In other words, social stimuli can activate some neurotransmitters in the patient's brain that bind to the same receptors to which pharmacological agents bind. Therefore, an interference between psychosocial context and drug action may take place, and this occurs on the basis of a cognitive-affective modulation of drug action.

7) All these mechanisms indicate that the ritual of the therapeutic act per se has a profound impact on the patient's brain, and every effort should be made by the clinician to enhance it. In addition, the clinician should be aware that reduced responses to a treatment may have different causes that are psychological in nature. For example, some patients respond poorly because of their weak expectations and lack of learning, although genetic factors must always be taken into consideration.

8) Understanding the biological underpinnings of the psychosocial effects on the patient's brain means to furnish scientific evidence of the intricate relationship between mental activity and different physiological functions. This should be taken into account in routine medical practice in order to avoid negative psychosocial influences on the therapeutic outcome. In fact, what we have learned today is that the response to a treatment very much depends on the psychosocial context around the patient.

6.1 **The ritual of the therapeutic act changes the patient's brain**

6.1.1 **The patient is deluged with social stimuli during the therapeutic act**

When a medical treatment, for example a drug, is given to a patient, it is not administered in a vacuum but within a complex set of psychological states that vary from patient to patient and from situation to situation. This complex set of psychosocial stimuli tell the patient that a benefit or worsening may occur shortly, and represent the context around the therapy and the patient, as shown in Fig 6.1. It can be as important as the specific pharmacodynamic effect of a drug. Di Blasi et al. (2001) listed a series of contextual factors that might affect the therapeutic outcome. These range from the treatment characteristics (colour and shape of a pill) to the patient's and provider's characteristics (treatment and illness beliefs, status, sex), and from the patient–provider relationship (suggestion, reassurance, and compassion) to the healthcare setting (home or hospital, and room layout). Thus, the context is made up of anything which

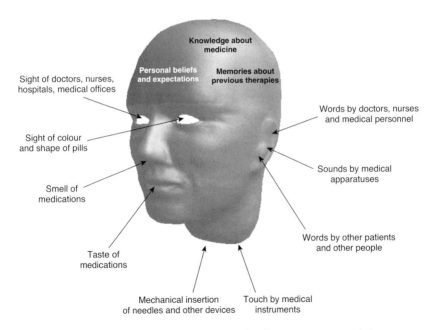

Fig 6.1 During a therapy, many social/sensory stimuli are present around the patient, and represent the psychosocial context, or the ritual of the therapeutic act. In addition, the patient's internal psychological states contribute to the psychosocial context as well. The placebo effect, or response, is the effect of this psychosocial context on the patient's brain.

surrounds the patient under treatment, like doctors, nurses, hospitals, syringes, pills, machines, and such like, but certainly doctors and nurses represent a very important component of the context, as they can transmit a lot of information to the patient through their words, attitudes, and behaviours (Benedetti 2002). Balint (1955) referred to this context as the whole atmosphere around the treatment.

Thomas (1987) found that positive and negative consultations in general practice have an important impact on patients who present with minor illness (see section 5.2.1). Likewise, Di Blasi et al. (2001) examined 25 randomized clinical trials whereby the context about the treatment and the patient's expectations about the therapeutic outcome were manipulated. A consistent finding was that those doctors who adopt a friendly and reassuring manner are more effective than those who are formal and do not offer reassurance.

Other complex factors, e.g. marketing, may affect the therapeutic outcome as well. In a study in 835 patients suffering from headache, the participants were randomized to branded aspirin, unbranded aspirin, branded placebos, and unbranded placebo (Branthwaite and Cooper 1981). Pills were dispensed in either a plain bottle or a bottle with a prominent brand name on the label. Results showed that branded aspirin was the most effective, followed by the unbranded aspirin, then by branded placebo, and finally by unbranded placebo. Waber et al. (2008) investigated the effects of price on analgesic response to placebo pills. After randomization, half of the participants were informed that the drug (actually a placebo) had a regular price of $2.50 per pill and half that the price had been discounted to $0.10 per pill. Overall, the participants in the regular price group experienced a larger pain reduction compared to the low-price (discounted) group. These results are consistent with described phenomena of commercial variables affecting patients' expectations, and expectations influencing therapeutic efficacy. This may explain the popularity of high-cost medical therapies over inexpensive, widely available alternatives, such as over-the-counter drugs (Waber et al. 2008).

During a treatment, a patient can be surrounded by a negative psychosocial context as well. For example, negative diagnoses may lead to symptom worsening because of negative expectations about the course of the disease. Likewise, distrust towards health professionals and therapies are common. In this latter case, unwanted effects and side effects may occur as a result of negative expectations, and these may reduce, or even conceal, the efficacy of some treatments. Another example is represented by health warnings in western societies, whereby negative warnings by the mass media may have an important impact on the perceived symptoms of many individuals as well as on the therapeutic outcome.

The ritual of the therapeutic act includes all the elements described above and must be taken into serious consideration whenever the doctor interacts with his patient. These social stimuli, which are indissociable from any medical treatment, begin to be understood in terms of biological mechanisms. In other words, the mechanisms through which the psychosocial context affects the patient's brain and the therapeutic outcome is today a fruitful field of research of neuroscience.

6.1.2 The placebo effect helps understand how social stimuli may be therapeutic

The study of the placebo effect has emerged as a crucial approach to understand the effects of the psychosocial context on the patient's brain, and particularly how it can lead to positive therapeutic outcomes. By definition, a placebo effect is the effect that follows the administration of a placebo, that is, of an inert treatment. As the inert treatment is given along with contextual stimuli, for example verbal suggestions of clinical improvement which make the patient believe that the treatment is real and effective, its study is basically the study of the context around the treatment and how it affects the patient's brain. When the context is positive and leads to positive outcomes, the term placebo effect is used. Conversely, when the context is negative and leads to negative outcomes, the term nocebo effect is adopted.

Therefore, the placebo effect is a psychobiological phenomenon, i.e. something active happening in the patient's brain. It has nothing to do with spontaneous remission, habituation, patients' and/or observers' biases, the effects of unidentified co-interventions, and many other factors, which are phenomena that are sometimes mistakenly taken for placebo effects.

There is not a single mechanism of the placebo effect and there is not a single placebo effect but many, so that we have to look for different mechanisms in different medical conditions and in different therapeutic interventions. Expectation and anticipation of clinical benefit play a crucial role when conscious physiological functions are involved, whereas classical conditioning takes place in unconscious physiological functions (Benedetti et al. 2003b). For example, expectations have no effect on hormone secretion, whereas a conditioning procedure can induce conditioned placebo hormonal responses. Therefore, different systems and apparatuses as well as different diseases and treatments are affected by placebos in different ways.

Most of the research on placebos has focused on expectations as the main factor involved in placebo responsiveness. Indeed, the literature is full of studies whereby expectations are analysed, and the terms 'effects of placebos' and 'effects of expectations' are frequently used interchangeably. In general, the expectation of a future outcome and of a future response, the so-called response expectancy, is held by an individual about one's own emotional and physiological responses such as pain, anxiety, and sexual arousal (Kirsch 1985, 1990, 1999). Expectation may lead to a cognitive readjustment of the appropriate behaviour. Thus, it is not surprising that positive expectations lead to adopt a particular behaviour, e.g. resuming a normal daily schedule, whereas negative expectations lead to its inhibition (Bandura 1977, 1997; Bootzin 1985). Otherwise, the effects of expectations may be mediated by changes in other cognitions, such as a decrease in self-defeating thoughts when expecting analgesia (Stewart-Williams and Podd 2004). Expectations are unlikely to operate alone, and several other factors have been identified and described, such as memory and motivation (Price and Barrell 2000; Price et al. 1985; Price et al. 2001, 2008; Geers et al. 2005a) and meaning of the illness experience (Pennebaker 1997; Brody 2000). According to Brody (2000), the meaning precedes other causal mechanisms, like expectation. In an attempt to explain the causal mechanisms of the placebo effect, Bootzin and Caspi (2002) and Caspi and Bootzin (2002) integrate multiple explanatory mechanisms in a model that involves factors that are both internal and external to the individual, including expectation.

Expectation can involve different factors and mechanisms. For example, Frank (1961, 1971, 1981) analysed the healing process within the context of patient's expectations, though he proposed that hope is the primary mechanism of change in folk tradition of healing and in psychotherapy. Indeed, hope can be defined as the desire and expectation that the future will be better than the present. Expectations may also play a role in the so-called Hawthorne effect. This consists of the clinical improvement in a group of patients in a clinical trial that is attributable to the fact of being under study (Last 1983). In other words, a patient who knows to be under study may expect a better therapeutic benefit because of the many exams he undergoes, the special attention by the medical personnel, and the trust in the new therapy under investigation. It appears therefore that expectation is a general term that can be described from many different perspectives.

From a neuroscientific point of view, expecting a future event may involve several brain mechanisms that are aimed at preparing the body to anticipate that event. For example, the expectation of a future positive outcome may reduce anxiety and/or activate the neuronal networks of reward mechanisms, whereas the expectation of a negative outcome is aimed at anticipating a possible threat, thus increasing anxiety (Fig 6.2A). Indeed, anxiety has been found to be reduced after placebo administration in some studies. In other words, if one expects a distressing symptom to subside shortly, anxiety tends to decrease. For example, McGlashan et al. (1969) and Evans (1977) studied experimental

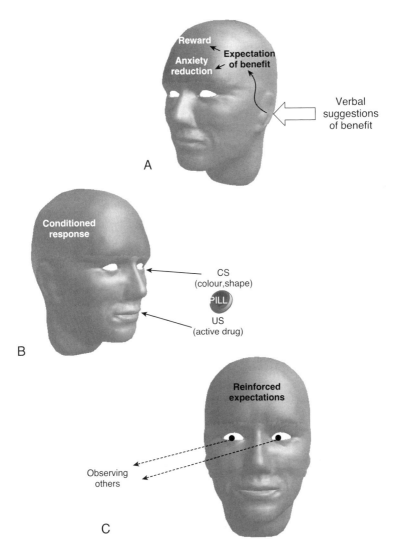

Fig 6.2 Three principal mechanisms of the placebo effect are presented. (A) Verbal suggestions of benefit induce expectations of clinical improvement which, in turn, may either reduce anxiety or activate reward mechanisms. It should be noted that the opposite is also true. Verbal suggestions of worsening induce negative expectations which, in turn, may increase anxiety. (B) When a pill is administered, its pharmacological agent is the unconditioned stimulus (US), whereas its colour and shape are the conditioned stimulus (CS). After repeated CS-US pairings, the CS can elicit the same response as the US. (C) Merely observing others who experience analgesia may reinforce expectations through social observational learning.

pain in both trait and state anxiety subjects. Trait anxiety represents a personality trait and thus can be found throughout life, whereas state anxiety may be present in specific stressful situations and represents an adaptive and transitory response to stress. These researchers gave the subjects a placebo which they believed to be a painkiller. Whereas there was no correlation between trait anxiety and pain tolerance after placebo administration, a strict correlation occurred between situational anxiety and pain tolerance during the placebo session. In fact, in those subjects who showed decreased anxiety there was a better pain tolerance than in those who experienced increased anxiety. Similar results were obtained more recently by Vase et al. (2005), who found decreased anxiety in patients with irritable bowel syndrome who received a placebo treatment. Moreover, brain imaging studies have found reduced activation of anxiety-related areas during a placebo response (Petrovic et al. 2005). The role of anxiety is also particularly evident in nocebo effects. Anxiety-induced hyperalgesia is a good example and has been described in section 3.3.3.

Expectations may also induce changes through reward mechanisms (Fig 6.2A), which ensure future reward acquisition, as we have already seen in Chapter 4. These mechanisms are mediated by specific neuronal circuits linking cognitive, emotional, and motor responses, and are traditionally studied in the context of the pursuit of natural (e.g. food), monetary, and drug rewards (Mogenson and Yang 1991; Kalivas et al. 1999). In animals, dopaminergic cells in the brainstem ventral tegmental area projecting to the nucleus accumbens of the ventral basal ganglia respond to both the magnitude of anticipated rewards and deviations from the predicted outcomes, thus representing an adaptive system modulating behavioural responses (Setlow et al. 2003; Tobler et al. 2005; Schultz 2006). A simplified schema of the reward circuitry is shown in Fig 4.2. The nucleus accumbens plays a central role in the dopamine-mediated reward mechanisms together with the ventral tegmental area. However, it should be noted that other regions are also involved, like the amygdala, the periacqueductal grey, and other areas in the thalamic, hypothalamic, and subthalamic (pallidum) regions.

Within the context of reward-seeking behaviour, we have seen in section 4.2.3 that de la Fuente-Fernandez et al. (2001, 2002), by using positron emission tomography, found dopamine activation in the nucleus accumbens following the administration of a placebo in patients with Parkinson's disease. Interestingly, no relationship was found between nucleus accumbens dopamine activity and the actual placebo effects on motor function, thus suggesting that dopamine activation was better related to the expectation of reward. Likewise, Mayberg et al. (2002) observed nucleus accumbens activation in depressed patients after one week of placebo treatment, and Petrovic et al. (2005)

described a correlation between ratings of negative affect improvement during preconditioning with a benzodiazepine and ventral basal ganglia synaptic activity after receipt of a placebo. In addition, Scott et al. (2007) found a correlation between the responsiveness to placebo and that to monetary reward by using a model of experimental pain in healthy subjects, and that placebo responsiveness was related to the activation of dopamine in the nucleus accumbens. All these studies seem to confirm an involvement of nucleus accumbens dopamine activity, and more in general of the reward circuitry, in the expectations induced by placebo administration.

Learning is another mechanism that is central to placebo responsiveness. Subjects who suffer from a painful condition, such as headache, and who regularly consume aspirin, can associate the shape, colour, and taste of the pill to pain decrease. After repeated associations, if they are given a sugar pill that looks like aspirin, pain can decrease. In place of the shape, colour, and taste of pills, several other stimuli can be associated to clinical improvement, such as syringes, stethoscopes, white coats, hospitals, doctors, nurses, and so on. As shown in Fig 6.2B, the mechanism that underlies this effect is conditioning, whereby a conditioned (neutral) stimulus, e.g. the colour and shape of a pill, can become effective in inducing the reduction of a symptom if repeatedly associated to an unconditioned stimulus, i.e. the drug inside the pill. This type of associative learning may represent the basis of many placebo effects, whereby the placebo is the conditioned (neutral) stimulus itself. Indeed, in the 1960s, Herrnstein (1962) found that an injection of scopolamine induced motor changes in the rat, and these motor changes also occurred following an injection of saline solution (placebo) that was performed after the scopolamine injection.

A sequence effect of this sort is also present in humans. For example, it has long been known that placebos given after drugs are more effective than when given for the first time (Sunshine et al. 1964; Batterman 1966; Batterman and Lower 1968; Laska and Sunshine 1973). If a placebo is given for the first time, the placebo response is present but small. If the placebo is administered after two prior administrations of an effective painkiller, the placebo analgesic response is much larger (Amanzio and Benedetti 1999), thus indicating that the placebo effect is a learning phenomenon.

These clinical and pharmacological observations are in keeping with studies in the laboratory setting by Voudouris et al. (1989, 1990), who showed that the placebo effect can indeed be conditioned. These investigators applied a neutral non-anaesthetic cream (placebo) to one group of subjects who were assured that it was a local anaesthetic; not surprisingly, some of these subjects showed a placebo response after painful electrical stimulation. In a second group, the application of the same placebo cream was associated to the surreptitious reduction of the intensity of stimulation, so as to make the subjects believe that it was a powerful painkiller. These subjects, who had experienced a 'true analgesic effect', became strong placebo responders. Voudouris et al. (1989, 1990) concluded that conditioning is the main mechanism that is involved in the placebo effect.

These experiments were replicated by some authors, however a cognitive component was found to contribute to the conditioning-induced placebo responses. For example, De Jong et al. (1996) found a correlation between the expected and the actual level of analgesia in a similar experimental situation, thus suggesting that expectation is involved. Montgomery and Kirsch (1997) used a design in which subjects were given cutaneous pain via iontophoretic stimuli. Subjects were surreptitiously given stimuli with reduced intensities in the presence of a placebo cream (conditioning procedure) and were divided into two groups. The first did not know about the stimulus manipulation whereas the second group was informed about the experimental design and learned that the cream was inert. There was no placebo analgesic effect in this second group, which suggests that conscious expectation is necessary for placebo analgesia. This is a very important point, as it suggests that expectation plays a major role, even in the presence of a conditioning procedure. In other words, expectation and conditioning are not mutually exclusive, as they may represent two sides of the same coin (Stewart-Williams and Podd 2004).

Early in the 1930s, Tolman (1932) dissented from the view that conditioning is an automatic nonconscious event that is due to the temporal contiguity between the conditioned and the unconditioned stimulus. Indeed, in the following years, conditioning was reinterpreted in cognitive terms on the basis that conditioned learning does not depend simply on the pairing of the conditioned and the unconditioned stimuli, but on the information that is contained in the conditioned stimulus (Rescorla 1988). In other words, conditioning would lead to the expectation that a given event will follow another event, and this occurs on the basis of the information that the conditioned stimulus provides about the unconditioned stimulus (Reiss 1980; Rescorla 1988; Kirsch et al. 2004).

Despite the reinterpretation of conditioning in cognitive terms, conditioning in humans is not always cognitively mediated, particularly by considering conditioned placebo responses (Stewart-Williams and Podd 2004). For example, there is experimental evidence that in humans unconscious conditioned placebo responses are present in the immune and endocrine system and in the cardiovascular and respiratory system (Benedetti 2008b). It has also been suggested that unconscious conditioning is important in those placebo responses that involve unconscious physiological functions, whereas it is cognitively mediated when conscious processes come into play (Benedetti et al. 2003b). According to this model, expectation has no effect on unconscious processes. It is also worth noting that even in placebo analgesia some non-cognitive unconscious components may be present. For example, Amanzio and Benedetti (1999) showed that a placebo analgesic response was still present, albeit reduced, in the absence of expectation after prior conditioning, thus suggesting that a small portion of the placebo effect may occur unconsciously. Therefore, as emphasized many times (Ader 1997; Siegel 2002), many placebo effects can be explained in the context of conditioning theories. In fact, a placebo is by definition a neutral stimulus with no therapeutic effects, in the same way as a conditioned stimulus is by definition neutral. Likewise, a placebo response is by definition elicited by a neutral stimulus, in the same way as a conditioned response is induced by a neutral stimulus.

Conditioning is not the only learning mechanism that may be involved in placebo phenomena. Social learning is another form of learning whereby people learn from one another by observation and imitation (Fig 6.2C). Placebo effects may involve social learning as well (Bootzin and Caspi 2002), and expectations of future outcomes may have a major effect in social learning. Colloca and Benedetti (2009) compared placebo analgesia induced through social observation with first-hand experience via a typical conditioning procedure and with verbal suggestion alone. In the social condition, subjects underwent painful stimuli and placebo treatment after they had observed a demonstrator (actually a simulator) showing analgesic effect when the painful stimuli were paired to a green light. In the conditioning experimental condition, subjects were conditioned according to a classical conditioning procedure, whereby a green light was associated to the surreptitious reduction of stimulus intensity, so as to make them believe that the treatment worked. In the verbal suggestion condition, subjects received painful stimuli and were verbally instructed to expect a benefit from a green light. It was found that observing the beneficial effects in the demonstrator induced substantial placebo analgesic responses which were positively correlated with empathy scores. Moreover, observational social learning produced placebo responses that were similar to those induced by directly experiencing the benefit through the conditioning procedure, whereas verbal suggestions alone produced significantly smaller effects. Thus, social observation is as powerful as conditioning in producing substantial placebo responses.

Although some inconsistency in the findings about the relationship between personality and placebo responsiveness does exist (Geers et al. 2005b), some recent studies indicate that there might be some personality traits that can predict placebo responsiveness. For example, De Pascalis et al. (2002) found that individual differences in suggestibility contribute significantly to the magnitude of placebo analgesia. The highest placebo effect was found in highly suggestible subjects who received suggestions presumed to elicit high expectations for drug efficacy. Geers et al. (2005b) found that personality and situational variables interact to determine placebo responding in a study whereby optimists and pessimists were randomly assigned to one of three groups. The subjects of the first group were told that they were to ingest a pill that would make them feel unpleasant (deceptive expectation). In the second group, the participants were told that they were to ingest either a real or an inactive pill (conditional expectation). The third group was told they were to ingest an inactive pill (control). Pessimists were more likely than optimists to follow a negative placebo (nocebo) expectation when given a deceptive expectation, but not when given a conditional expectation, which suggests that the personality variable 'optimism-pessimism' relates to placebo responding when individuals are given a deceptive but not a conditional expectation. Thus, personality and situational variables seem to interact to determine placebo responding. In a subsequent study, Geers et al. (2007) tested individuals varying in their level of optimism. In a first condition, participants were given the expectation that a placebo sleep treatment would improve their sleep quality. In the second condition, the subjects underwent the same sleep treatment but were not given the positive placebo expectation. In the third condition, the subjects received neither the positive placebo expectation nor underwent the placebo sleep treatment. Optimism was positively associated with better sleep quality in the first condition, thus suggesting that optimism relates to placebo responding.

6.1.3 How the ritual of the therapeutic act changes brain chemistry and circuitry

In searching for specific brain mechanisms generating the placebo response, scientists and clinician scientists have focused on a number of medical conditions, which represent today the main targets of placebo research. These conditions include pain, Parkinson's disease, depression, anxiety, immune responses, hormone secretion, as well as physical performance (Benedetti 2008a, b; Enck et al. 2008; Price et al. 2008; Zubieta and Stohler 2009; Finniss et al. 2010).

It was in the field of placebo analgesia that neuropharmacological evidence of a chemical substrate for the placebo phenomenon was first obtained (Levine et al. 1978). Much subsequent work has corroborated the model whereby the secretion of endogenous opioids in the brain is the central event of the pain modulation by a placebo, with the activation of the descending antinociceptive pathway as its anatomical substrate (Fields and Levine 1984; Grevert et al. 1983; Amanzio and Benedetti 1999; Benedetti et al. 1999). In fact, in many of these studies, placebo analgesia was reversed by naloxone, although the presence of some naloxone-insensitive effects points to the involvement of other antinociceptive mechanisms as well, our understanding of which is still scarce (Gracely et al. 1983; Amanzio and Benedetti 1999; Vase et al. 2005). Enhancing effects on placebo analgesia have been obtained with proglumide, a cholecystokinin (CCK) antagonist (Benedetti et al. 1995; Benedetti 1996), thereby suggesting that placebo analgesia is under the opposing actions of promoting endogenous opioids and inhibiting endogenous CCK. These two systems show overlapping distribution of brain receptors (see section 3.3.3 and Fig 3.10), the opposing role of which has been suggested also for the emotional modulation of other incoming signals, like visual input (Gospic et al. 2008).

Brain imaging and mapping techniques, such as positron emission tomography, functional magnetic resonance imaging, magnetoelectroencephalography, and electroencephalography have brought important contributions to the understanding of where and when placebo analgesia is generated in the central nervous system (Colloca et al. 2008a). A positron emission tomography study first showed that brain areas activated during opioid- or placebo-induced analgesia largely overlapped, involving part of the anatomical substrate of this system, i.e. the rostral anterior cingulate cortex, the orbitofrontal cortex and the periaqueductal grey (Petrovic et al. 2002). Subsequently, direct evidence for endogenous opioid release during a placebo intervention was provided by another positron emission tomography study, measuring μ-opioid receptor availability (Zubieta et al. 2005). In this study, $[^{11}C]$ carfentanil was displaced by the activation of opioid neurotransmission, showing significant binding decrease after placebo in pregenual rostral anterior cingulate cortex, insula, nucleus accumbens and dorsolateral prefrontal cortex. In all areas except dorsolateral prefrontal cortex, this decrease was correlated with placebo reduction of pain intensity reports. A number of other studies brought more contributions, by reporting different activation and deactivation patterns during placebo analgesia in brain areas of the pain matrix, like thalamus, anterior insula, caudal rostral anterior cingulate cortex, as well as the hypothalamus, periaqueductal grey, and rostroventromedial medulla (Wager et al. 2004; Bingel et al. 2005; Kong et al. 2006; Price et al. 2007; Eippert et al. 2009a). Scalp laser-evoked potential amplitude was also found to be reduced during the placebo analgesic response, e.g. in the N2-P2 components, thought to be originated in the bilateral insula and in the cingulate gyrus (Wager et al. 2006; Watson et al. 2007; Colloca et al. 2008b).

In a combined positron emission tomography and functional magnetic resonance imaging study, Scott et al. (2007) found a correlation between individual responsiveness to placebo analgesia and monetary reward (see section 4.2.3). The stronger the nucleus accumbens activation is during the placebo response, the larger the activation of the same nucleus during the monetary task. In a within-subject design positron emission tomography study using both [^{11}C] carfentanil and [11C]raclopride, both opioid and dopamine neurotransmission were found to be coupled with the placebo response, with changes of activity induced in several brain regions associated with the opioid and dopamine networks (Scott et al. 2008). As emphasized in section 4.2.3, this suggests the involvement of reward mechanisms.

There is also compelling experimental evidence that the spinal cord is also affected by placebos (Matre et al. 2006; Goffaux et al. 2007; Eippert et al. 2009b). For example, in a functional magnetic resonance imaging study, Eippert et al. (2009b) were able to show that pain-induced activation in the dorsal horn of the spinal cord was reduced by placebo administration, thus indicating that placebos activate a neural network that, starting from cortical areas, goes down to subcortical regions and brainstem, reaching the spinal cord. As shown in Fig 6.3, the activation of this cortical-brainstem network can be blocked by the opioid antagonist naloxone, which indicates that it is an opioidergic system. Most importantly, naloxone abolishes placebo-induced coupling between the rostral anterior cingulate cortex and the periaqueductal grey, which predicts both neural and behavioural placebo effects as well as activation of the rostroventromedial medulla (Fig 6.3D) (Eippert et al. 2009a).

In the anticipatory phase of the placebo analgesic response, increased activity in the dorsolateral prefrontal cortex and other frontal regions was positively correlated with increase in a midbrain region containing the periacqueductal grey, and negatively correlated with the signal reduction in pain regions and with reported pain intensity. The interpretation could be that just before the onset of placebo analgesia, prefrontal cortical evaluation could drive the activation of the descending antinociceptive system (Wager et al. 2004). Similarly, a comparison of high and low expectations before a painful stimulus showed changes in activity in many areas of the descending inhibitory pathway (Keltner et al. 2006). In order to discriminate whether expectation exerts its psychophysical effect through changes of the perceptual sensitivity of early cortical processes (i.e. in the primary and secondary somatosensory areas) or on later evaluative elaborations, such as stimulus identification and response selection (represented in the anterior cingulate cortex), Lorenz et al. (2005) used a combined application of the high temporal resolution techniques of electroencephalography and magnetoencephalography. They found that the amplitude of the laser-evoked magnetic fields in the secondary somatosensory area was

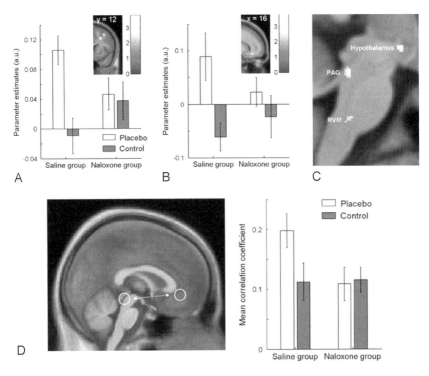

Fig 6.3 Activations of (A) the dorsolateral prefrontal cortex (DLPFC) and (B) the subgenual rostral anterior cingulate cortex (rACC) are significantly stronger under placebo compared to control in the saline group. This difference is strongly reduced in the naloxone group. (C) The sagittal slice shows placebo-enhanced responses in the hypothalamus, the periaqueductal grey (PAG), and the rostroventromedial medulla (RVM), all of which are significantly reduced by naloxone. (D) The midline sagittal slice depicts the approximate location of rACC and PAG. The intraindividual coupling between rACC and PAG is significantly stronger under placebo than under control in the saline group, whereas this difference is abolished in the naloxone group. Error bars indicate SEM. See colour plate 14.
Source: From Eippert et al. 2009a with permission from Elsevier and Cell Press, Copyright 2009.

highly correlated to the expected stimulus intensity as signalled by an auditory cue, while the ensuing evoked responses with source in the caudal anterior cingulate cortex varied with stimulus intensity (requiring a varying level of task engagement) but failed to show any cue validity effects.

As occurs with pain and analgesia, the placebo effect in Parkinson's disease is usually obtained through the administration of an inert substance which the patient believes to be an effective anti-Parkinsonian drug. The assessment of the ensuing motor performance improvement is somewhat more objective than the self-reported variation of pain, as it can be evaluated by a blinded examiner with the Unified Parkinson's Disease Rating Scale (UPDRS). However, recent experimental work has also exploited the technique of subthalamic nucleus-deep brain stimulation, manipulating the electrode activity to configure different expectation and conditioning protocols. In an early such study, patients with the stimulator turned off showed faster hand movements when they mistakenly believed it to be on than when they were correctly informed (Pollo et al. 2002). An influence of expectation on UPDRS scores was also found by Mercado et al. (2006) comparing aware and unaware conditions of the stimulator status, both for the on and off situations. Thus, expectation plays an important role not only for placebo effects affecting sensory input but also motor output. Subsequently, intraoperative recording of single neuron activity in the subthalamic nucleus in patients conditioned with apomorphine showed that placebo responders exhibited a significant decrease of neuronal firing rate associated to a shift from a bursting to a non-bursting pattern of discharge (Benedetti et al. 2004b). These changes in the subthalamic nucleus have been found to be associated to changes in neuronal activity in the substantia nigra pars reticulata and in the thalamus, as shown in Fig 6.4 in a representative patient, which suggest that most of the basal ganglia and thalamic circuit is affected by placebos (Benedetti et al. 2009). In addition, these neurophysiological changes were found to be related to both muscle rigidity reduction and subjective reports of well-being. These studies demonstrated for the first time a link between a placebo intervention and single-cell activity, proving the influence of an expectation-inducing procedure on a specific neuronal population. Furthermore, the study by Benedetti et al. (2009) was able to characterize part of the neuronal circuit that is involved in the placebo effect in Parkinson patients (Fig 6.4C).

In a positron emission tomography study employing the D_2-D_3 dopamine receptor agonist [^{11}C]raclopride as a radiotracer, de la Fuente-Fernández et al. (2001) obtained the first evidence that endogenous dopamine is released in the striatum after placebo administration. Their finding was later corroborated by similar results obtained with the use of sham transcranial magnetic stimulation as a placebo (Strafella et al. 2006). As described in section 4.2.3, dopamine has been proposed as a possible mediator also of placebo effects not strictly pertaining to the motor context. Its release has in fact been observed not only in the dorsal but also in the ventral striatum (nucleus accumbens), an area known to be involved in the reward circuitry (de la Fuente-Fernández et al. 2002). According to the authors, while dorsal striatum release is directly linked to performance improvement, ventral release could rather be connected to expectation of reward, i.e. of clinical benefit. As such, it could well be

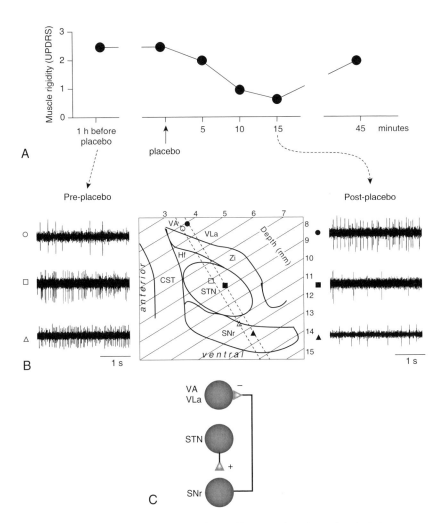

Fig 6.4 Data from a single representative Parkinson patient from the study by Benedetti et al. (2009). (A) Decreased scores of the Unified Parkinson's Disease Rating Scale (UPDRS) after placebo administration, showing specifically the decrease in muscle rigidity at the wrist. (B) Representative recordings from single neurons one hour before placebo and during the maximal placebo response, in the ventral anterior (VA) and anterior ventral lateral (VLa) thalamus (circles), in the subthalamic nucleus (STN) (squares), and in the substantia nigra pars reticulata (SNr) (triangles). The location of the neurons and the electrode tracks (broken lines) are shown in the middle. Note that during the placebo response there is an increase in firing rate in VA-VLa and a decrease in STN and SNr. (C) The pattern of neuronal firing after placebo supports the involvement of the circuit in which there is an excitatory connection between STN and SNr, and an inhibitory connection between SNr and VA-VLa.
Source: Data from Benedetti et al. (2009).

implicated also in other types of placebo effect, including placebo analgesia. In fact, some of the cortical and subcortical areas activated during sustained pain are known to receive dopaminergic projections (Zubieta et al. 2001). In support of the role of reward mechanisms in generating placebo responses, there is for example the study by Scott et al. (2007) on placebo analgesia, in which a correlation between individual responsiveness to placebo analgesia and monetary reward was found (see above).

The relevance of motor placebo responses is not confined to damaged systems as in Parkinson's disease, but it can be extended to intact motor systems. In a recent study testing ergogenic placebos, muscle performance of healthy subjects was improved and their subjective rate of perceived exertion lessened, following a conditioning and expectation procedure (Pollo et al. 2008). As the subjects were required to perform leg extensions until complete exhaustion, it is possible that the placebo effect could be exerted on a putative central governor of fatigue, which integrates peripheral and central signals to determine maximal exercise (St Clair Gibson et al. 2006).

As far as depression is concerned, clinical trials for antidepressants show very high rates of placebo responses, with an increasing trend over time (Walsh et al. 2002). In an attempt to differentiate the therapeutic effect of antidepressants from the placebo response in patients with major depressive disorder, Leuchter et al. (2002) used quantitative electroencephalography to show changes in brain function of placebo responders (increase in frontal cordance) that are distinct from those associated with antidepressant medication (decrease), and from those observed in nonresponders to either placebo or medication (no change). In a positron emission tomography study on the serotonin reuptake inhibitor fluoxetine, Mayberg et al. (2002) reported a pattern of activity changes (including increases in prefrontal, anterior cingulate, and other cortical and subcortical regions) which is similar for placebo and drug responders, with the latter exhibiting more pronounced changes. However, drug responders also showed additional subcortical and limbic variations which were not seen after placebo. Interestingly, there were unique ventral striatal (nucleus accumbens) and orbital frontal changes in both placebo and drug responders at one week of treatment, that is, well before clinical benefit. Thus these changes are not associated to the clinical response, but rather to expectation and anticipation of the clinical benefit. Such changes were seen neither in the eventual drug non-responders nor at six weeks when the antidepressant response was well established, consistent with an expectation pattern of response (Mayberg et al. 2002; Benedetti et al. 2005). This is in keeping with other brain imaging studies in which an involvement of the ventral striatum (nucleus accumbens) was found after placebo administration in Parkinson's disease (de la Fuente-Fernandez et al. 2001) and in pain (Scott et al. 2007). This pattern of activation of the ventral striatum is in agreement with an involvement of reward mechanisms in some types of placebo response.

6.1.4 Placebo effects can be completely unconscious

The ritual of the therapeutic act can affect the patient's brain through completely unconscious processes. In other words, one needs not believe in the treatment and trust his doctor in order to respond to a placebo treatment. Immune and hormonal responses represent two good examples of unconscious placebo responses, whereby the underlying mechanism is likely to be classical, or Pavlovian, conditioning, as we have seen in section 6.1.2 (see also Fig 6.2B). This aspect of placebo responsiveness is important because it goes in a different direction compared to expectation of reward or anxiety reduction. In fact, in these latter cases cognitive/affective processes are crucial and the patient must be aware of what is going on. By contrast, conditioned placebo responses take place regardless of what the patient expects. For example, conditioned hormonal increases can be obtained even if the subject expects hormonal decreases (see below and Benedetti et al. 2003b).

Some of the first compelling evidences that immunological responses can be behaviourally conditioned was obtained by a long series of experiments performed in the 1970s and 1980s. By using a taste aversion conditioning paradigm in rats, Ader and Cohen (1975) paired a flavoured drinking solution (saccharin) with the immunosuppressive drug, cyclophosphamide. The rats were subsequently immunized with sheep red blood cells. Those rats that were re-exposed to saccharin at the time of antigenic stimulation were found to have lower hemagglutinating antibodies six days after the injection of the sheep red blood cells compared to conditioned animals that were not re-exposed to saccharin, non-conditioned animals given saccharin and a placebo group. Thus, saccharin was capable of mimicking the immunosuppressive action of cyclophosphamide.

Behavioural conditioning has also been found in a graft-versus-host response, a phenomenon that is suppressed by low-dose injections of cyclophosphamide (Whitehouse et al. 1973). In fact, three low-dose injections of cyclophosphamide are capable of reducing the weight of lymph nodes following the injection of a cellular graft. By contrast, a single low-dose is much less effective. However, if the single low-dose of cyclophosphamide is paired to saccharin in rats that had previously been conditioned with saccharin, the single low dose is capable of inducing graft-versus-host responses that are similar to those obtained with three doses. A conditioned enhancement of antibody production is also possible using an antigen as unconditioned stimulus of the immune system. Gorczynski et al. (1982) grafted skin tissue from C57BL/6J mice to CBA mice many times. Although the recipient mice were then re-exposed to the grafting procedures but without receiving the allogenic tissue, there was nonetheless an increase in the number of cytotoxic lymphocyte precursor cells in response to the conditioned stimulus. In another study, mice were given repeated immunizations with keyhole limpet hemocyanin paired with a gustatory conditioned stimulus (chocolate milk). A classically conditioned enhancement of anti-keyhole limpet hemocyanin antibodies was observed when the mice were re-exposed to the gustatory stimulation along with a low-dose injection of keyhole limpet hemocyanin (Ader et al. 1993). Subsequently, Alvarez-Borda et al. (1995) found an increase in IgG and IgM in animals re-exposed to a conditioned stimulus previously paired with an antigen (hen egg lysosome). These behaviourally conditioned immune responses have been found to undergo extinction, thus lending support to the notion that associative processes are involved in the behavioural alteration of immune responses (Gorczynski et al. 1982; Bovbjerg et al. 1984).

Conditioned immune responses can also be obtained in humans. Some early studies produced contrasting results. Smith and McDaniels (1983) described a conditionally reduced delayed type hypersensitivity response, which however was not elicited by a conditioned stimulus previously paired with tuberculin. These findings were not confirmed in a subsequent study (Booth et al. 1995). Contrasting results were also obtained in other human studies on conditioned increase in natural killer cell activity (Kirschbaum et al. 1992), on allergic rhinitis patients (Gauci et al. 1994), and on recombinant interferon-gamma as unconditioned stimulus (Longo et al. 1999). More recently, a study provided convincing evidence that behavioural conditioning of immunosuppression is possible in humans (Goebel et al. 2002). Repeated associations between cyclosporine A and a flavoured drink induced conditioned immunosuppression in healthy male volunteers, in which the flavoured drink alone produced a suppression of the immune functions, as assessed by means of interleukin-2 (IL-2) and interferon-γ (IFN-γ) mRNA expression, *in vitro* release of IL-2 and IFN-γ, as well as lymphocyte proliferation. It is interesting to note that the effects of the conditioned stimulus were the same as those of the specific effects of cyclosporine A. In fact, cyclosporine A binds to cyclophilins, which leads to intracellular phosphatase calcineurin inhibition, then selectively reducing the expression of some cytokines, such as IL-2 and IFN-γ, which finally results in the suppression of T-cell function. A subsequent study by the same group suggested that more than a single associative learning trial would be necessary in order to produce immune conditioned effects (Goebel et al. 2005), thus emphasizing the important role of learning in placebo responsiveness.

There is some experimental evidence that these conditioned immune responses have a biological and clinical relevance. Ader and Cohen (1982) paired a conditioned stimulus (a solution of saccharin) with an unconditioned stimulus (cyclophosphamide) in NZB/NZW hybrid mice, a standard model for systemic lupus erythematosus in humans (Steinberg et al. 1981; Theofilopoulos and Dixon 1981). These mice develop a lethal glomerulonephritis at 8–14 months of age, and the progression of the disease can be delayed by means of cyclophosphamide (Casey 1968; Morris et al. 1976). Ader and Cohen (1982) found that those mice that were conditioned by pairing saccharin and cyclophosphamide, showed less severe glomerulonephritis, as assessed through proteinuria measurements, and longer survival times compared with non-conditioned mice. Similarly, the severity of adjuvant-induced arthritis in rats was found to be reduced by conditioned stimuli that had been previously associated with immunosuppressive stimuli (Klosterhalfen and Klosterhalfen 1983; Lysle et al. 1992). The possible clinical implications of behavioural conditioning is also evident in transplantation models of graft reject. On the basis of the fact that A/J mice reject skin grafts from BALB/c or C57BL/6 donors and that cyclophosphamide promotes survival of the allograft, Gorczynski (1990) paired saccharin with cyclophosphamide and subsequently re-exposed conditioned A/J mice to saccharin alone. Survival of the skin allograft was prolonged by saccharin. Similar findings were also obtained in other studies (Grochowicz et al. 1991; Exton et al. 1998).

A clinical case study of a child with lupus erithematosus has been described by Olness and Ader (1992). The child received cytoxan paired with taste and smell stimuli, according to the conditioning procedure used in animals. During the course of twelve months a clinically successful outcome was obtained by using taste and smell stimuli alone on half the monthly chemotherapy sessions. In another study, multiple sclerosis patients received four monthly intravenous treatments with cyclophosphamide paired with anise-flavoured syrup (Giang et al. 1996). After six months of administering the placebo treatment paired with the drink, eight out of ten patients displayed decreased peripheral leucocyte counts, an effect that mimics that of cyclophosphamide. In another clinical study, Goebel et al. (2009) investigated whether the effects of a histamine 1 (H1) receptor antagonist are inducible in patients suffering from house-dust mite allergy using a behavioural conditioning procedure. During the association phase, patients with allergic house-dust mite rhinitis received a novel-tasting drink once daily, followed by a standard dose of the H1 receptor antagonist, desloratadine, on five consecutive days. After nine days of drug washout, the evocation trial commenced. The first group of patients received water together with an identically looking placebo pill.

The second group was re-exposed to the novel-tasting drink and received a placebo pill. The third group received water and desloratadine. During the association phase, desloratadine decreased the subjective total symptom scores, attenuated the effects of the skin prick test for histamine and reduced basophil activation *ex vivo* in all groups. During the evocation trial, the first group, that was not re-exposed to the gustatory stimulus, showed a reduction in subjective total symptom scores and skin prick test results, but no inhibition of basophil activation. In the second group, re-exposure to the novel-tasting drink decreased basophil activation, the skin prick test result and the subjective symptom score to a degree that was similar to the effects of desloratadine in the third group. Thus, behaviourally conditioned effects in humans are not only able to relieve subjective rhinitis symptoms and allergic skin reactions, but they can induce changes in immune functions as well.

Conditioning of immune placebo responses represents an example of the intimate relationship between the brain and the immune system. Part of the mechanisms underlying the brain-immune interaction and the pathways responsible for behavioural conditioning of immune responses have been partially elucidated. Some experimental evidence for neural networks that are involved in immune placebo effects comes from lesion studies. Lesions of the insular cortex in rats have been found to disrupt the acquisition of conditioned immunosuppression by taste aversion (Ramirez-Amaya et al. 1996). Likewise, the lesion of the amygdala interferes with the acquisition of conditioned immunosuppressive responses but has no effect on the performance of pre-existing conditioned responses when the experimental model is the pairing of saccharine taste with cyclophosphamide administration (Ramirez-Amaya et al. 1998). In addition, the insular cortex and the amygdala, but not the hippocampus, have been found to be involved in conditioned enhancement of antibody production when taste or smell stimuli are paired with antigenic stimulation (Ramirez-Amaya and Bermudez-Rattoni 1999; Chen et al. 2004).

By using the association between saccharin as conditioned stimulus and cyclosporine A as unconditioned stimulus, it has been demonstrated that lesions of specific and discrete brain regions affect the conditioned reduction of splenocyte responsiveness and the conditioned decrease of cytokine production, such as IL-2 and IFN-γ (Pacheco-Lopez et al. 2005). The insular cortex is essential for acquiring and evoking these conditioned placebo responses, whereas the amygdala is likely to mediate the input of visceral information necessary at the time of acquisition. By contrast, the ventromedial hypothalamic nucleus seems to participate in the output pathway to the immune system, which is necessary to evoke the behaviourally conditioned immune response (Pacheco-Lopez et al. 2005, 2006).

In the endocrine system, similar effects can be found. The hypoglycaemic effects of insulin can be conditioned by pairing insulin with a conditioned stimulus in animals (Alvarez-Buyalla and Carrasco-Zanini 1960; Alvarez-Buyalla et al. 1961). This conditioned hypoglycaemia was analysed in detail by Woods and collaborators in a long series of experiments in animals. In a typical experiment, in the experimental groups of rats a conditioned stimulus was paired with insulin whereas in the control group the conditioned stimulus was paired with saline solution. After repeated pairings, the experimental group showed a significant decrease of blood glucose compared to the control group (Woods et al. 1968), a conditioned effect that underwent extinction (Woods et al. 1969). Conditioned hypoglycaemia was found to be mediated by the vagus nerve, as both vagotomy and pharmacological blockade with atropine abolished it (Woods 1972). By performing a conditioning procedure with tolbutamide, a drug that stimulates insulin release, Woods et al. (1972) also showed a conditioned insulin secretion that was mediated by the vagus nerve. Interestingly, conditioned insulin secretion was also found by using food as an unconditioned stimulus (Morrell et al. 1988).

Hypoglycaemia can also be conditioned in humans (Stockhorst et al. 1999, 2000). The first human observations were performed in schizophrenic patients who underwent insulin shock therapy, whereby high doses of insulin are administered. When insulin was replaced with a placebo, symptoms of hypoglycaemia, like sweating, tiredness, heart rate, and blood pressure changes, occurred (Lichko 1959). Subsequent studies gave contrasting results (Fehm-Wolfsdorf et al. 1993a, b) and the number of acquisition trials was found to be a possible explanation for these discrepant findings (Fehm-Wolfsdorf et al. 1999). In fact, a substantial change of blood glucose was found in 9 of 16 subjects after 4 acquisition trials, whereas only 2 of 16 subjects showed substantial changes after 2 acquisition trials. This difference emphasizes once again the important role of learning in the placebo effect and the reason why sometimes the inter-individual variability in placebo responsiveness may be high. Another study that used a placebo control group provided evidence that conditioned hypoglycaemia can be obtained in humans (Stockhorst et al. 1999, 2000). Although in this study the conditioned placebo response was not large, the response pattern was consistent. In this study, a trend for a conditioned insulin increase was also found. In addition, there was a first hint that cortisol increased as part of a counter-regulatory response.

In order to assess whether conditioning on the one hand and expectation on the other affect hormone secretion, one study was aimed at differentiating the effects of conditioning and expectation on plasma levels of growth hormone and cortisol (Benedetti et al. 2003b). In the first experimental condition, verbal suggestions of growth hormone increase and cortisol decrease were delivered to healthy volunteers, so as to make them expect hormonal changes. These verbal instructions did not have any effect on both hormones, and in fact no plasma concentration change was detected. In the second experimental condition, sumatriptan, a serotonin 5-HT$_{1B/1D}$ receptor agonist that stimulates growth hormone and inhibits cortisol secretion (Rainero et al. 2001), was administered for two days in a row and then replaced with a placebo on the third day. A significant increase of growth hormone and decrease of cortisol plasma concentrations were found after placebo administration. These conditioned effects occurred regardless of the verbal suggestions the subjects received. In other words, the placebo mimicked the sumatriptan-induced growth hormone increase, even though the subjects expected a growth hormone decrease. Likewise, the placebo mimicked the sumatriptan-induced cortisol decrease, even though the subjects expected a cortisol increase. It can be assumed that in this case the conditioned stimulus was represented by the act of injecting the pharmacological agent (i.e. the context around the treatment). The experiment by Benedetti et al. (2003b) clearly shows that sometimes it is not necessary to expect anything in order for a placebo response to occur. These represent the best examples of unconscious placebo effects that take place even in the absence of the patient's expectations and beliefs (see also section 6.3.3).

6.1.5 Different genetic variants may alter placebo responsiveness

The patient's brain can be affected differently by the ritual of the therapeutic act on the basis of genetic inter-individual differences. Some genetic variants have been found that are particularly responsive to placebo treatment, thereby emphasizing the important role of genetic factors. For example, Furmark et al. (2008) used functional neuroimaging to examine neural correlates of anxiety reduction resulting from placebo treatment in patients with social anxiety disorder (Fig 6.5). Brain activity was assessed during a stressful public speaking task by means of positron emission tomography before and after an eight-weeks treatment period. The patients were genotyped with respect to the serotonin transporter-linked polymorphic region (5-HTTLPR) and the G-703T polymorphism in the tryptophan hydroxylase-2 (TPH2) gene promoter. It was found that the placebo response was accompanied by reduced activity in the amygdala only in subjects who were homozygous for the long allele of the 5-HTTLPR or the G variant of the TPH2 G-703T polymorphism, and not in carriers of short or T alleles. In addition, the TPH2 polymorphism was a significant predictor of clinical placebo response, homozygosity for the G allele being associated with greater improvement in anxiety symptoms.

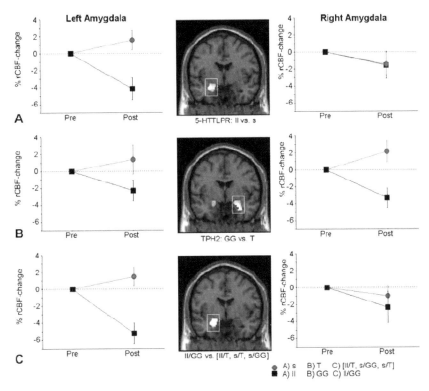

Fig 6.5 Changes in functional magnetic resonance imaging activity in the left and right amygdala after placebo administration during public speaking in different genetic subgroups. A significantly greater reduction of amygdala activity from pre- to post-placebo treatment was observed in the following: (A) long allele (ll) homozygotes compared with short (s) allele carriers of the serotonin transporter gene (5-HTTLPR), (B) G allele (GG) homozygotes compared with T allele carriers of the TPH2 G-703T polymorphism; and (C) long and G allele homozygous patients (ll/GG group) compared with patients carrying s and/or T alleles (ll/T, s/GG, s/T group). See colour plate 15. Source: From Furmark et al. 2008, with permission from the Society for Neuroscience, Copyright 2008.

On the basis of the action of placebos on monoamines of the reward circuitry and because monoaminergic signalling is under strong genetic control, Leuchter et al. (2009) examined the relationship between placebo responses and polymorphisms in genes encoding the catabolic enzymes catechol-O-methyltransferase and monoamine oxidase A in subjects with major depressive disorder. Subjects with monoamine oxidase A G/T polymorphisms (rs6323) coding for the highest activity form of the enzyme (G or G/G) had a significantly lower magnitude of placebo response than those with other genotypes. Subjects with ValMet catechol-O-methyltransferase polymorphisms coding for a lower activity form of the enzyme (2 Met alleles) showed a statistical trend towards a lower magnitude of placebo response. These data support the possible role of genes in some types of placebo responses, for example a genetically controlled serotoninergic modulation of amygdala activity, which is linked to placebo-induced anxiety relief, and a genetically controlled monoaminergic tone, which is related to degree of placebo responsiveness in major depressive disorder.

6.2 The global effect of drugs is influenced by cognition and emotions

6.2.1 Knowledge and non-knowledge about treatments affect the therapeutic outcome

Any medical treatment that is performed in routine medical practice has two components, one related to the specific effects of the treatment itself and the other related to the perception that the therapy is being administered (Fig 6.6A). The latter represents the placebo effect. The placebo component of a treatment is usually studied by simulating a therapy through the administration of a dummy treatment (the placebo), in order to eliminate the specific effects of the therapy itself (Fig 6.6B). This approach is typically used in clinical trials and has also revealed the underlying biological mechanisms of the placebo effect in a variety of medical conditions (Benedetti 2008b).

In recent years, a radically different approach to analysing placebo effects has been implemented, in which placebo effects are assessed without placebo groups. This experimental approach consists in eliminating the placebo component and maintaining the specific effects of the treatment. In order to eliminate the placebo component the patient is made completely unaware that a medical therapy is being carried out (Fig 6.6C). Then hidden therapies are compared with open ones. The difference between the hidden and the open treatment represents the placebo component, even though no placebo has been given. The importance of this approach resides in the fact that open therapies are expected whereas hidden therapies are unexpected. Therefore, the study of the open–hidden (expected–unexpected) paradigm gives us information on the role of expectations in the therapeutic outcome (Colloca et al. 2004).

Typically, the subjects who participate in these studies are told that they could receive either an 'active drug' or a 'placebo' or 'nothing', thus giving their informed consent to receiving different treatments. Therefore, when a hidden infusion of a drug is performed, these subjects believe that 'nothing' is being administered. Another approach that is used is an unknown temporal sequence of drug administration. In this case, the subjects know that a medical

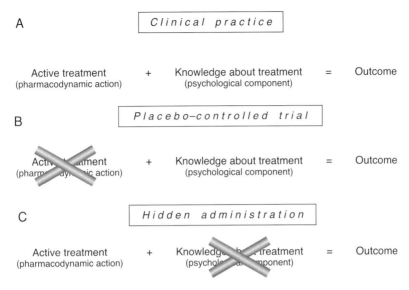

Fig 6.6 Any therapy has a specific effect (pharmacodynamic action for drugs) and a placebo psychological component, that derives from the knowledge about the therapy itself. (A) In routine clinical practice, the therapeutic outcome is the sum of these two components. (B) In placebo-controlled trials, the effectiveness of the active treatment is assessed by eliminating the specific component. (C) In a hidden administration paradigm, the effectiveness of the treatment is assessed by eliminating the knowledge about the therapy.

procedure will be administered but they do not know 'when'. For example, the patient is in a bed with an intravenous line and the drug can be delivered at the first or second or third hour through a pre-programmed infusion machine, but he does not know this temporal sequence. If the drug is really effective, symptom reduction should be temporally correlated with drug administration.

In the 1980s and 1990s, some studies were performed in which analgesic drugs were administered by machines through hidden infusions (Levine et al. 1981; Gracely et al. 1983; Levine and Gordon 1984; Benedetti et al. 1995). It is possible to perform a hidden infusion of a drug by means of a computer-controlled infusion pump that is pre-programmed to deliver the drug at the desired time. The essential point is that the patient does not know that any drug is being injected. This hidden procedure is relatively easy to carry out in the postoperative phase, in which the computer-controlled infusion pump can deliver a painkiller automatically, without any doctor or nurse in the room, and with the patient being completely unaware that an analgesic treatment has been started. In postoperative pain following the extraction of the third molar, Levine et al. (1981) and Levine and Gordon (1984) found that a hidden injection of a 6–8 mg intravenous dose of morphine corresponds to an open intravenous injection of saline solution in full view of the patient (placebo). In other words, telling the patient that a painkiller is being injected (actually a placebo) is as powerful as 6–8 mg of morphine. An explanation might be that an open injection of morphine in full view of the patient, which represents routine medical practice, is more effective than a hidden one because in the latter the placebo component is absent.

An analysis of the differences between open (expected) and hidden (unexpected) injections of analgesics was performed by Amanzio et al. (2001). The effects of four widely used painkillers (buprenorphine, tramadol, ketorolac, metamizol) in the postoperative setting were analysed by using either open or hidden administrations. A doctor carried out the open administration at the bedside by telling the patient that the injection was a powerful analgesic and that the pain would subside in a few minutes. By contrast, the hidden injection of the same analgesic dose was performed by an automatic infusion machine that started the painkilling infusion without any doctor or nurse in the room. Thus these patients were completely unaware that an analgesic therapy had been started. It was found that the analgesic dose needed to reduce the pain by 50% (AD_{50}) was much higher with hidden infusions than with open ones for all four painkillers, indicating that a hidden administration is less effective than an open one. Likewise, the time course of post-surgical pain was significantly different between open and hidden injections. In fact, during the first hour after the injection, pain ratings were much higher with a hidden injection than with an open one.

These effects have also been found with morphine, for both open–hidden administration and interruption (Benedetti et al. 2003a). In fact, the relapse of pain occurs faster and the pain intensity is higher with an open interruption of morphine compared with a hidden one, which indicates that the hidden interruption prolongs the post-interruption analgesia. The faster relapse of pain after the open interruption might be due to a nocebo effect, whereby the knowledge that the therapy has been stopped leads to an increase in anxiety and fear of pain relapse.

Pain is not a special case. Another study was carried out in postoperative patients with high scores of State-Trait Anxiety Inventory–State (STAI-S) after surgery (Benedetti et al. 2003a). In order to reduce state anxiety, some of them were treated with open (expected) administrations of diazepam whereas other patients were given hidden (unexpected) infusions of diazepam. The open and hidden administrations were given with the same procedures as those described above for pain. Likewise, the same open–hidden procedure was used to interrupt the diazepam therapy either overtly or covertly. The difference between the open and the hidden administration of diazepam was highly significant at

2 hr after the injection, such that in the open group there was a clear-cut decrease of the STAI-S, whereas in the hidden group diazepam was totally ineffective. As to diazepam interruption, in the open condition the STAI-S increased significantly after 4 and 8 hr whereas in the hidden condition it did not change. In this case also, the anxiety relapse after the open interruption of diazepam might be due to the expectation and fear of anxiety relapse because anti-anxiety drugs are no longer provided.

The open–hidden paradigm has also been applied to deep brain stimulation of the subthalamic nucleus for the treatment of Parkinson's disease. There are at least two lines of evidence indicating that hidden deep brain stimulation is less effective than open stimulation. The first comes from the stimulation with macroelectrodes in the postoperative phase (Pollo et al. 2002; Benedetti et al. 2003b). By using a hand movement analyser to assess bradykinesia, Parkinson patients performed a visual directional-choice task in which the right index finger was positioned on a central sensor and moved towards a target when a light was turned on. Each patient was tested twice, with an overt and covert stimulation, on different days. In the open condition, the subthalamic stimulus intensity was overtly reduced to 20% of the optimal stimulation, and the patient was told that motor performance would worsen. After 2 hr, the stimulus intensity was overtly increased to optimal stimulation, and the patients were told that motor performance would return to normal. By contrast, in the hidden condition, the stimulus reduction to 20% and the subsequent stimulus increase to optimal stimulation were performed covertly, with the patients completely unaware that such changes were being performed. The open interruption of subthalamic nucleus stimulation induced a larger reduction of movement velocity at 30 min than the hidden one. Similarly, when the stimulation returned to normal, the open procedure was more effective than the hidden one at 10 min. Therefore, the hidden unexpected interruption induced a lesser worsening of motor performance, while the hidden stimulus increase produced smaller therapeutic effects.

The second line of evidence that hidden deep brain stimulation is less effective than open stimulation comes from the analysis of autonomic and emotional responses to intraoperative stimulation with microelectrodes (Benedetti et al. 2004a; Lanotte et al. 2005). The stimulation of the most dorsal portion of the subthalamic region, which includes the zona incerta and the dorsal pole of the subthamic nucleus, produced autonomic responses that did not differ in the hidden and the open conditions. By contrast, the stimulation of the most ventral region, which includes the ventral pole of the subthalamic nucleus and the substantia nigra pars reticulata, produced autonomic and emotional responses that were inconstant over time and varied according to the open or hidden condition of stimulation (see also section 3.3.2). The minimum stimulus intensity to produce a response (threshold) increased from 2.25 ± 1.4 Volts in the open condition to 4.1 ± 0.9 Volts in the hidden condition. In other words, the hidden unexpected stimulation was less effective, so that an increase of the stimulus intensity was necessary in order to induce an autonomic response. It is worth pointing out that this ventral portion of the subthalamic region is likely to be involved in limbic-associative functions (Alexander et al. 1986, 1990; Limousin et al. 1997; Bejjani et al. 1999; Krack et al. 2001).

These studies show that the patient's knowledge about a therapy affects the therapy outcome. Thus, in the open condition the patient knows the details of the therapy, why it is being carried out and what outcomes to expect. By contrast, in the hidden condition the patient is completely unaware that a therapy is being given. In this covert situation, no doctors or nurses are in the room and the treatment is started by a pre-programmed machine. Although many factors and variables may contribute to the differences between the two situations, certainly the awareness of the treatment, the presence of the therapist, and the expectation of the outcome are likely to play a crucial role. Since all these factors are strongly influenced by the doctor–patient interaction (e.g. the doctor's words), the patient's knowledge about a therapy appears to be fundamental to produce the optimal therapeutic effects. Another important point is represented by the interruption of a therapy. Interestingly, and paradoxically, the awareness of the patient about a treatment is advantageous only when the therapy is being administered. By contrast, if the therapy has to be interrupted, such awareness might be deleterious for the patient. In fact, the open interruption of morphine, diazepam and subthalamic stimulation produces a greater worsening of the symptoms compared to a hidden one. Therefore, the expectation of worsening may counteract the beneficial effects that are present after the treatment interruption.

In clinical practice, all efforts should be made in order to make the patient aware of what is going on, why a procedure is being carried out and what kind of outcome should be expected. The differences between open and hidden administrations of therapies should induce doctors, nurses, psychologists, and all other medical and paramedical personnel to further increase their interaction with patients. Even when a treatment has to be stopped, what the therapist tells his patient is essential. The way in which drugs and brain stimulation are delivered or interrupted plays an important role in the therapeutic outcome.

6.2.2 The patient's psychological state interferes with the action of drugs

Drugs are not injected into a vacuum but into a complex living organism that may be in different states. In particular, human beings continuously switch from one psychological, cognitive, and emotional state to another, and this has been found to affect the global action of a pharmacological agent. In the previous section, we have seen that one of the best examples of the role of expectations in the therapeutic outcome is represented by the hidden unexpected administration of drugs. If the patient does not know that a drug is being administered, and thus he does not expect any effect, the action of the drug is reduced. There are a number of studies that show that the global effect of a drug can be modified, or even reversed, by manipulating the psychological state of the subject. For example, Dworkin et al. (1983) found that verbal suggestions can change the direction of nitrous oxide action from analgesia to hyperalgesia, with a reduction of both pain threshold and tolerance following electrical tooth-pulp stimulation. Kirk et al. (1998) found that, in drug abusers, the response to a drug is more pleasurable when subjects expect to receive the drug than when they do not. Likewise, Flaten et al. (1999) showed that carisoprodol, a centrally acting muscle relaxant, resulted in different outcomes, either relaxant or stimulant, depending on the combination of verbal suggestion and drug administration.

In this regard, the balanced placebo design is an interesting paradigm because it allows the study of cognitive modulation of drug action. It has been developed to better understand the role of suggestion in the therapeutic outcome, and refers to a methodology for studying many aspects of human behaviour and drug effects, orthogonally manipulating instructions (told drug versus told placebo) and drug administered (received drug versus received placebo) (Ross et al. 1962). It has been used in many conditions such as alcohol research (Marlatt et al. 1973; Rohsenow and Bachorowski 1984; Wilson et al. 1985; Epps et al. 1998), smoking (Sutton 1991), and amphetamine effects (Mitchell et al. 1996).

In one study on the effects of methylphenidate on brain glucose metabolism, Volkow et al. (2003) adopted a balanced placebo design. In one condition, cocaine abusers expected to receive the drug, and indeed received the drug. In a second condition, they expected the drug but received a placebo. In a third condition, they expected to receive a placebo but actually received the drug. In a fourth condition, they expected a placebo and indeed they received a placebo. This paradigm is rather similar to the open–hidden design, as in the first case methylphenidate is expected, while in the third case its administration is unexpected. The increases in brain glucose metabolism were about 50% larger, particularly in the cerebellum and the thalamus, when methylphenidate was expected than when it was not. By contrast, methylphenidate induced larger increases in left lateral orbitofrontal cortex when it was unexpected compared with when it was expected. In addition, the self-reports of 'high' were also 50%

greater when methylphenidate was expected than when it was not. Volkow et al. (2003) also found a correlation between the subjectively reported 'high' and the metabolic activity in the thalamus but not in the cerebellum. This study indicates that the psychological state of the patient makes a big difference; it can either enhance or reduce the drug effects, and the thalamus may mediate this drug enhancement by expectations, whereas the orbitofrontal cortex mediates the unexpected response to the drug.

The same research group, by using the same balanced placebo design, repeated a similar experiment in non-drug abusing subjects who had minimal prior experience with stimulant drugs (Volkow et al. 2006). It was found that methylphenidate induced decreases in the striatum that were larger when the subjects expected it than when they did not. In addition, when the subjects expected to receive methylphenidate but actually received a placebo, the researchers found increases in the ventral cingulate gyrus and in the nucleus accumbens. The involvement of the nucleus accumbens following placebo administration, along with expectation to receive methylphenidate, is in agreement with the other studies in pain (Scott et al. 2007), Parkinson's disease (de la Fuente-Fernandez et al. 2001), and depression (Mayberg et al. 2002), in which the reward circuitry in the ventral striatum (nucleus accumbens) was found to be involved following placebo administration (see section 4.2.3). The work by Volkow and colleagues (Volkow et al. 2003, 2006) shows that expectation, and indeed any psychological state, is an important variable to be considered whenever reinforcing and therapeutic effects of drugs are tested both in subjects who assume drugs of abuse and in subjects who have no previous experience of drugs.

6.2.3 It is not possible to fully understand how therapies work

The fact that the ritual of the therapeutic act triggers a variety of biological events in the patient's brain and that the psychological state of the patient, such as the expectation of therapeutic benefit, may interfere with drug action, leads to an important implication. Is the therapy that the doctor is administering really effective? Or, in other words, does it act through a specific action? Or, rather, does the patient's brain and psychological state modify (either increasing or reducing) its effects?

In 1995, Benedetti et al. (1995) found that the cholecystokinin (CCK) antagonist proglumide was better than placebo, and placebo was better than no-treatment in relieving postoperative pain. According to the methodology used in classical clinical trials, these results would indicate that proglumide is a good analgesic which acts on the pain pathways, whereas placebo reduces pain by inducing expectations of analgesia, thus activating expectation pathways.

However, this conclusion proved to be erroneous, as a hidden injection of proglumide was totally ineffective. In fact, if proglumide had a specific pharmacodynamic effect, there should be no difference between open and hidden administration. Therefore, the likely interpretation of the mechanism of action of proglumide is that it does not act on pain pathways at all, but rather on expectation pathways, thus enhancing the placebo analgesic response. In other words, proglumide induces a reduction of pain if, and only if, it is associated with a placebo procedure. Now we know that proglumide is not a painkiller, but it acts on placebo-activated opioid mechanisms. By borrowing the Heisenberg uncertainty principle from physics, which imposes limits on the precision of a measurement (Wheeler and Zurek 1983), we can apply a similar principle to outcomes of clinical trials. As noted by Colloca and Benedetti (2005), in the same way as the uncertainty principle of physics states that a dynamical disturbance is necessarily induced on a system by a measurement, in clinical trials a dynamical disturbance might be induced on the brain by virtually any kind of drug. The very nature of this disturbance is the interference of the injected drug with the expectation pathways, which affects both the outcome measures and the interpretation of the data. Therefore, as occurs in the Heisenberg principle, the disturbance is the cause of the uncertainty. For example, a pharmacological analgesic agent has its own specific pharmacodynamic effect on the pain pathways, but an interference with the mechanisms of top-down control of pain might occur. We have no a priori knowledge of which substances act on pain pathways and which on expectation mechanisms. Indeed, virtually all drugs might interfere with the top-down mechanisms, thus this uncertainty cannot be solved with the standard clinical trial design. The only way to partially solve this problem is to make the expectation pathways, so to speak, silent. To do this, the treatment has to be given covertly (unexpectedly), so that the subject does not have expectations. In this way, a drug may be really given, at least in part, in a vacuum, free of any psychologically-induced activation of biochemical pathways.

Therefore, different psychological states and social stimuli can activate neurotransmitters and neuromodulators that bind to the same receptors to which drugs bind, and can trigger biochemical pathways that are similar to those activated by pharmacological agents (Fig 6.7). Today we know that whenever a medical treatment is carried out, a complex biochemical matrix is activated by several social stimuli. This biochemical cascade of events will inevitably interfere with any drug that is given. In other words, drugs are not administered in a vacuum but rather in a complex biochemical environment that varies according to the patient's cognitive/affective state and to the previous exposure to other pharmacological agents (conditioning). Any drug, which will be eventually given

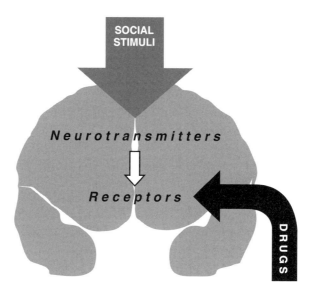

Fig 6.7 A variety of social stimuli can activate a number of neurotransmitters in the patient's brain that, in turn, bind to the same receptors to which different drugs bind. Thus, cognitive and affective factors can interfere with the action of drugs. When a drug is given, the act of administering it (i.e. the social stimuli around the patient) may perturb the system and change the response to the drug.

for a specific condition, may act on a set of receptors that could have been modified by the therapeutic context, as depicted in Fig 6.7. It appears clear that, if we want to test a new drug for relieving pain, the act of its administration may interfere with its real pharmacodynamic effects. On the basis of all these considerations, complex cognitive/affective factors are capable of modulating the action of drugs through the activation of the very same receptors to which drugs bind. Therefore, a drug that is tested according to the classical methodology of clinical trials can paradoxically be better than a placebo even though it has no analgesic properties (Benedetti et al. 1995). This should be taken into account whenever a new treatment is tested, because the very act of its administration may interfere with its real pharmacodynamic effects.

6.3 **A closer look into unconscious conditioning and conscious expectation**

6.3.1 Pavlovian conditioning is due to the temporal contiguity of the stimuli

The role of Pavlovian conditioning and expectation in the therapeutic setting is particularly interesting because it is related to an important debate in neuroscience, that is, whether conditioning is really unconscious or rather it is attributable to a cognitive component. In the original formulation, classical Pavlovian conditioning is a form of associative learning whereby a pairing between two stimuli occurs. The process is totally unconscious and the crucial point for the pairing, or association, between the two stimuli is their temporal contiguity. If an unconditioned stimulus (US), e.g. food, inducing an unconditioned response (UR), e.g. salivation, is paired with a neutral, or conditioned stimulus (CS), e.g. a sound, after repeated pairings the neutral CS, i.e. the sound alone, will be capable of inducing a conditioned response (CR), i.e. salivation (Fanselow 1998).

The CS is also called neutral because a sound per se does not produce salivation. The central point in Pavlovian conditioning is that the neutral stimulus (the CS) will eventually acquire the capability of inducing salivation if, and only if, it is temporally paired with the US, i.e. the food. According to this view, the conditioning phenomenon is completely unconscious. It only requires pairing and contiguity. In this regard, the cellular substrate of associative learning, for example long-term potentiation, is based only on a sort of contiguity detectors, which would guarantee the emergence of learning after repeated pairings between the CS and the US.

6.3.2 Cognition may be at work during conditioning

The first challenge to the notion of temporal contiguity in Pavlovian conditioning was provided by Kamin (1968) in the rat, according to the experimental paradigm depicted in Fig 6.8. In a pre-training Phase 1, in one group of rats (blocking) a noise was paired with an aversive electric shock, whereas in the other group (control) no such pairing was performed. In Phase 2, both groups received the same eight pairings of a light (the CS) and a noise with an aversive electric shock (the US). The control rats with no experience with the noise in Phase 1 showed near maximal conditioned fear to the light in Phase 3, but those that had received noise-shock pairings in the pre-training Phase 1 ('blocking' group) exhibited virtually no conditioned fear. It is important to note that both groups received exactly the same experience with the light and they differed only with how the noise was treated. As the pre-training to the noise 'blocked' conditioning to the light, this effect is called 'blocking'. The critical point in Kamin's experiment is that conditioning in the two groups was very different, although both experienced identical temporal contiguity between the light and shock. Therefore, contiguity does not seem to be a sufficient requirement of conditioning.

Kamin (1968) suggested the important role of surprise or, in other words, the difference between what the rats get and what they expect to get. In Phase 2, the

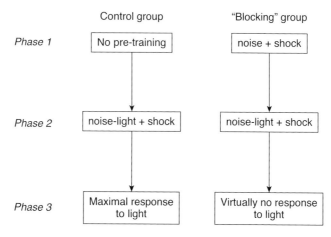

Fig 6.8 The blocking paradigm in rats, as performed in the experiment by Kamin (1968). The 'blocking' group is trained with several pairings of a noise stimulus and an electric shock in Phase 1, whereas the control group does not undergo this training. Both the control and the 'blocking group' undergo the pairing of an electric shock and a noise+light stimulus in Phase 2. When the light is presented in Phase 3, the control group shows a maximal fear response, whereas the 'blocking' group shows virtually no response to the light.

'blocking' rats expected a shock because of their previous learning about the noise. They got that shock, so they were not surprised and did not learn about the light. This suggests that the US supports increases in associative strength proportional to the degree that it exceeds what the environment already predicts (Rescorla and Wagner 1972; Fanselow 1998).

As already discussed in section 6.1.2, the notion that conditioning is a mere automatic unconscious event had already been questioned by Tolman (1932). The information content of the CS is crucial during the pairing with the US. In fact, the crucial point of such a pairing is not so much the CS-US temporal contiguity, but rather the expectation that a given event will follow another event, and this occurs on the basis of the information that the CS provides about the US (Reiss 1980; Rescorla 1988; Kirsch et al. 2004). Thus, the CS induces expectations.

6.3.3 Both conscious expectation and unconscious conditioning take place in the patient's brain

The effects of the therapeutic act on the patient's brain are attributable to both conscious expectation mechanisms and unconscious conditioning mechanisms. In some circumstances, expectation can override a conditioning procedure, whereas in some other conditions, conditioning overrides conscious expectations. In this regard, the experiment by Benedetti et al. (2003b) was aimed at inducing conflicting expectation and conditioning outcomes. In other words, while the conditioning procedure went towards a given direction, expectation was manipulated in the opposite direction. In this study, which is shown in Fig 6.9A, in one group of subjects a pharmacological preconditioning with ketorolac, a nonopioid analgesic, was performed for two days in a row and then ketorolac was replaced with a placebo on the third day along with verbal suggestions of analgesia. This procedure induced a strong placebo analgesic response. In order to see whether this placebo response was due to the pharmacological preconditioning, in a second group of subjects the same preconditioning procedure with ketorolac was carried out but the placebo was given on the third day along with verbal suggestions that the drug was a hyperalgesic agent. These verbal instructions were enough not only to block placebo analgesia completely, but also to produce hyperalgesia. These findings clearly show that expectation of hyperalgesia can antagonize the pharmacological conditioning completely.

In the same study (Benedetti et al. 2003b), which is shown in Fig 6.9B, patients implanted for deep brain stimulation were tested for the velocity of movement of their right hand according to a double-blind experimental design in which neither the patient nor the experimenter knew whether the stimulator was turned off. The velocity of hand movement was assessed by means of a movement analyser, characterized by a rectangular surface where the patients performed a visual directional-choice task. To do this, the right index finger was positioned on a central sensor with a green light. After a random interval of a few seconds, a red light turned on randomly in one of three sensors placed 10 cm away from the green-light sensor. The patients were instructed to move their hand as quickly as possible in order to reach the target red-light sensor. As shown in Fig 6.9B, the stimulator was turned off several times (at 4 and 2 weeks) before the test session. Each time the velocity of movement was measured just before the stimulator was turned off and 30 min later. Thus the measurement at 30 min reflects the worsening of motor performance. On the day of the experimental session, the stimulator was maintained on but the patients were told that it had been turned off, so as to induce negative expectations of motor performance worsening (nocebo procedure). It can be seen that, although the stimulator was on, motor performance worsened and mimicked the worsening of the previous days. In Fig 6.9B, it can also be seen that this nocebo bradykinesia could be prevented completely by verbal suggestions of good motor performance (placebo procedure). Therefore, as occurs for pain, in this case also, motor performance can be modulated in two opposite directions on the basis of positive and negative expectations about motor performance.

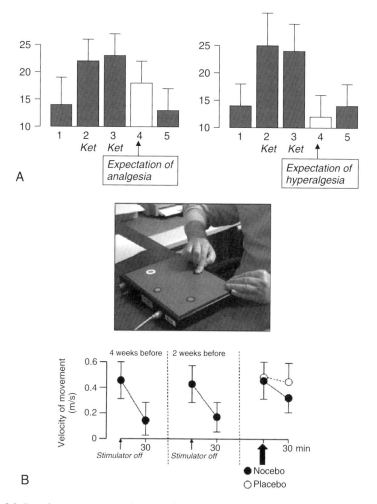

Fig 6.9 Experiments to assess the contribution of expectation and conditioning in the placebo effect. (A) Placebo administration (left panel), along with suggestion of analgesia, on day 4 after a two days preconditioning with ketorolac (Ket) induces a robust placebo analgesic response, as shown by the increase in pain tolerance (white column) compared to baseline (days 1 and 5). The same ketorolac preconditioning is totally ineffective if placebo is given on day 4 along with suggestion of hyperalgesia (right panel). Indeed, a moderate hyperalgesic effect occurs (white column).

Source: From Benedetti et al. 2003b with permission from the Society for Neuroscience, Copyright 2003.

(B) Top panel: the movement analyser to assess movement velocity in Parkinson patients is shown (from Benedetti et al. 2007 with permission from Elsevier, Copyright 2007). Bottom panel: after the stimulator for deep brain stimulation had

Fig 6.9 (*Cont'd*) been turned off at 4 and 2 weeks before the experimental session, nocebo suggestions of clinical worsening were given but the stimulator was maintained on. Each time the velocity of movement was measured just before the stimulator was turned off and 30 min later. Thus the measurement at 30 min reflects the worsening of motor performance. Note that, despite the stimulator was still on, nocebo induced worsening. Placebo suggestions of improvement antagonized this nocebo effect completely, in spite of the nocebo preconditioning at week 4 and 2 before the experimental session.
Source: From Benedetti et al. 2003b with permission from the Society for Neuroscience, Copyright 2003.

Besides pain and motor performance in Parkinson's disease, the same study (Benedetti et al. 2003b) also tested hormone secretion (Fig 6.10). Verbally induced expectations of hormonal changes did not produce any effect on growth hormone and cortisol secretion (Fig 6.10 A, B). Then, the serotonin 5-HT$_{1B/1D}$ receptor agonist, sumatriptan, that produces growth hormone increase, was administered for two consecutive days and then replaced with a placebo on the third day, along with the verbal suggestion of growth hormone decrease (Fig 6.10C). A significant increase of growth hormone plasma concentrations was found after placebo administration, regardless of the verbally induced expectation of decrease. In other words, the placebo mimicked the sumatriptan-induced growth hormone increase, even though the subjects expected a growth hormone decrease. The same effect was observed with cortisol. After conditioning with sumatriptan, which induced cortisol decrease, the placebo mimicked the sumatriptan-induced cortisol decrease, even though the subjects expected a cortisol increase. Therefore, in contrast to pain and Parkinson's disease, whereby expectation modulates the direction of the conditioning procedure, in hormonal secretion the direction of conditioning cannot be modulated by conscious expectations.

These data suggest that conscious expectation and unconscious conditioning may be at work in different conditions. In particular, conscious expectation of a future outcome seems to be important in the modulation of conscious processes, like pain and motor performance, whereas unconscious conditioning appears to be involved in unconscious physiological processes, such as hormone secretion. It is worth remembering that the immune system is amenable to classical conditioning both in animals and in humans (see section 6.1.4). Therefore, the conditioned placebo hormonal and immune responses indicate that unconscious conditioning is possible in humans, and cognitive components do not need to be always present (Stewart-Podd and Williams 2004).

By definition, a symptom is consciously perceived by the patient, thus expectation plays a crucial role here. For example, pain, which can be considered as

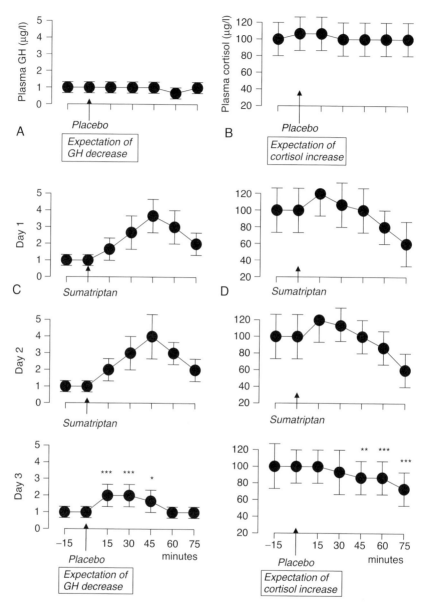

Fig 6.10. Verbal suggestions of growth hormone (GH) increase (A) and cortisol decrease (B) have no effect on GH and cortisol plasma concentration. (C) After two days of sumatriptan preconditioning, a placebo mimics the GH-increasing effects of sumatriptan, even though verbal suggestions of GH decrease are given. *$p < 0.05$; ***$p < 0.01$. (D) Likewise, after two days of sumatriptan preconditioning, a placebo mimics the cortisol-decreasing effects of sumatriptan, even though verbal suggestions of cortisol increase are given. **$p < 0.02$; ***$p < 0.01$.
Source: From Benedetti et al. 2003b with permission of the Society for Neuroscience, Copyright 2003.

the prototype of conscious experience, is amenable to modulation of conscious expectation (see above). This is also shown by the socially learned placebo responses, whereby merely observing others who experience analgesia leads to robust placebo responses that are as large as those obtained by the first-hand experience of a classical conditioning procedure (Colloca and Benedetti 2009) (see also section 6.1.2). In the case of pain, thus, conditioning relies on a fundamental cognitive component, which can be better conceptualized as reinforced expectations rather than mere contiguity-dependent learning. One should not forget, however, that Pavlovian conditioning mechanisms coexist and may take place unconsciously in different systems and apparatuses.

References

Ader R (1997). The role of conditioning in pharmacotherapy. In: A Harrington, ed., *The placebo effect: an interdisciplinary exploration*, pp. 138–65. Harvard University Press, Cambridge, MA.

Ader R and Cohen N (1975). Behaviorally conditioned immunosuppression. *Psychosomatic Medicine*, **37**, 333–40.

—— (1982). Behaviorally conditioned immunosuppression and murine systemic lupus erythematosus. *Science,* **215**, 1534–6.

Ader R, Kelly K, Moynihan JA, Grota LJ and Cohen N (1993). Conditioned enhancement of antibody production using antigen as the unconditioned stimulus. *Brain, Behavior and Immunity*, **7**, 334–43.

Alexander GE, DeLong MR, Strick PL (1986). Parallel organization of functionally segregated circuits linking basal ganglia and cortex. *Annual Review of Neuroscience*, **9**, 357–81.

Alexander GE, Crutcher MD and DeLong MR (1990). Basal ganglia-thalamocortical circuits: parallel substrates for motor, oculomotor, 'prefrontal' and 'limbic' functions. *Progress in Brain Research*, **85**, 119–46.

Alvarez-Borda B, Ramirez-Amaya V, Pèrez-Montfort R and Bermùdez-Rattoni F (1995). Enhancement of antibody production by a learning paradigm. *Neurobiology of Learning and Memory*, **64**, 103–5.

Alvarez-Buyalla R and Carrasco-Zanini J (1960). A conditioned reflex which reproduces the hypoglycemic effect of insulin. *Acta Physiologica Latino Americana*, **10**, 153–8.

Alvarez-Buyalla R, Segura ET and Alvarez-Buyalla ER (1961). Participation of the hypophysis in the conditioned reflex which reproduces the hypoglycemic effect of insulin. *Acta Physiologica Latino Americana*, **11**, 113–9.

Amanzio M and Benedetti F (1999). Neuropharmacological dissection of placebo analgesia: expectation-activated opioid systems versus conditioning-activated specific subsystems. *Journal of Neuroscience,* **19**, 484–94.

Amanzio M, Pollo A, Maggi G and Benedetti F (2001). Response variability to analgesics: a role for non-specific activation of endogenous opioids. *Pain,* **90**, 205–15.

Balint M (1955). The doctor, his patient, and the illness. *Lancet,* **1**, 683–8.

Bandura A (1977). Self efficacy: toward a unifying theory of behavior change. *Psychological Review,* **84**, 191–215.

Bandura A (1997). *Self efficacy: the exercise of control.* Cambridge University Press, New York.

Batterman RC (1966). Persistence of responsiveness with placebo therapy following an effective drug trial. *Journal of New Drugs*, **6**, 137–41.

Batterman RC and Lower WR (1968). Placebo responsiveness – influence of previous therapy. *Current Therapeutic Research*, **10**, 136–43.

Bejjani BP, Damier P, Arnulf I, Thivard L, Bonnet AM, Dormont D et al. (1999). Transient acute depression induced by high-frequency deep-brain stimulation. *New England Journal Medicine*, **340**, 1476–80.

Benedetti F (1996). The opposite effects of the opiate antagonist naloxone and the cholecystokinin antagonist proglumide on placebo analgesia. *Pain,* **64**, 535–43.

—— (2002). How the doctor' s words affect the patient' s brain. *Evaluation & Health Professions*, **25**, 369–86.

—— (2008a). Mechanisms of placebo and placebo-related effects across diseases and treatments. *Annual Review of Pharmacology and Toxicology*, **48**, 33–60.

—— (2008b). *Placebo effects: understanding the mechanisms in health and disease.* Oxford University Press, Oxford.

Benedetti F, Amanzio M and Maggi G (1995). Potentiation of placebo analgesia by proglumide. *Lancet*, **346**, 1231.

Benedetti F, Arduino C and Amanzio M (1999). Somatotopic activation of opioid systems by target-expectations of analgesia. *Journal of Neuroscience,* **9**, 3639–48.

Benedetti F, Colloca L, Lanotte M, Bergamasco B, Torre E and Lopiano L (2004a). Autonomic and emotional responses to open and hidden stimulations of the human subthalamic region. *Brain Research Bulletin*, **63**, 203–11.

Benedetti F, Colloca L, Torre E, Lanotte M, Melcarne A, Pesare M et al. (2004b). Placebo-responsive Parkinson patients show decreased activity in single neurons of subthalamic nucleus. *Nature Neuroscience*, **7**, 587–8.

Benedetti F, Lanotte M, Colloca L, Ducati A, Zibetti M and Lopiano L (2009). Electrophysiological properties of thalamic, subthalamic and nigral neurons during the anti-parkinsonian placebo response. *Journal of Physiology*, **587**, 3869–83.

Benedetti F, Maggi G, Lopiano L, Lanotte M, Rainero I, Vighetti S et al. (2003a). Open versus hidden medical treatments: the patient's knowledge about a therapy affects the therapy outcome. *Prevention & Treatment*, http://content2.apa.org/journals/pre/6/1/1

Benedetti F, Mayberg HS, Wager TD, Stohler CS and Zubieta JK (2005). Neurobiological mechanisms of the placebo effect. *Journal of Neuroscience,* **25**, 10390–402.

Benedetti F, Pollo A, Lopiano L, Lanotte M, Vighetti S and Rainero I (2003b). Conscious expectation and unconscious conditioning in analgesic, motor and hormonal placebo/ nocebo responses. *Journal of Neuroscience*, **23**, 4315–23.

Bingel U, Lorenz J, Schoell E, Weiller C and Büchel C (2005). Mechanisms of placebo analgesia: rACC recruitment of a subcortical antinociceptive network. *Pain,* **120**, 8–15.

Booth RJ, Petrie KJ and Brook RJ (1995). Conditioning allergic skin responses in humans: a controlled study. *Psychosomatic Medicine*, **57**, 492–5.

Bootzin RR (1985). The role of expectancy in behavior change. In: L White, B Tursky and GE Schwartz, eds., *Placebo: theory, research, and mechanisms*, pp. 196–210. Guilford Press, New York, NY.

Bootzin RR and Caspi O (2002). Explanatory mechanisms for placebo effects: cognition, personality and social learning. In: HA Guess, A Kleinman, JW Kusek and LW Engel, eds, pp. 108–32. British Medical Journal Books, London.

Bovbjerg D, Ader R and Cohen N (1984). Acquisition and extinction of conditioned suppression of a graft-versus-host response in the rat. *Journal of Immunology*, **132**, 111–3.

Branthwaite A and Cooper P (1981). Analgesic effects of branding in treatment of headaches. *British Medical Journal*, **282**, 1576–8.

Brody H (2000). *The placebo response*. Harper-Collins, New York, NY.

Casey TP (1968). Immunosuppression by cyclophosphamide in NZB/NZW mice with lupus nephritis. *Blood*, **32**, 436–44.

Caspi O and Bootzin RR (2002). Evaluating how placebos produce change. *Evaluation & the Health Professions*, **25**, 436–64.

Chen J, Lin W, Wang W, Shao F, Yang J, Wang B et al. (2004). Enhancement of antibody production and expression of c-Fos in the insular cortex in response to a conditioned stimulus after a single-trial learning paradigm. *Behavioral Brain Research*, **154**, 557–65.

Colloca L and Benedetti F (2005). Placebos and painkillers: is mind as real as matter? *Nature Reviews Neuroscience*, **6**, 545–52.

—— (2009). Placebo analgesia induced by social observational learning. *Pain*, **144**, 28–34.

Colloca L, Benedetti F and Porro CA (2008a). Experimental designs and brain mapping approaches for studying the placebo analgesic effect. *European Journal of Applied Physiology*, **102**, 371–80.

Colloca L, Lopiano L, Lanotte M and Benedetti F (2004). Overt versus covert treatment for pain, anxiety and Parkinson's disease. *Lancet Neurology*, **3**, 679–84.

Colloca L, Tinazzi M, Recchia S, Le Pera D, Fiaschi A, Benedetti F et al. (2008b). Learning potentiates neurophysiological and behavioral placebo analgesic responses. *Pain*, **139**, 306–14.

de la Fuente-Fernandez R, Ruth TJ, Sossi V, Schulzer M, Calne DB and Stoessl AJ (2001). Expectation and dopamine release: mechanism of the placebo effect in Parkinson's disease. *Science*, **293**, 1164–6.

de la Fuente-Fernández R, Phillips AG, Zamburlini M, Sossi V, Calne DB, Ruth TJ et al. (2002). Dopamine release in human ventral striatum and expectation of reward. *Behavioural. Brain Research*, **136**, 359–63.

De Jong PJ, van Baast R, Arntz A and Merkelbach H (1996). The placebo effect in pain reduction: the influence of conditioning experiences and response expectancies. *International Journal of Behavioral Medicine*, **3**, 14–29.

De Pascalis V, Chiaradia C and Carotenuto E (2002). The contribution of suggestibility and expectation to placebo analgesia phenomenon in an experimental setting. *Pain*, **96**, 393–402.

Di Blasi Z, Harkness E, Ernst E, Georgiou A and Kleijnen J (2001). Influence of context effect on health outcomes: a systematic review. *Lancet*, **357**, 757–62.

Dworkin SF, Chen AC, LeResche L and Clark DW (1983). Cognitive reversal of expected nitrous oxide analgesia for acute pain. *Anesthesia and Analgesia*, **62**, 1073–7.

Eippert F, Bingel U, Schoell ED, Yacubian J, Klinger R, Lorenz J et al. (2009a). Activation of the opioidergic descending pain control system underlies placebo analgesia. *Neuron*, **63**, 533–43.

Eippert F, Finsterbusch J, Bingel U and Buchel C (2009b). Direct evidence for spinal cord involvement in placebo analgesia. *Science*, **326**, 404.

Enck P, Benedetti F and Schedlowski M (2008). New insights into the placebo and nocebo responses. *Neuron*, **59**, 195–206.

Epps J, Monk C, Savage S and Marlatt GA (1998). Improving credibility of instruction in the balanced placebo design: a misattribution manipulation. *Addictive Behaviors*, **23**, 426–35.

Evans FJ (1977). The placebo control of pain: a paradigm for investigating non-specific effects in psychotherapy. In: JP Brady, J Mendels, WR Reiger and MT Orne, eds, *Psychiatry: areas of promise and advancement*, pp. 249–71. Plenum Press, New York, NY.

Exton MS, von Hörsten S, Schult M, Vöge J, Strubel T, Donath S et al. (1998). Behaviourally conditioned immunosuppression using cyclosporine A: central nervous system reduces IL-2 production via splenic innervation. *Journal of Neuroimmunology*, **88**, 182–91.

Fanselow MS (1998). Pavlovian conditioning, negative feedback, and blocking: mechanisms that regulate association formation. *Neuron*, **20**, 625–7.

Fehm-Wolfsdorf G, Beermann U, Kern W and Fehm HL (1993a). Failure to obtain classical conditioned hypoglycemia in man. In: Lehnert H, Murison R, Weiner H, Hellhammer D and Beyer J Jr, eds, *Neuronal control of bodily function: basic and clinical aspects. Endocrine and nutritional control of basic biological functions*, pp. 257–61. Hogrefe & Huber Publishers, Seattle, WA.

Fehm-Wolfsdorf G, Gnadler M, Kern W, Klosterhalfen W and Kerner W (1993b). Classically conditioned changes of blood glucose level in humans. *Physiology and Behavior*, **54**, 155–60.

Fehm-Wolfsdorf G, Pohl J and Kerner W (1999). Classically conditioned changes of blood glucose level in humans. *Integrative Physiological and Behavioral Sciences*, **34**, 132.

Fields HL and Levine JD (1984). Placebo analgesia-a role for endorphins? *Trends in Neurosciences*, **7**, 271–3.

Finniss DG, Kaptchuk TJ, Miller F and Benedetti F (2010). Biological, clinical and ethical advances of placebo effects. *Lancet*, **375**, 686–95.

Flaten MA, Simonsen T and Olsen H (1999). Drug-related information generates placebo and nocebo responses that modify the drug response. *Psychosomatic Medicine*, **61**, 250–5.

Frank JD (1961). *Persuasion and healing: a comparative study of psychotherapy*. Schocken Books, New York (rev. ed.: Johns Hopkins University Press, Baltimore, 1973).

—— (1971). Therapeutic factors in psychotherapy. *American Journal of Psychotherapy*, **25**, 350–61.

—— (1981). Therapeutic components shared by all psychotherapies. In: JH Hawey and MM Parks, eds, *Psychotherapy research and behavior change*, pp. 00. American Psychological Association, Washington, DC.

Furmark T, Appel L, Henningsson S, Ahs F, Faria V, Linnman C et al. (2008). A link between serotonin-related gene polymorphisms, amygdala activity, and placebo-induced relief from social anxiety. *Journal of Neuroscience*, **28**, 13066–74.

Gauci M, Husband AJ, Saxarra H and King MG (1994). Pavlovian conditioning of nasal tryptase release in human subjects with allergic rhinitis. *Physiology and Behavior*, **55**, 823–5.

Geers AL, Weiland PE, Kosbab K, Landry SJ and Helfer SG (2005a). Goal activation, expectations, and the placebo effect. *Journal of Personality and Social Psychology*, **89**, 143–59.

Geers AL, Helfer SG, Kosbab K, Weiland PE and Landry SJ (2005b). Reconsidering the role of personality in placebo effects: dispositional optimism, situational expectations, and the placebo response. *Journal of Psychosomatic Research*, **58**, 121–7.

Geers AL, Kosbab K, Helfer SG, Weiland PE and Wellman JA (2007). Further evidence for individual differences in placebo responding: an interactionist perspective. *Journal of Psychosomatic Research,* **62**, 563–70.

Giang DW, Goodman AD, Schiffer RB, Mattson DH, Petrie M, Cohen N et al. (1996). Conditioning of cyclophosphamide-induced leukopenia in humans. *Journal of Neuropsychiatry and Clinical Neuroscience,* **8**, 194–201.

Goebel MU, Trebst AE, Steiner J, Xie YF, Exton MS, Frede S et al. (2002). Behavioral conditioning of immunosuppression is possible in humans. *FASEB Journal,* **16**, 1869–73.

Goebel MU, Hübell D, Kou W, Janssen OE, Katsarava Z, Limmroth V et al. (2005). Behavioural conditioning with interferon beta-1a in humans. *Physiology and Behavior,* **84**, 807–14.

Goebel MU, Meykadeh N, Kou W, Schedlowski M and Hengge UR (2009). Behavioral conditioning of antihistamine effects in patients with allergic rhinitis. *Psychotherapy and Psychosomatics,* **77**, 227–34.

Goffaux P, Redmond WJ, Rainville P and Marchand S (2007). Descending analgesia – when the spine echoes what the brain expects. *Pain,* **130**, 137–43.

Gorczynski RM (1990). Conditioned enhancement of skin allograft in mice. *Brain, Behavior, and Immunity,* **4**, 85–92.

Gorczynski RM, Macrae S and Kennedy M (1982). Conditioned immune response associated with allogeneic skin grafts in mice. *Journal of Immunology,* **129**, 704–9.

Gospic K, Gunnarsson T, Fransson P, Ingvar M, Lindefors N and Petrovic P (2008). Emotional perception modulated by an opioid and a cholecystokinin agonist. *Psychopharmacology,* **197**, 295–307.

Gracely RH, Dubner R, Wolskee PJ and Deeter WR (1983). Placebo and naloxone can alter postsurgical pain by separate mechanisms. *Nature,* **306**, 264–5.

Grevert P, Albert LH and Goldstein A (1983). Partial antagonism of placebo analgesia by naloxone. *Pain,***16**,129–43.

Grochowicz P, Schedlowski M, Husband AJ, King MG, Hibberd AD and Bowen KM (1991). Behavioral conditioning prolongs heart allograft survival in rats. *Brain, Behavior, and Immunity,* **5**, 349–56.

Herrnstein RJ (1962). Placebo effect in the rat. *Science,* **138**, 677–8.

Kalivas PW, Churchill L and Romanides A (1999). Involvement of the pallidal-thalamocortical circuit in adaptive behavior, *Annals of the New York Academy of Sciences,* **877**, 64–70.

Kamin LJ (1968). 'Attention-like' processes in classical conditioning. In: MR Jones, ed., *Miami symposium on the prediction of behavior: aversive stimulation,* pp. 9–31. University of Miami Press, Miami, FL.

Keltner, JR, Furst, A, Fan, C, Redfern, R, Inglis, B and Fields HL (2006). Isolating the modulatory effect of expectation on pain transmission: a functional magnetic imaging study. *Journal of Neuroscience,* **26**, 4437–43.

Kirk JM, Doty P and De Wit H (1998). Effects of expectancies on subjective responses to oral delta9-tetrahydrocannabinol. *Pharmacology, Biochemistry and Behavior,* **59**, 287–93.

Kirsch I (1985). Response expectancy as determinant of experience and behavior. *American Psychologist,* **40**, 1189–202.

—— (1990). *Changing expectations: a key to effective psychotherapy.* Brooks-Cole, Pacific Grove, CA.

—— (1999). *How expectancies shape experience.* American Psychological Association, Washington, DC.

Kirsch I, Lynn SJ, Vigorito M and Miller RR (2004). The role of cognition in classical and operant conditioning. *Journal of Clinical Psychology*, **60**, 369–92.

Kirschbaum C, Jabaaij L, Buske-Kirschbaum A, Hennig J, Blom M, Dorst K et al. (1992). Conditioning of drug-induced immunomodulation in human volunteers: a European collaborative study. *British Journal of Clinical Psychology*, **31**, 459–72

Klosterhalfen W and Klosterhalfen S (1983). Pavlovian conditioning of immunosuppression modifies adjuvant arthritis in rats. *Behavioral Neuroscience*, **97**, 663–6.

Kong J, Gollub RL, Rosman IS, Webb JM, Vangel MG, Kirsch I et al. (2006). Brain activity associated with expectancy-enhanced placebo analgesia as measured by functional magnetic resonance imaging. *Journal of Neuroscience*, **26**, 381–8.

Krack P, Kumar R, Ardouin C, Dowsey PL, McVicker JM, Benabid AL et al. (2001). Mirthful laughter induced by subthalamic nucleus stimulation. *Movement Disorders*, **16**, 867–75.

Lanotte M, Lopiano L, Torre E, Bergamasco B, Colloca L and Benedetti F (2005). Expectation enhances autonomic responses to stimulation of the human subthalamic limbic region. *Brain Behavior Immunity*, **19**, 500–9.

Laska E and Sunshine A (1973). Anticipation of analgesia a placebo effect. *Headache*, **13**, 1–11.

Last JM (1983). *A dictionary of epidemiology*. Oxford University Press, New York.

Leuchter AF, Cook IA, Witte EA, Morgan M and Abrams M (2002). Changes in brain function of depressed subjects during treatment with placebo. *Americal Journal of Psychiatry*, **159**, 122–9.

LeuchterAF, McCracken JT, Hunter AM, Cook IA and Alpert JE (2009). Monoamine oxidase a and catechol-o-methyltransferase functional polymorphisms and the placebo response in major depressive disorder. *Journal of Clinical Psychopharmacology*, **29**, 372–7.

Levine JD and Gordon NC (1984). Influence of the method of drug administration on analgesic response. *Nature*, **312**, 755–6.

Levine JD, Gordon NC and Fields HL (1978). The mechanisms of placebo analgesia. *Lancet*, **2**, 654–7.

Levine JD, Gordon NC, Smith R and Fields HL (1981). Analgesic responses to morphine and placebo in individuals with postoperative pain. *Pain*, **10**, 379–89.

Lichko AE (1959). Conditioned reflex hypoglycaemia in man. Pavlovian *Journal of High Nervous Activity*, **9**, 731–7.

Limousin P, Greene J, Pollak P, Rothwell J, Benabid AL and Frackowiak R (1997). Changes in cerebral activity pattern due to subthalamic nucleus or internal pallidum stimulation in Parkinson's disease. *Annals of Neurology*, **42**, 283–91.

Longo DL, Duffey PL, Kopp WC Heyes MP, Alvord WG, Sharfman WH et al. (1999). Conditioned immune response to interferon-γ in humans. *Clinical Immunology*, **90**, 173–81.

Lorenz J, Hauck M, Paur RC et al. (2005). Cortical correlates of false expectations during pain intensity judgments – a possible manifestation of placebo/nocebo cognitions. *Brain, Behavior and Immunity*, **19**, 283–95.

Lysle DT, Luecken LJ and Maslonek KA (1992). Suppression of the development of adjuvant arthritis by a conditioned aversive stimulus. *Brain, Behavior, and Immunity*, **6**, 64–73.

Marlatt GA, Demming B and Reid JB (1973). Loss of control drinking in alcoholics: an experimental analogue. *Journal Abnormal Psychology*, **81**, 223–41.

Matre D, Casey KL and Knardahl S (2006). Placebo-induced changes in spinal cord pain processing. *Journal of Neuroscience,* **26**, 559–63.

Mayberg HS, Silva JA, Brannan SK, Tekell JL, Mahurin RK, McGinnis S et al. (2002). The functional neuroanatomy of the placebo effect. *American Journal of Psychiatry,* **159**, 728–37.

McGlashan TH, Evans FJ and Orne MT (1969). The nature of hypnotic analgesia and placebo response to experimental pain. *Psychosomatic Medicine*, **31**, 227–46.

Mercado R, Constantoyannis C, Mandat T, Kumar A, Schulzer M, Stoessl AJ et al. (2006). Expectation and the placebo effect in Parkinson's disease patients with subthalamic nucleus deep brain stimulation. *Movement Disorders*, **21**, 1457–61.

Mitchell SH, Laurent CL and de Wit H (1996). Interaction of expectancy and the pharmacological effects of d-amphetamine: subjective effects and self-administration. *Psychopharmacology*, **125**, 371–8.

Mogenson GJ and Yang CA (1991). The contribution of basal forebrain to limbic-motor integration and the mediation of motivation to action. *Advances in Experimental Medicine and Biology*, **295**, 267–90.

Montgomery GH and Kirsch I (1997). Classical conditioning and the placebo effect. *Pain,* **72**, 107–13.

Morrell EM, Surwit RS, Kuhn CM, Feinglos MN and Cochrane C (1988). Classically conditioned enhancement of hyperinsulinemia in the ob/ob mouse. *Psychosomatic Medicine*, **50**, 586–90.

Morris AD, Esterly J, Chase G and Sharp GC (1976). Cyclophosphamide protection in NZB/NZW disease. *Arthritis and Rheumatism*, **19**, 49–55.

Olness K and Ader R (1992). Conditioning as an adjunct in the pharmacotherapy of lupus erythematosus. *Journal of Developmental and Behavioral Pediatrics*, **13**, 124–5.

Pacheco-Lopez G, Niemi MB, Kou W, Harting M, Fandrey J and Schedlowski M (2005). Neural substrates for behaviourally conditioned immunosuppression in the rat. *Journal of Neuroscience*, **25**, 2330–7.

Pacheco-Lopez G, Engler H, Niemi MB and Schedlowski M (2006). Expectations and associations that heal: immunomodulatory placebo effects and its neurobiology. *Brain, Behavior, and Immunity*, **20**, 430–46.

Pennebaker JW (1997). Writing about emotional experiences as a therapeutic process. *Psychological Science*, **8**, 162–6.

Petrovic P, Kalso E, Petersson KM and Ingvar M (2002). Placebo and opioid analgesia-imaging a shared neuronal network. *Science,* **295**, 1737–40.

Petrovic P, Dietrich T, Fransson P, Andersson J and Carlsson K (2005). Placebo in emotional processing-induced expectations of anxiety relief activate a generalized modulatory network. *Neuron,* **46**, 957–69.

Pollo A, Torre E, Lopiano L, Rizzone M, Lanotte M, Cavanna A et al. (2002). Expectation modulates the response to subthalamic nucleus stimulation in Parkinsonian patients. *Neuroreport,* **13**, 1383–6.

Pollo A, Carlino E and Benedetti F (2008). The top-down influence of ergogenic placebos on muscle work and fatigue. *European Journal of Neuroscience*, **28**, 379–88.

Price DD and Barrell JJ (2000). Mechanisms of analgesia produced by hypnosis and placebo suggestions. *Progress in Brain Research,* **122**, 255–71.

Price DD, Barrell JE and Barrell JJ (1985). A quantitative-experiential analysis of human emotions. *Motivation and Emotion,* **9**, 19–38.

Price DD, Riley J and Barrell JJ (2001). Are lived choices based on emotional processes? *Cognition and Emotion,* **15**, 365–79.

Price DD, Craggs J, Verne GN, Perlstein WM and Robinson ME (2007). Placebo analgesia is accompanied by large reductions in pain-related brain activity in irritable bowel syndrome patients. *Pain,* **127**, 63–72.

Price DD, Finniss DG and Benedetti F (2008). A comprehensive review of the placebo effect: recent advances and current thought. *Annual Review of Psychology,* **59**, 565–90.

Rainero I, Valfrè W, Savi L, Gentile S, Pinessi L, Gianotti L et al. (2001). Neuroendocrine effects of subcutaneous sumatriptan in patients with migraine. *Journal of Endocrinological Investigation,* **24**, 310–5.

Ramirez-Amaya V and Bermudez-Rattoni F (1999). Conditioned enhancement of antibody production is disrupted by insular cortex and amygdale but not hippocampal lesions. *Brain, Behavior, and Immunity,* **13**, 46–60.

Ramirez-Amaya V, Alvarez-Borda B, Ormsby C, Martinez R, Pèrez-Montfort R and Bermudez-Rattoni F (1996). Insular cortex lesions impair the acquisition of conditioned immunosuppression. *Brain, Behavior, and Immunity,* **10**, 103–14.

Ramirez-Amaya V, Alvarez-Borda B and Bermudez-Rattoni F (1998). Differential effects of NMDA-induced lesions into the insular cortex and amigdala on the acquisition and evocation of conditioned immunosuppression. *Brain, Behavior, and Immunity,* **12**, 149–60.

Reiss S (1980). Pavlovian conditioning and human fear: an expectancy model. *Behavioral Therapy,* **11**, 380–96.

Rescorla RA (1988). Pavlovian conditioning: it's not what you think it is. *American Psychologist,* **43**, 151–60.

Rescorla RA and Wagner AR (1972). A theory of Pavlovian conditioning: variation in the effectiveness of reinforcement and non-reinforcement. In: AH Black and WF Prokasy, eds, *Classical conditioning II: current theory and research,* pp. 65–99. Appleton Century Crofts, New York, NY.

Rohsenow DJ and Bachorowski J (1984). Effects of alcohol and expectancies on verbal aggression in men and women. *Journal Abnormal Psychology,* **93**, 418–32.

Ross S, Krugman AD, Lyerly SB and Clyde DJ (1962). Drugs and placebos: a model design. *Psychological Reports,* **10**, 383–92.

Schultz W (2006). Behavioral theories and the neurophysiology of reward. *Annual Review Psychology,* **57**, 87–115.

Scott DJ, Stohler CS, Egnatuk CM, Wang H, Koeppe RA and Zubieta J-K (2007). Individual differences in reward responding explain placebo-induced expectations and effects. *Neuron,* **55**, 325–36.

—— (2008). Placebo and nocebo effects are defined by opposite opioid and dopaminergic responses. *Archives of General Psychiatry,* **65**, 220–31.

Setlow B, Schoenbaum G and Gallagher M (2003). Neural encoding in ventral striatum during olfactory discrimination learning, *Neuron,* **38**, 625–36.

Siegel S (2002). Explanatory mechanisms for placebo effects: Pavlovian conditioning. In: HA Guess, A Kleinman, JW Kusek, LW Engel, eds, *The science of the placebo: toward an interdisciplinary research agenda*, pp. 133–57. BMJ Books, London.

Smith GR and McDaniels SM (1983). Psychologically mediated effect on the delayed hypersensitivity reaction to tuberculin in humans. *Psychosomatic Medicine*, **45**, 65–70.

St Clair Gibson A, Lambert EV, Rauch LH, Tucker R, Baden DA, Foster C et al. (2006). The role of information processing between the brain and peripheral physiological systems in pacing and perception of effort. *Sports Medicine*, **36**, 705–22.

Steinberg AD, Huston DP, Taurog JD, Cowdery JS and Raveche ES (1981). The cellular and genetic basis of murine lupus. *Immunology Reviews*, **55**, 121–54.

Stewart-Williams S and Podd J (2004). The placebo effect: dissolving the expectancy versus conditioning debate. *Psychological Bulletin*, **130**, 324–40.

Stockhorst U, Gritzmann E, Klopp K, Schottenfeld-Naor Y, Hübinger A, Berresheim HW et al. (1999). Classical conditioning of insulin effects in healthy humans. *Psychosomatic Medicine*, **61**, 424–35.

Stockhorst U, Steingruber HJ and Scherbaum WA (2000). Classically conditioned responses following repeated insulin and glucose administration in humans. *Behavioural Brain Research*, **110**, 143–59.

Strafella AP, Ko JH and Monchi O (2006). Therapeutic application of transcranial magnetic stimulation in Parkinson's disease: the contribution of expectation. *Neuroimage*, **31**, 1666–72.

Sunshine A, Laska E, Meisner M and Morgan S (1964). Analgesic studies of indomethacin as analyzed by computer techniques. *Clinical Pharmacology and Therapeutics*, **5**, 699–707.

Sutton SR (1991). Great expectations: some suggestions for applying the balanced placebo design to nicotine and smoking. *British Journal Addiction*, **86**, 659–62.

Theofilopoulos AN and Dixon FJ (1981). Etiopathogenesis of murine SLE. *Immunology Reviews*, **55**, 179–216.

Thomas KB (1987). General practice consultations: is there any point in being positive? *British Medical Journal*, **294**, 1200–2.

Tobler PN, Fiorillo CD and Schultz W (2005). Adaptive coding of reward value by dopamine neurons, *Science*, **307**, 1642–5.

Tolman EC (1932). *Purposive behavior in animals and men*. Appleton-Century-Crofts, New York.

Vase L, Robinson ME, Verne GN and Price DD (2005). Increased placebo analgesia over time in irritable bowel syndrome (IBS) patients is associated with desire and expectation but not endogenous opioid mechanisms. *Pain*, **115**, 338–47.

Volkow ND, Wang GJ, Ma Y, Fowler JS, Zhu W, Maynard L et al. (2003). Expectation enhances the regional brain metabolic and the reinforcing effects of stimulants in cocaine abusers. *Journal of Neuroscience*, **23**, 11461–8.

Volkow ND, Wang GJ, Ma Y, Fowler JS, Wong C, Jayne M et al. (2006). Effects of expectation on the brain metabolic responses to methylphenidate and to its placebo in non-drug abusing subjects. *Neuroimage*, **32**, 1782–92.

Voudouris NJ, Peck CL and Coleman G (1989). Conditioned response models of placebo phenomena: further support. *Pain*, **38**, 109–16.

—— (1990). The role of conditioning and verbal expectancy in the placebo response. *Pain*, **43**,121–28.

Waber RL, Shiv B, Carmon Z and Ariely D (2008). Commercial features of placebo and therapeutic efficacy. *Journal of American Medical Association*, **299**, 1016–7.

Wager TD, Matre D and Casey KL (2006). Placebo effects in laser-evoked pain potentials. *Brain Behavior and Immunity*, **20**, 219–30.

Wager TD, Rilling, JK, Smith EE, Sokolik A, Casey KL, Davidson RJ et al. (2004). Placebo-induced changes in fMRI in the anticipation and experience of pain. *Science*, **303**, 1162–6.

Walsh BT, Seidman SN, Sysko R and Gould M (2002). Placebo response in studies of major depression: variable, substantial, and growing. *Journal of the American Medical Association*, **287**, 1840–7.

Watson A, El-Dereby W, Vogt BA and Jones AK (2007). Placebo analgesia is not due to compliance or habituation: EEG and behavioural evidence. *Neuroreport*, **18**, 771–5.

Wheeler JA and Zurek H, eds (1983). *Quantum theory and measurement*. Princeton University Press, Princeton, NJ.

Whitehouse MW, Levy L and Beck FJ (1973). Effect of cyclophosphamide on a local graft-versus-host reaction in the rat: influence of sex, disease and different dosage regimens. *Agents and Actions*, **3**, 53–60.

Wilson GT, Niaura RS and Adler JL (1985). Alcohol: selective attention and sexual arousal in men. *Journal of Studies on Alcohol*, **46**, 107–15.

Woods SC (1972). Conditioned hypoglycemia: effect of vagotomy and pharmacological blockade. *American Journal of Physiology*, **223**, 1424–7.

Woods SC, Makous W and Hutton RA (1968). A new technique for conditioned hypoglycemia. *Psychonomic Science*, **10**, 389–90.

—— (1969). Temporal parameters of conditioned hypoglycemia. *Journal of Comparative Physiology and Psychology*, **69**, 301–7.

Woods SC, Alexander KR and Porte D Jr (1972). Conditioned insulin secretion and hypoglycemia following repeated injections of tolbutamide in rats. *Endocrinology*, **90**, 227–31.

Zubieta JK and Stohler CS (2009). Neurobiological mechanisms of placebo responses. *Annals of New York Academy of Science*, **1156**, 198–210.

Zubieta JK, Bueller JA, Jackson LR, Scott DJ, Xu Y, Koeppe RA et al. (2005). Placebo effects mediated by endogenous opioid activity on μ-opioid receptors. *Journal of Neuroscience*, **25**, 7754–62.

Zubieta JK, Smith YR, Bueller JA, Xu Y, Kilbourn MR, Jewett DM et al. (2001). Regional mu opioid receptor regulation
of sensory and affective dimensions of pain. *Science*, **293**, 311–5.

Chapter 7

The brain of the demented patient

Summary and relevance to the clinician

1) The purpose of this chapter is to describe the brain of the patient with dementia in relation to the doctor–patient relationship. The crucial point here is that the four steps that have been described throughout the book, i.e. 'feeling sick', 'seeking relief', 'meeting the therapist', and 'receiving the therapy' are all modified, or totally absent, in the demented patient. Whereas this is true in many medical conditions, like dementia, autism and vegetative state, and in some patients populations, like children, this chapter focuses on patients suffering from dementia as an example of the effects of impaired doctor–patient communication.

2) In relation to 'how the demented patient feels sick', different types of dementia may lead to changes in the perception of some symptoms. Most research has been performed in the field of pain. For example, patients with Alzheimer's disease can discriminate between a tactile and a painful stimulus, though their tolerance to pain is increased in some circumstances. Despite Alzheimer patients can recognize a painful stimulus, their autonomic responses to pain, such as heart rate and blood pressure, are blunted, thereby indicating that autonomic assessment is not reliable to understand whether a demented patient feels pain or not.

3) Patients with vascular dementia may experience pain in a completely different way. In fact, subcortical ischemic vascular dementia with white matter lesions may lead to hyperalgesia, which is attributable to deafferentation of the cortex, because of the interruption of thalamocortical pathways.

4) Frontotemporal dementia with hypoperfusion of frontal and temporal lobes leads to reduced pain perception. This is mainly due to the heavy neuronal degeneration and malfunctioning of the frontal lobes which play a critical role in the awareness of pain and in the global experience of pain.

5) As to 'seeking relief', the demented patient does not have a purposive behavioural repertoire that is aimed at seeking a doctor for relieving his

own symptoms. Dementia has a powerful impact on cognitive functions, thus the demented patient does not have expectations of future rewards, for example, of future positive therapeutic outcomes, as we have seen in Chapter 4.

6) Similarly, in 'meeting the therapist' the cognitively impaired patient cannot interact with health professionals. All the complex functions that have been analysed in Chapter 5, such as trust and hope, are not present in dementia, thus they do not take part in the doctor–patient relationship. As in any condition whereby communication is not present, the central point of the interaction is based on the doctor's inference of the symptoms through observation. This is done through the use of observation scales that are aimed at understanding the suffering and the needs of the demented non-communicative patient.

7) As far as 'receiving the therapy' is concerned, there is compelling evidence that demented patients are undertreated in the presence of painful conditions. This is attributable to several factors, including impaired communication. In other words, although the demented patient may suffer from a painful condition, he is not able to communicate his own suffering.

8) When undergoing a therapeutic intervention, placebo and expectation effects are reduced, or even absent, in Alzheimer patients. This is due to the disruption of prefrontal executive functions and to the functional disconnection of the prefrontal lobes from the rest of the brain. The disruption of placebo and expectation mechanisms underscores the need of considering a possible revision of some therapies in Alzheimer patients in order to compensate for this disruption.

9) As the prefrontal cortex can be severely affected in other neurodegenerative conditions, the neuroanatomical localization of placebo- and expectation-related mechanisms in prefrontal regions should alert us to the potential disruption of placebo and expectation mechanisms in all those conditions whereby the prefrontal lobes are involved.

10) In relation to the disruption of placebo responses in a clinical condition such as Alzheimer's disease, there is today compelling evidence that the experimental inactivation of prefrontal functioning in the laboratory setting in healthy subjects disrupts the placebo response. In fact, blockade of opioid neurotransmission in the prefrontal cortex or its inactivation by means of transcranial magnetic stimulation abolish placebo responsiveness. Therefore, if there is no prefrontal control, there is no placebo response.

7.1 Many patients cannot communicate their discomfort

7.1.1 Who cannot communicate

There are a variety of conditions in which communication is impaired, thus the doctor–patient interaction is lost. A situation of this kind is of particular interest because the four steps that have been described throughout this volume are not present, i.e. 'feeling sick', 'seeking relief', 'meeting the therapist', and 'receiving the therapy'. It goes without saying that one of these conditions is represented by newborns and children, or otherwise by patients who are in coma or in a vegetative state. These patients may feel sick and seek relief differently. For example, children may exaggerate pain while coma patients may not respond to pain at all. Likewise, newborns and children may seek relief through the contact with their parents, while vegetative state patients may seek relief by adopting specific postures as well as behavioural repertoires. Needless to say, this kind of patients neither meet the therapist with a conscious act nor expect any benefit from the treatment that is being administered. There is no real relationship among these patients and doctors, thus they will not be discussed further in this volume.

There are many other conditions in which communication is impaired. In all the conditions with impaired cognition, the lack of an adequate doctor–patient interaction raises major clinical and ethical problems. Very often it is not clear what the patient actually feels, and this lack of understanding poses important clinical dilemmas, particularly as far as the therapy is concerned. For example, in some autistic children self-injurious behaviour is common but its meaning is not clear at all. Does the autistic child feel pain due to self-injury? Or, rather, is self-injury behaviour triggered by an altered sensory input? The therapeutic dilemma is emphasized by the several attempts to prevent self-injury. For example, opioid antagonists, both naloxone and naltrexone, have been used on the ground that self-injury might be due to endorphin-induced anaesthesia (Barrett et al. 1989; Walters et al. 1990). Thus, it was supposed that by blocking endorphins with naloxone, the autistic child would feel pain and would inhibit the self-injurious behaviour. The unclear therapeutic outcomes underscore the important clinical and ethical dilemma of interacting with the non-communicative patient.

One of the most studied medical conditions in which impaired communication leads to altered symptom perception and impaired doctor–patient interaction is dementia. The four steps 'feeling sick', 'seeking relief', 'meeting the therapist', and 'receiving the therapy' are all impaired, and several attempts to understand how they are impaired have been made. Therefore, this chapter is about the brain of the demented patient only, which is representative of many other less-known conditions in which the patient's communication is impaired.

7.1.2 **Dementia is a major medical problem**

Dementia affects about 7% of the general population above 65 years and 30% of the population older than 80 years (Robertson et al. 1989; Hofman et al. 1991; Rocca et al. 1991; White et al. 1996; Lobo et al. 2000). More than 50% is represented by Alzheimer's disease, about 30% by vascular dementia, and the remaining 20% includes other types of dementia, like frontotemporal dementia, Parkinson's disease, dementia with Lewy bodies, sporadic and variant Creutzfeldt-Jakob disease.

Dementia is a major medical problem for several reasons. For example, the increased age of the population in western societies is invariably associated with the risk of developing a type of dementia, and this poses several clinical and social problems, such as caregiving and hospice organization. The increased risk of developing dementia is also associated to new and so far unrecognized clinical problems. For example, ample evidence shows that ageing is associated with a high rate of painful conditions, regardless of cognitive status (Horgas and Elliott 2004). Thus the number of patients with dementia who will experience painful conditions is likely to increase. This raises a crucial question, i.e. whether and how patients with dementia perceive pain. Patients with dementia may express their pain in ways that are quite different from those of elderly people without dementia (Herr and Decker 2004). Particularly in the more severe stages of dementia, the complexity and consequent inadequacy of pain assessment may lead to the undertreatment of pain (Scherder et al. 2005, 2009).

Within the context of this volume, that is, by considering the four steps 'feeling sick', 'seeking relief', 'meeting the therapist', and 'receiving the therapy', a better understanding of some of these aspects has been achieved in the past few years. In particular, how the demented patient feels sick and how he reacts to the therapeutic act has furnished important information for both assessment and management of pain.

7.2 **How the demented patient feels sick**

7.2.1 **The lateral and medial pain systems are affected differently in Alzheimer's disease**

Dementia of the Alzheimer's type is the best-known condition whereby pain processing has been investigated. As we have seen in section 3.2, pain is one of the most common symptoms and, moreover, its sensory pathways, mechanisms and pathophysiology are better understood compared to other symptoms, like nausea, vomiting, fatigue, tiredness, and the like. Therefore, it is not surprising that pain has been investigated in some detail in different types of dementia.

Alzheimer's disease is particularly interesting to be investigated in this regard because of the pattern of neuronal degeneration. In fact, the lateral and medial pain systems are affected differently (see section 3.2 for a detailed description of the pain systems). Both the primary somatosensory cortex and some thalamic nuclei, which belong to the lateral pain system, are relatively unaffected by the histological changes that characterize Alzheimer's disease (Farrell et al. 1996; Rudelli et al. 1984), thus indicating that a preserved sensory-discriminative function should be expected. By contrast, the intralaminar thalamic nuclei, which represent an important component of the affective/emotional medial pain system, are early and progressively affected by the Alzheimer's disease-related cellular pathology (Rub et al. 2002). Therefore, the emotional-affective function should be expected to be affected, as also suggested by the conspicuous neuronal and synaptic loss in the prefrontal and limbic regions (Mountjoy et al. 1983; Hyman et al. 1984; Scheff and Price 2001).

In a detailed study on the dynamics of grey matter loss in Alzheimer's disease, Thompson et al. (2003) observed three main features. First, the heaviest neuronal loss is found in the temporal and frontal regions. Second, the left hemisphere degenerates faster than the right and this asymmetric loss rate increases the existing asymmetry in cortical grey matter found in healthy elderly subjects. Third, some regions, particularly the sensorimotor regions, are spared late in the disease. Figure 7.1 shows the pattern of neuronal degeneration in the Alzheimer patient. It can be seen that, whereas the frontal, temporal, and medial portions are heavily affected, there is a relative sparing of the sensorimotor cortices both at the initial stage and after 1.5 years. In general, virtually all the regions that belong to the medial pain system are affected by Alzheimer's disease, whereas the regions of the lateral pain system, like the primary somatosensory cortex, are preserved (Scherder et al. 2003a).

As expected from this pattern of degeneration, several studies have found a dissociation between the sensory-discriminative component of pain, which is processed in the lateral pain system, and the affective-emotional component, which is processed in the medial system. For example, some studies aimed at assessing pain thresholds in demented patients did not reveal significant differences compared with normal subjects, suggesting that the sensory-discriminative component of pain is preserved in dementia (Cornu 1975; Jonsson et al. 1977). In addition, Porter et al. (1996) found altered heart rate responses prior to, during, and following venipuncture in elderly patients with poor cognitive abilities and in demented patients, indicating altered emotional responses. Although these studies may suggest some possible differences in pain processing in the lateral and medial system in demented patients, they were not aimed at addressing this issue.

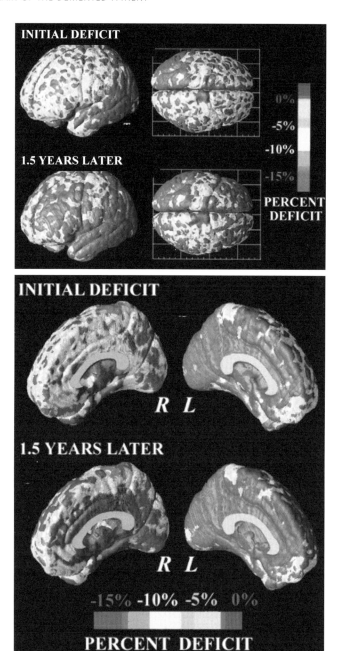

Fig 7.1 Average percentage loss of grey matter in Alzheimer's disease. Note the heavy loss in the frontal and temporal regions (top panel) as well of the medial portion of the hemispheres (bottom panel). Also note the asymmetric deficits and the relative sparing of the sensorimotor regions with virtually no grey matter loss (blue). See colour plate 16. Source: From Thompson et al. 2003 with permission from the Society for Neuroscience, Copyright 2003.

A systematic and detailed analysis of pain processing started with the study by Benedetti et al. (1999), which was specifically designed to investigate sensory and affective components of pain in patients with a diagnosis of probable or possible Alzheimer's disease based on the NINCDS-ADRDA criteria, as proposed by McKhann et al. (1984), thus limiting the investigation of pain to a restricted population of demented patients. In this study, Benedetti et al. (1999) tested both pain thresholds and pain tolerance in Alzheimer patients by means of phasic and tonic noxious stimuli. In the first case, electrical stimulation was used, whereas in the second case experimental arm ischemia was studied. By comparing Alzheimer patients with normal subjects of the same age, no difference was found in stimulus detection and pain thresholds, whereas a clear-cut increase in pain tolerance was present in Alzheimer patients. Furthermore, the severity of the disease was assessed by means of the Mini Mental State Examination test (MMSE) and the spectral analysis of the electroencephalogram. The authors found a straightforward correlation between MMSE scores and pain tolerance, such that the more severe the cognitive impairment was, the higher was the tolerance to pain. The analysis of the electroencephalographic power spectra indicated that patients with low alpha and high delta peaks showed an increase in pain tolerance to both electrical stimulation and ischemia. Therefore, whereas the sensory-discriminative component of pain was maintained in Alzheimer patients, pain tolerance was altered and depended on cognitive and affective factors.

In a subsequent study by the same group (Rainero et al. 2000), the effects of electrical noxious stimulation on the autonomic nervous system of Alzheimer's disease patients were analysed. To do this, electrical stimuli at two different intensities were used, just above pain threshold and twice pain threshold, and heart rate and systolic blood pressure were recorded. When a pain stimulus just above threshold was delivered, Alzheimer patients were found to have blunted autonomic responses compared to controls of the same age. Similarly, pre-stimulus expectation produced a less pronounced increase of the responses in Alzheimer patients compared to the controls. However, when the painful stimulus was increased to twice the pain threshold, the systolic blood pressure increase of Alzheimer patients did not differ from the controls, whereas heart rate increase was still slightly diminished. By contrast, pain perception was similar in the two groups when the stimulus was at pain threshold, whereas it was blunted in Alzheimer patients when the stimulus was twice the pain threshold. Therefore, in Alzheimer patients, a mild noxious stimulation produces blunted autonomic responses and normal pain perception, whereas strong noxious stimulation produces quasi-normal autonomic responses and blunted pain perception, which indicates that Alzheimer patients have an increased threshold for both autonomic activation and pain tolerance.

A detailed correlation between these changes in pain responses and different degrees of cognitive impairment was performed by Benedetti et al. (2004), who studied patients with Alzheimer's disease whose cognitive status was assessed through the MMSE test and whose brain electrical activity was measured by means of quantitative electroencephalography. After assessment of both cognitive impairment and brain electrical activity deterioration, these patients underwent sensory measurements in which the minimum stimulus intensity for both stimulus detection and pain sensation was determined. In addition, heart rate responses to pain threshold X 1.5 were recorded. Neither stimulus detection nor pain threshold were found to be correlated to cognitive status and brain electrical activity decline. Conversely, a correlation between heart rate responses and deterioration of both cognitive functions and brain electrical activity was found. In particular, the heart rate increase after pain stimulation was correlated to the presence of slow brain electrical activity (delta and theta frequencies), and this correlation was also found for the anticipatory heart rate increase just before pain stimulation. Therefore, pain anticipation and reactivity depend on both the cognitive status and the frequency bands of the electroencephalogram, whereas both stimulus detection and pain threshold are not affected by the progression of Alzheimer's disease. These findings indicate that, whereas the sensory-discriminative components of pain are preserved even in advanced stages of Alzheimer's disease, the cognitive and affective functions, which are related to both anticipation and autonomic reactivity, are severely affected.

An example of an Alzheimer patient with mild-moderate cognitive impairment (MMSE = 21/30) and normal electroencephalographic pattern is shown in Fig 7.2. In A the distribution of delta, theta, alpha-1, alpha-2, beta-1, beta-2 bands (relative power) is represented on a 3D reconstruction of a standard head volume. It can be seen that this patient showed a normal electroencephalographic pattern with a peak in the alpha-1 domain in the occipital and posterior parietal regions. In Fig 7.2B the global relative power spectrum, obtained by averaging all the 19 channels, shows the peak in the alpha-1 range and the lack of low frequencies below 8 Hz. Figure 7.2C shows that heart rate increased after the warning (anticipation of pain) and after the delivery of the pain stimulus. This increase was about 7% and 18%, respectively. The stimulus detection and the pain threshold of this patient was 3 mA and 19 mA, respectively. An example of a patient with severe cognitive impairment (MMSE = 9/30) and an abnormal electroencephalographic pattern is shown in Fig 7.3. In A, it can be seen that the low frequencies (delta and theta bands) were distributed in the frontal, parietal, and temporal regions, whereas a small alpha-1 activity was present in the occipital region. Figure 7.3B shows the mean relative power

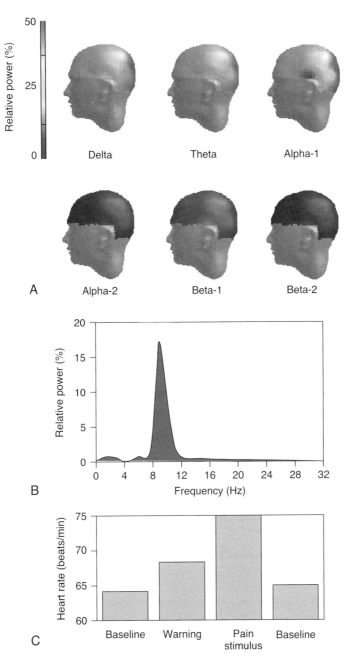

Fig 7.2 Alzheimer patient with mild-moderate cognitive impairment (MMSE = 21), and with stimulus detection = 3 mA, and pain threshold = 19 mA. (A) 3D mapping of the distribution of the relative powers of the delta, theta, alpha-1, alpha-2, beta-1, and beta-2 bands over the scalp. (B) Mean relative power spectrum obtained by averaging the relative powers of all the 19 electrodes. (C) Heart rate responses to warning (pain anticipation) and to pain stimulation. Note the normal electroenephalogram with an alpha-1 peak in the occipital and posterior parietal region, and the heart rate response to both warning and pain. See colour plate 17.

Source: From Benedetti et al. 2004 with permission from the International Association for the Study of Pain, Copyright 2004.

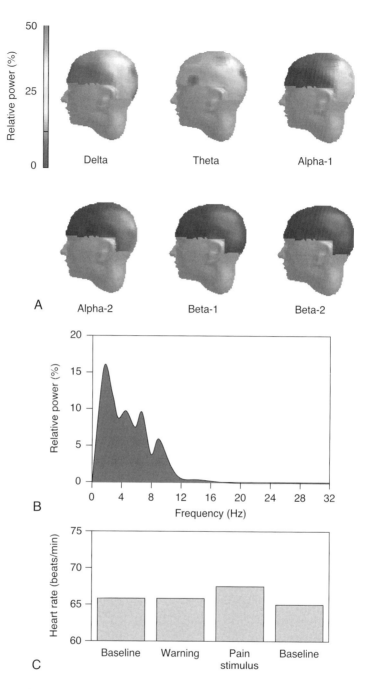

Fig 7.3 As in Fig 7.2, but this Alzheimer patient has severe cognitive impairment (MMSE =9), and stimulus detection = 4 mA, and pain threshold = 20 mA. Note the distribution of the delta and theta frequencies on the frontal, temporal, and parietal regions, and the small alpha-1 activity in the occipital region (A). Also note the prevalence of delta and theta rhythms (below 8 Hz) in the spectrum (B), the absence of the heart rate response to warning and the small heart rate response to pain (C). See colour plate 18.

Source: From Benedetti et al. 2004 with permission from the International Association for the Study of Pain, Copyright 2004.

spectrum averaged across all 19 electrodes, in which it is possible to see that the low frequencies below 8 Hz prevailed. Figure 7.3C shows that in this patient no anticipatory heart rate increase occurred (following the warning), and that the pain-induced heart rate increase was very small (about 3%). The stimulus detection and the pain threshold of this patient was 4 mA and 20 mA, respectively, that is, not different from the patient with mild cognitive impairment of Fig 7.2.

The two patients of Figs 7.2 and 7.3 are two representative patients who clearly show that stimulus detection and pain threshold do not depend on the degree of cognitive impairment and brain electrical activity deterioration, whereas autonomic responses do. In the study by Benedetti et al. (2004), this was true for all the patients who were examined. Figure 7.4 shows the regression analysis and correlation between the MMSE and stimulus intensity (A), and MMSE and heart rate change (B). In A it can be seen that neither stimulus detection nor pain threshold depended on the MMSE scores. By contrast, Fig 7.4B shows that a highly significant positive correlation was present between MMSE and heart rate increase in pain anticipation, and between MMSE and heart rate increase after painful stimulation. Thus, stimulus detection and pain threshold were not correlated with cognitive impairment, whereas heart rate increases after warning and after pain were positively correlated with cognitive status.

Therefore, whereas severely cognitively impaired individuals may show blunted autonomic responses, they can still distinguish a painful from a tactile stimulus. Needless to say, this is very important in clinical practice, for blunted autonomic responses do not mean increased pain thresholds. In other words, autonomic responses cannot be taken as a reliable index of pain perception.

It is also worth pointing out that the severity of the disease is likely to impact dramatically on the functioning of the medial and lateral pain system. For example, Cole et al. (2006) measured pain ratings and brain responses by means of functional magnetic resonance imaging following mechanical pressure stimulation in patients in the early stages of Alzheimer's disease (mean MMSE = 19.4). They found that activity in the medial and lateral pain pathways was preserved in Alzheimer patients, and was similar to that in the controls. Therefore, in the early stages of the disease, both pain systems show a normal functioning, which points to the importance of the severity of cognitive impairment when assessing pain perception.

7.2.2 Vascular dementia may be associated to hyperalgesia

In contrast to Alzheimer's disease, in which the degeneration pattern is constant, vascular dementia is a highly heterogeneous disorder. In fact, the

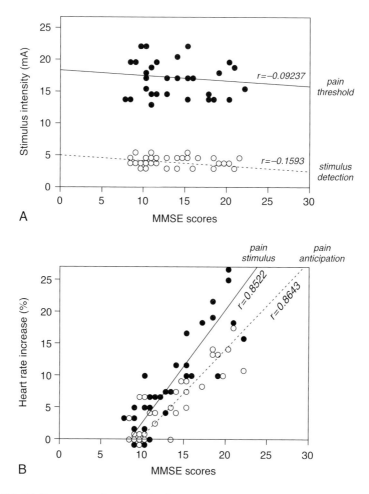

Fig 7.4 (A) Linear regression analysis of MMSE scores versus stimulus detection (white circles, broken line) and pain threshold (black circles, bold line). (B) Linear regression analysis of MMSE scores versus heart rate response to anticipation of pain (white circles, broken line) and to pain stimulation (black circles, bold line). Note that whereas stimulus detection and pain threshold do not depend on the severity of cognitive impairment, as assessed by means of MMSE, autonomic responses are smaller when cognitive impairment is more severe.
Source: From Benedetti et al. 2004 with permission from the International Association for the Study of Pain, Copyright 2004.

vascular lesions can be localized in different regions and, accordingly, may produce different effects on pain perception. Therefore, it is not possible to generalize how a patient with vascular dementia perceives pain. None the less, it is interesting to note that vascular dementia is characterized by white matter lesions in most cases (Romàn et al. 2002; O'Brien et al. 2003; Scherder et al. 2003a). As shown in Fig 7.5, a lesion in the white matter interrupts afferent pathways, for example the thalamocortical projections, and may cause a deafferentation syndrome with hyperalgesia.

There is some clinical evidence that hyperalgesia may indeed be present in vascular dementia. For example, Scherder et al. (2003b) found that vascular dementia patients show an increase in pain affect in a variety of painful conditions, such as arthrosis, arthritis, osteoporosis, bone fractures and diabetic neuropathy. In a different study on white matter hyperintensities, Oosterman et al. (2006) found that periventricular hyperintensities were the strongest predictors of increase in pain affect but not of pain intensity. This increase may be attributable to a deafferented cortex (see also Scherder et al. 2003a, 2005). Therefore, patients with vascular dementia may feel pain differently, with an increase in its affective/emotional component.

7.2.3 Frontotemporal dementia leads to reduced pain responses

In frontotemporal dementia, a heavy degeneration of the frontal and temporal lobes occurs. As the frontal lobes play a central role in pain processing, the global experience of pain should be expected to be altered. Indeed, in one study, Bathgate et al. (2001) compared a wide array of behavioural changes in Alzheimer's disease, vascular dementia, and frontodemporal dementia. Loss of

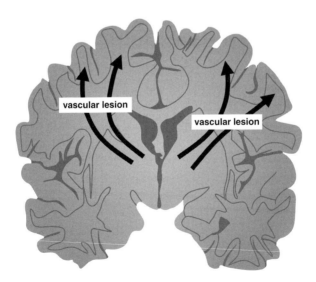

Fig 7.5 Subcortical vascular lesions in the white matter may interrupt afferent pathways, and may induce a deafferentation syndrome with hyperalgesia.

pain awareness was included among the behavioural disturbances best able to discriminate frontotemporal dementia from other types of dementia. In another study, Snowden et al. (2001) compared semantic dementia, a variant of frontotemporal dementia, with the apathetic and the disinhibited forms of frontotemporal dementia. It was found that loss of pain awareness was quite frequent, with a peak of 45% in the apathetic form. In addition, more than half semantic dementia patients showed exaggerated responses to pain and other sensory stimuli.

In contrast to these clinical studies, a more recent study examined pain processing in frontotemporal dementia patients in the experimental setting (Carlino et al. 2010). Both pain threshold and pain tolerance were assessed. If the patients were selected on the basis of the neuropsychological diagnosis, as assessed by means of the Frontal Assessment Battery test, they showed increased pain threshold but normal pain tolerance. Conversely, if the patients were selected on the basis of frontotemporal hypoperfusion, as assessed by means of Single Positron Emission Computerized Tomography (SPECT), pain tolerance was increased as well. Since pain threshold is a sensory-discriminative aspect of pain sensation, which is mediated by the lateral pain system, while pain tolerance represents the emotional aspect of pain, which is mediated by the medial pain system (see sections 3.2 and 7.2.1), this study suggests that hypoperfusion analysis can detect more specific changes compared to neuropsychological analysis. Figure 7.6 shows two SPECT images from two different frontotemporal dementia patients, one with frontal hypoperfusion (left), the other with frontal and anterior temporal hypoperfusion (right). An increase in pain tolerance may better reflect these neuroanatomical changes, with the disruption of the medial pain system, including the anterior cingulate cortex, the insula, and the prefrontal cortex, all of which show atrophy in frontotemporal dementia (Rosen et al. 2002).

7.3 The demented patient cannot seek relief

7.3.1 Purposive behaviour is impaired in dementia

Needless to say, the patient who suffers from dementia cannot seek relief, with the exception of some behavioural repertoires that are more automatic than purposive. For example, the severely demented patient can adopt some postures that aim to reduce pain, and can seek the contact with other people and even with objects. Of course, the degree of cognitive impairment plays a key role in this sense, and the amount of either automatic or purposive behaviours that the demented patient adopts very much depend on his cognitive status. In general, however, the demented patient does not have a purposive behavioural

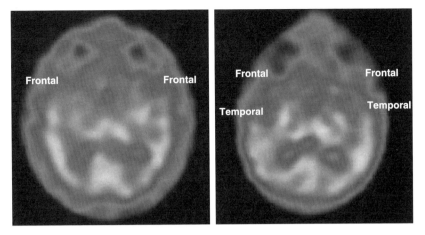

Fig 7.6 Single Photon Emission Computerized Tomography (SPECT) of two fronto-temporal dementia patients who show hypoperfusion of the frontal lobes (patient on the left), and frontal and anterior temporal lobes (patient on the right). Both patients show increased pain threshold and pain tolerance. See colour plate 19.

repertoire that is aimed at seeking a doctor for relieving his own symptoms, such as pain. Dementia has a powerful impact on cognitive functions, thus the demented patient does not have expectations of future rewards, for example, of future positive therapeutic outcomes, as we have seen in Chapter 4.

In different types of dementia, such as Alzheimer's disease, subcortical ischemic vascular dementia, frontotemporal dementia, the functions of the frontal, and particularly the prefrontal lobes are severely impaired. The set of frontal functions that control purposive behaviour are named executive functions, or executive control. Frontal executive functions control volition, planning, pro-gramming, anticipation, inhibition of inappropriate behaviours, and monitor-ing of complex goal-directed, purposeful activities (Wolfe et al. 1990; Cummings 1993; Romàn and Royall 1999; Royall 2000; Romàn et al. 2002). The impair-ment of frontal lobes implies the loss of executive control, with the disruption of planning capacity, working memory, attention, stimuli discrimination, abstrac-tion, and capacity of initiating the required behaviour (Romàn et al. 2002).

Not only are executive functions related to the functioning of the frontal lobes, but also to subcortical regions that belong to cortical-subcortical loops (Cummings 1993). For example, dementia affecting the striatum, globus pallidus, thalamus and white matter may interrupt prefrontal-subcortical loops that are involved in executive control. In addition, it should be noted that these cortical-subcortical loops also involve the limbic system, thereby influencing emotional behaviour as well, like uninhibited behaviours and impulsivity

(Romàn et al. 2002). Therefore, it is not surprising that motivational and reward behaviours may be profoundly affected by different types of dementia.

7.4 **The demented patient meets the therapist**

7.4.1 **There is no real interaction between the demented patient and the doctor**

It goes without saying that the cognitively impaired patient cannot interact with his therapist. All the complex functions that have been analysed in Chapter 5, such as trust and hope, are not present in dementia, thus they do not take part in the doctor–patient relationship. As in any condition whereby communication is not present, the central point of the interaction is based on the doctor's inference of the symptoms from observation.

In clinical practice, self-report pain rating scales are administered to patients who can still communicate about their pain. These scales generally target only the sensory-discriminative aspects of pain (that is, presence and intensity), instead of the important motivational/affective aspects (Horgas and Elliott 2004). For example, verbal, visual, and numerical rating scales are often used in communicative patients, but they can hardly be considered reliable in all conditions, for a symptom like pain can change from patient to patient and in different types of dementia (see section 7.2 and Scherder et al. 2005, 2009).

The approach is completely different, and is actually a challenge in medical practice, when communication is lacking. In fact, pain assessment in non-communicative patients relies primarily on observation scales (Herr and Decker 2004). Such scales may provide information about the motivational-affective aspects of pain, as shown by both physiological signs (e.g. frequency of breathing) and physical signs (e.g. facial expressions). One disadvantage of typical observation scales is the necessary assumption that signs that are normally indicative of pain (such as guarding, bracing, moaning) are also representative of pain in elderly patients with dementia. This assumption is doubtful, however, given the identification of less obvious or atypical behavioural presentations in some people with dementia. For example, 'absence of a relaxed body posture', one of the items of the discomfort scale-dementia of Alzheimer type (DSDAT), may also be a reflection of the extrapyramidal symptoms that can occur in Alzheimer's disease (Caligiuri et al. 2001). On the other hand, assessing for pain only with tools that include typical pain behaviours but do not recognize subtle behaviours and changes in usual activities may result in under-recognition of pain in this population.

Assessing autonomic responses does not seem to be useful, as these responses do not provide an accurate reflection of the perceived intensity of pain.

We have seen in section 7.2.1 that Alzheimer patients show reduced autonomic responses but they can still distinguish between tactile and painful stimuli, thus indicating that pain perception is hardly related to autonomic responsiveness (Benedetti et al. 1999; Rainero et al. 2000; Benedetti et al. 2004).

Interestingly, caregiving can cause pathology. Both professional and lay carers of dementia patients have high rates of physical and mental disorders (Brodaty and Hadzi-Pavlovic 1990; Schultz and Williamson 1997; Ritchie and Lovestone 2002). In addition, high rates of abuse both of and by the demented patient have been found (Homer and Gilleard 1990; Pillemer and Suitor 1992; Cahill and Shapiro 1993). Therefore, the stress-inducing interaction with the demented patient may have a substantial impact on the carer, and this represents an important and timely major social problem. This issue is of particular interest because it shows that a bad, stress-inducing interaction between the demented patient and the health professional can cause behavioural changes and pathology even in the latter. Little, if any, is known about the biological changes that occur during this negative interaction, and this should stimulate future research in this direction.

7.5 How the demented patient responds to treatments

7.5.1 Demented patients are often undertreated for their symptoms such as pain

There is compelling evidence that patients with dementia and who suffer from a painful condition receive less treatment than non-demented patients (Scherder et al. 2005, 2009). In one study, demented patients recovering from hip fracture surgery received only 1/3 the amount of morphine sulphate equivalents administered to non-demented adults, and 76% of demented patients had no standing order for post-operative analgesia (Morrison and Siu 2000). In another study, only 33% of Alzheimer patients received appropriate analgesic medication compared to 64% of non-demented adults and this was true for non-steroidal anti-inflammatory drugs (NSAIDs) as well as other classes of analgesics (e.g. opioids), even though the need for pain relief was judged equivalent according to the treating physician (Scherder and Bouma 1997). Likewise, Parkinson's disease is characterized by chronic pain, but only part of the patients receive analgesics (Négre-Pagés et al. 2008). These findings suggest undertreatment of pain. The risk for undertreatment of pain is further enhanced in non-communicative patients with white matter lesions, as these may cause an increase in the suffering due to deafferentiation (see section 7.2.2).

There might be several causes for pain undertreatment in patients with dementia (Scherder et al. 2005, 2009). For example, recognizing pain and suffering is not always easy in the demented patient, due to the lack of specificity of several assessment scales (see section 7.4.1). The lack of communication and the impaired doctor–patient relationship plays a critical role in this sense.

7.5.2 Placebo and expectation effects are reduced in Alzheimer's disease

The hidden administration of a medical treatment reduces or completely abolishes the efficacy of the treatment itself (see section 6.2.1). This is due to the lack of the patient's expectations about the outcome when a therapy is given covertly (unexpectedly). A natural situation whereby expectations are absent is represented by clinical conditions in which cognitive impairment is present. For example, in Alzheimer's disease, there is an impairment of prefrontal executive control. This executive control by the prefrontal regions has been found to be correlated with specific areas, for example, abstract reasoning with dorsolateral frontal regions and inhibitory control with orbital and medial frontal areas (Berman et al. 1995; Nagahama et al. 1996; Rolls et al. 1996; Konishi et al. 1998, 1999a, b). Interestingly, similar regions have been found to be activated by placebo-induced expectation of benefit, such as pain reduction (Petrovic et al. 2002; Wager et al. 2004; Zubieta et al. 2005). Alzheimer's disease is known to severely affect the frontal lobes, with a neuronal degeneration in those areas involved in the placebo analgesic effect, for example, the dorsolateral prefrontal cortex, the orbitofrontal cortex, and the anterior cingulate cortex (Thompson et al. 2003).

By taking all these aspects into account, administration of therapies to patients with prefrontal impairment and administrations of hidden therapies

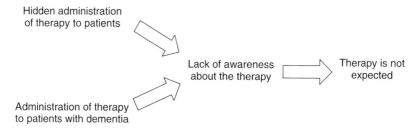

Fig 7.7 The hidden administration of a therapy to non-demented patients and the normal administration of a therapy to demented patients have a common characteristic, i.e. in both cases there is a lack of awareness about the therapy. In other words, in both cases the patients do not know that a therapy is being administered, in the first case because the therapy is given covertly, in the second case because there is cognitive impairment. Therefore, in both cases the therapy is unexpected.

to non-demented patients should be expected to produce the same effects, as shown in Fig 7.7. In other words, the hidden administration of a therapy to non-demented patents and the normal open administration of a therapy (in full view) to demented patients have a common feature, that is, in both cases there is a lack of awareness about the therapy. In fact, in both cases the patients do not know that a therapy is being administered, in the first case because the therapy is given unbeknownst to the patient, in the second case because there is cognitive impairment. Thus, in both cases the therapy is unexpected.

Benedetti et al. (2006) studied Alzheimer patients at the initial stage of the disease and after one year. They were treated with either open (expected) or hidden (unexpected) local lidocaine to reduce pain following venipuncture, in order to see whether the placebo component of the therapy, which is represented by the difference between the overt and covert application, was affected by the disease. In this study, the placebo component of the analgesic therapy was correlated with both cognitive status, as assessed by means of the Frontal Assessment Battery (FAB) test, and functional connectivity among different brain regions, as assessed by means of electroencephalographic connectivity analysis. In fact, it was found that Alzheimer patients with reduced FAB scores showed reduced placebo component of the analgesic treatment. In addition, the disruption of the placebo component occurred when reduced connectivity of the prefrontal lobes with the rest of the brain was present (Fig 7.8). The loss of these placebo-related mechanisms reduced the overall effectiveness of the treatment (lidocaine), and indeed a dose increase was necessary to produce adequate analgesia.

This was the first study showing that a disruption of the placebo-psychological component of a treatment may occur in a clinical condition that affects the brain, specifically the prefrontal lobes, and that the loss of these prefrontal expectation-related mechanisms makes an analgesic treatment less effective. According to this view, the impairment of prefrontal connectivity would reduce the communication between the prefrontal lobes and the rest of the brain, so that no placebo and expectation mechanisms would be triggered.

There are at least two important clinical implications that emerge from the disruption of placebo and expectation mechanisms in Alzheimer's disease. First, the reduced efficacy of the open analgesic treatment with lidocaine underscores the need of considering a possible revision of some therapies in Alzheimer patients in order to compensate for the loss of placebo- and expectation-related mechanisms. By considering that many of these patients are likely to show severe impairment of the prefrontal lobes, and thus a loss of placebo- and expectation-related mechanisms, low doses of analgesics can be totally inadequate to relieve any kind of pain. Therefore, the analgesic

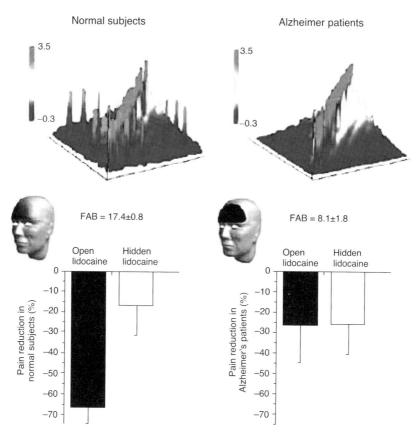

Fig 7.8 Correlation between electroencephalographic connectivity analysis (assessed by means of 'mutual information analysis': top panel), cognitive status (assessed by means of Frontal Assessment Battery or FAB) and the placebo component of open (black bars) and hidden (white bars) application of the local analgesic lidocaine. Note the differences between normal subjects (on the left) and Alzheimer patients (on the right). Alzheimer patients show reduced electroencephalographic connectivity, as shown by the disappearance of the orange peaks (top panel), reduced FAB scores, and reduced effects of open lidocaine. See colour plate 20. Source: From Benedetti et al. 2006 and Colloca et al. 2008 with permission from Springer, Copyright 2008.

treatments should be increased in order to compensate for the loss of these mechanisms. Second, as the prefrontal cortex can be severely affected in other neurodegenerative conditions, the neuroanatomical localization of placebo- and expectation-related mechanisms in the prefrontal areas should alert us to the potential disruption of placebo mechanisms in all those conditions whereby the prefrontal lobes are involved, for example, vascular dementia, frontotemporal dementia, or any lesion that involves the prefrontal cortex.

7.6 **If there is no prefrontal control, there is no placebo response**

7.6.1 **Blocking opioidergic transmission in the prefrontal cortex abolishes the placebo response**

As discussed in the previous section and shown in Fig 7.8, a functional disconnection of the prefrontal lobes from the rest of the brain is associated to a loss of placebo responsiveness. Interestingly, in recent years this notion has been supported by the deactivation of the prefrontal cortex in the experimental setting. On the basis of previous experiments on the blockade of placebo analgesia by the opioid antagonist naloxone (e.g. Amanzio and Benedetti 1999), Eippert et al. (2009) conducted a study to investigate where naloxone acts. By combining naloxone administration with functional magnetic resonance imaging, these authors found that naloxone reduced both behavioural and neural placebo effects as well as placebo-induced responses in pain-modulatory cortical structures, such as the dorsolateral prefrontal cortex and the rostral anterior cingulate cortex. In a brainstem-specific analysis, a similar naloxone modulation of placebo-induced responses in key structures of the descending pain control system, including the hypothalamus, the periaqueductal grey and the rostral ventromedial medulla, was found. Most importantly, naloxone abolished placebo-induced coupling between the rostral anterior cingulate cortex and the periaqueductal grey, which predicted both neural and behavioural placebo effects as well as activation of the rostral ventromedial medulla. Therefore, as occurs for prefrontal degeneration in Alzheimer's disease (Fig 7.9A and section 7.5.2), placebo analgesic responses are disrupted by the pharmacological blockade of prefrontal opioidergic functioning in the experimental setting (Fig 7.9B).

7.6.2 **Inactivating the prefrontal cortex with transcranial magnetic stimulation abolishes the placebo response**

Prefrontal degeneration in Alzheimer's disease and pharmacological blockade of prefrontal opioidergic transmission are not the only conditions whereby placebo responses are disrupted. Recently, transcranial magnetic stimulation has been used to inactivate the prefrontal cortex, particularly the dorsolateral prefrontal cortex, during a placebo analgesic response (Krummenacher et al. 2010). Repetitive transcranial magnetic stimulation is known to depress cortical excitability of the targeted cortical region, thus it represents an excellent experimental approach to investigate how loss of prefrontal control may affect complex cognitive functions, such as expectation-induced placebo responses. In a heat pain paradigm, Krummenacher et al. (2010) employed non-invasive low-frequency, repetitive transcranial magnetic stimulation to transiently disrupt the left and right dorsolateral prefrontal cortex function or used the

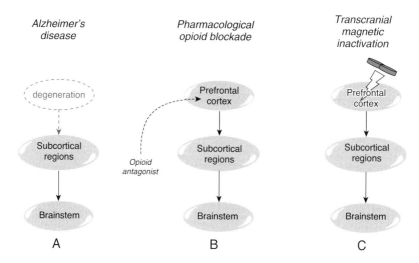

Fig 7.9 No prefrontal control, no placebo response. There are at least three conditions in which it is not possible to evoke placebo responses because of the disruption of the prefrontal cortex and the descending pain control system with which it is connected. (A) Prefrontal degeneration in Alzheimer's disease. (B) Pharmacological blockade of opioid receptors, included opioidergic transmission in the dorsolateral prefrontal cortex. (C) Inactivation of the prefrontal cortex by repetitive transcranial magnetic stimulation. Source: From Benedetti 2010 with permission from the International Association for the Study of Pain, Copyright 2010.

transcranial stimulation device itself as a placebo, before applying an expectation-induced placebo analgesia procedure. It was found that, whereas placebo significantly increased pain threshold and pain tolerance, repetitive transcranial magnetic stimulation completely blocked placebo analgesia.

Therefore, the inactivation of prefrontal regions by transcranial magnetic stimulation has the same effects as those induced by pharmacological blockade or prefrontal degeneration in Alzheimer's disease (Fig 7.9C). On the basis of all these studies, a normal functioning of prefrontal areas, as well as of the descending pain modulating network with which it is connected (Basbaum and Fields 1984), appears to be critical for placebo responsiveness. If there is a loss of prefrontal control, there also is a loss of placebo response (Benedetti 2010). This concept is summarized in Fig 7.9, where in A the disruption of placebo responses is attributable to degeneration and functional disconnection of prefrontal regions, as occurs in Alzheimer's disease, in B the loss of placebo responsiveness is induced through pharmacological opioid blockade with an opioid antagonist, and in C placebo responses are lost when the prefrontal cortex is inactivated by means of repetitive transcranial magnetic stimulation.

References

Amanzio M and Benedetti F (1999). Neuropharmacological dissection of placebo analgesia: expectation-activated opioid systems versus conditioning-activated specific subsystems. *Journal of Neuroscience,* **19**, 484–94.

Barrett RP, Feinstein C and Hole WT (1989). Effects of naloxone and naltrexone on self injury: a double-blind placebo controlled analysis. *American Journal of Mental Retardation*, **93**, 644–51.

Basbaum AI and Fields HL (1984). Endogenous pain control systems: brainstem spinal pathways and endorphin circuitry. *Annual Review of Neuroscience*, **7**, 309–38.

Bathgate D, Snowden JS, Varma A, Blackshow A and Neary (2001). Behaviour in frontotemporal dementia, Alzheimer's disease and vascular dementia. *Acta Neurologica Scandinavica*, **103**, 367–78.

Benedetti F (2010). No prefrontal control, no placebo response. *Pain*, **148**, 357–8.

Benedetti F, Vighetti S, Ricco C, Lagna E, Bergamasco B, Pinessi L et al. (1999). Pain threshold and tolerance in Alzheimer's disease. *Pain*, **80**, 377–82.

Benedetti F, Arduino C, Vighetti S, Asteggiano G, Tarenzi L and Rainero I (2004). Pain reactivity in Alzheimer patients with different degrees of cognitive impairment and brain electrical activity deterioration. *Pain*, **111**, 22–9.

Benedetti F, Arduino C, Costa S, Vighetti S, Tarenzi L, Rainero I et al. (2006). Loss of expectation-related mechanisms in Alzheimer's disease makes analgesic therapies less effective. *Pain,* **121**: 133–44.

Berman KF, Ostrem JL, Randolph C, Gold J, Goldberg TE, Coppola R et al. (1995). Physiological activation of a cortical network during performance of the Wisconsin Card Sorting Test: a positron emission tomography study. *Neuropsychologia*, **33**, 1027–46.

Brodaty H and Hadzi-Pavlovic D (1990). Psychosocial effects on carers of living with persons with dementia. *Australian and New Zealand Journal of Psychiatry*, **24**, 351–61.

Cahill S and Shapiro M (1993). I think he might have hit me once: aggression towards caregivers in dementia care. *Australian Journal of Ageing*, **12**, 10–15.

Caligiuri MP, Peavy G and Galasko DR (2001). Extrapyramidal signs and cognitive abilities in Alzheimer's disease. *International Journal of Geriatric Psychiatry,* **16**, 907–11.

Carlino E, Rainero I, Asteggiano G, Vighetti S, Cappa G, Tarenzi L et al. (2010). Pain perception and tolerance in patients with frontotemporal dementia. 13th World Congress of Pain, Montreal, Canada.

Cole LJ, Farrell MJ, Duff EP, Barber JB, Egan GF and Gibson SJ (2006). Pain sensitivity and fMRI pain-related brain activity in Alzheimer's disease. *Brain*, **129**, 2957–65.

Colloca L, Benedetti F and Porro CA (2008). Experimental designs and brain mapping approaches for studying the placebo analgesic effect. *European Journal of Applied Physiology*, **102**, 371–80.

Cornu F (1975). Perturbations de la perception de la doleur chez les dements degeneratifs. *Journal du Psychologie Normale et Pathologique*, **72**, 81–96.

Cummings JL (1993). Frontal-subcortical circuits and human behaviour. *Archives of Neurology*, **50**, 873–80.

Eippert F, Bingel U, Schoell CD et al. (2009). Activation of the opioidergic descending pain control system underlies placebo analgesia. *Neuron*, **63**, 533–43.

Farrell MJ, Katz B and Helme RD (1996). The impact of dementia on the pain experience. *Pain*, **67**, 7–15.

Herr K and Decker S (2004). Assessment of pain in older adults with severe cognitive impairment. *Annals of Long Term Care,* **12**, 46–52.

Hofman A, Rocca WA and Brayne C (1991). The prevalence of dementia in Europe: a collaborative study of 1980–1990 findings – European Prevalence Research Group. *International Journal of Epidemiology*, **20**, 736–48.

Homer A and Gilleard C (1990). Abuse of elderly people by their carers. *British Medical Journal*, **301**, 1359–62.

Horgas AL and Elliott AF (2004). Pain assessment and management in persons with dementia. *Nursing Clinic of North America*, **39**, 593–606.

Hyman BT, Van HGW, Damasio AR and Barnes CL (1984). Alzheimer's disease: cell-specific pathology isolates the hippocampal formation. *Science*, **225**, 1168–70.

Jonsson CO, Malhammar G and Waldton S (1977). Reflex elicitation thresholds in senile dementia. *Acta Psychiatrica Scandinavica*, **55**, 81–96.

Konishi S, Nakajima K, Uchida I, Kameyama M, Nakahara K, Sekihara K et al. (1998). Transient activation of inferior prefrontal cortex during cognitive set shifting. *Nature Neuroscience*, **1**, 80–4.

Konishi S, Kawazu M, Uchida I, Kikyo H, Asakura I and Miyashita Y (1999a). Contribution of working memory to transient activation in human inferior prefrontal cortex during performance of the Wisconsin Card Sorting Test. *Cerebral Cortex*, **9**, 745–53.

Konishi S, Nakajima K, Uchida I, Kikyo H, Kameyama M and Miyashita Y (1999b). Common inhibitory mechanism in human inferior prefrontal cortex revealed by event-related functional MRI. *Brain*, **122**, 981–91.

Krummenacher P, Candia V, Folkers G, Schedlowski M and Schönbächler G (2010). Prefrontal cortex modulates placebo analgesia. *Pain*, **148**, 368–74.

Lobo A, Launer LJ and Fratiglioni L (2000). Prevalence of dementia and major subtypes in Europe: a collaborative study of population-based cohorts – Neurologic Diseases in the Elderly Research Group. *Neurology*, **54** (suppl), 4–9.

McKhann G, Drachman D, Folstein M, Katzman R, Price D and Stadlan EM (1984). Clinical diagnosis of Alzheimer's disease. *Neurology*, **34**, 939–44.

Morrison RS and Siu AL (2000). A comparison of pain and its treatment in advanced dementia and cognitively intact patients with hip fracture. *Journal of Pain and Symptom Management*, **19**, 240–8.

Mountjoy CQ, Roth M, Evans NJR and Evans HM (1983). Cortical neuronal counts in normal elderly controls and demented patients. *Neurobiology of Aging*, **4**, 1–11.

Nagahama Y, Fukuyama H, Yamauchi H, Matsuzaki S, Konishi J, Shibasaki H et al. (1996). Cerebral activation during performance of a card sorting test. *Brain*, **119**, 1667–75.

Nègre-Pagès L, Regragui W, Bouhassira D, Grandjean H, Rascol O and DoPaMiP Study Group (2008). Chronic pain in Parkinson's disease: the cross-sectional French DoPaMiP survey. *Movement Disorders*, **23**, 1361–9.

O'Brien JT, Erkinjuntti T, Reisberg B, Roman G, Sawada T, Pantoni L et al. (2003). Vascular cognitive impairment. *Lancet Neurology*, **2**, 89–98.

Oosterman JM, van Harten B, Weinstein HC, Scheltens P and Scherder EJ (2006). Pain intensity and pain affect in relation to white matter changes. *Pain*, **125**, 74–81.

Petrovic P, Kalso E, Petersson KM and Ingvar M (2002). Placebo and opioid analgesia-imaging a shared neuronal network. *Science,* **295**, 1737–40.

Pillemer K and Suitor J (1992). Violence and violent feelings: what causes them among family care-givers? *Journal of Gerontology*, **47**, 165–72.

Porter FL, Malhotra KM, Wolf CM, Morris JC, Miller JP and Smith MC (1996). Dementia and response to pain in the elderly. *Pain*, **68**, 413–21.

Rainero I, Vighetti S, Bergamasco B, Pinessi L and Benedetti F (2000). Autonomic responses and pain perception in Alzheimer's disease. *European Journal of Pain*, **4**, 267–74.

Ritchie K and Lovestone S (2002). The dementias. *Lancet*, **360**, 1759–66.

Robertson D, Rockwood K and Stolee P (1989). The prevalence of cognitive impairment in an elderly Canadian population. *Acta Psychiatrica Scandinava*, **80**, 303–9.

Rocca WA, Hofman A and Brayne C (1991). Frequency and distribution of Alzheimer's disease in Europe: a collaborative study of 1980–1990 prevalence findings: the EURODEM-Prevalence Research Group. *Annals of Neurology*, **30**, 381–90.

Rolls ET, Critchley HD, Mason R and Wakeman EA (1996). Orbitofrontal cortex neurons: role in olfactory and visual association learning. *Journal of Neurophysiology*, **75**, 1970–81.

Romàn GC and Royall DR (1999). Executive control function: a rational basis for the diagnosis of vascular dementia. *Alzheimer Disease and Associated Disorders*, **13** (suppl 3), S69–80.

Romàn GC, Erkinjuntti T, Wallin A, Pantoni L and Chui HC (2002). Subcortical ischaemic vascular dementia. *Lancet Neurology*, **1**, 426–36.

Rosen HJ, Gorno-Tempini ML, Goldman WP Perry RJ, Schuff N, Weiner M, et al. (2002). Patterns of brain atrophy in frontotemporal dementia and semantic dementia. *Neurology*, **58**, 198–208.

Royall DR (2000). Executive cognitive impairment: a novel perspective on dementia. *Neuroepidemiology*, **19**, 293–9.

Rub U, Del Tredici K, Del Turco D and Braak H (2002). The intralaminar nuclei assigned to the medial pain system and other components of this system are early and progressively affected by the Alzheimer's disease-related cytoskeletal pathology. *Journal of Chemical Neuroanatomy*, **23**, 279–90.

Rudelli RD, Ambler MW and Wisniewski HM (1984). Morphology and distribution of Alzheimer neuritic (senile) and amyloid plaques in striatum and diencephalon. *Acta Neuropathologica*, **64**, 273–81.

Scheff SW and Price DA (2001). Alzheimer's disease-related synapse loss in the cingulate cortex. *Journal of Alzheimer Disease*, **3**, 495–505.

Scherder EJ and Bouma A (1997). Is decreased use of analgesics in Alzheimer disease due to a change in the affective component of pain? *Alzheimer Disease and Associated Disorders*, **11**, 171–4.

Scherder EJ, Sergeant JA and Swaab DF (2003a). Pain processing in dementia and its relation to neuropathology. *Lancet Neurology*, **2**, 677–86.

Scherder EJ, Slaets J, Deijen JB, Gorter Y, Ooms ME, Ribbe M et al. (2003b). Pain assessment in patients with possible vascular dementia. *Psychiatry*, **66**, 133–45.

Scherder E, Oosterman J, Swaab D, Herr K, Ooms M, Ribbe M et al. (2005). Recent developments in pain in dementia. *British Medical Journal*, **330**, 461–4.

Scherder E, Herr K, Pickering G, Gibson S, Benedetti F and Lautenbacher S (2009). Pain in dementia. *Pain*, **145**, 276–8.

Schultz R and Williamson G (1997). A two-year longitudinal study of depression amongst Alzheimer's care-givers. *Alzheimer Disease and Associated Disorders*, **11**, 117–24.

Snowden SJ, Bathgate D, Varma A, Blackshaw A, Gibbons ZC and Neary D (2001). Distinct behavioural profiles in frontotemporal dementia and semantic dementia. *Journal of Neurology, Neurosurgery and Psychiatry*, **70**, 323–32.

Thompson PM, Hayashi KM, de Zubicaray G, Janke AL, Rose SE, Semple J et al. (2003). Dynamics of gray matter loss in Alzheimer's disease. *Journal of Neuroscience*, **23**, 994–1005.

Wager TD, Rilling, JK, Smith EE, Sokolik A, Casey KL, Davidson RJ et al. (2004). Placebo-induced changes in fMRI in the anticipation and experience of pain. *Science,* **303**, 1162–6.

Walters AS, Barrett RP, Feinstein C, Mercurio A and Hole WT (1990). A case report of naltrexone treatment of self-injury and social withdrawal in autism. *Journal of Autism and Developmental Disorders*, **20**, 169–76.

White L, Petrovitch H and Ross GW (1996). Prevalence of dementia in older Japanese-American men in Hawaii: the Honolulu-Asia Aging study. *Journal of the American Medical Association*, **276**, 955–60.

Wolfe N, Linn R, Babikian VL, Knoefel JE and Albert ML (1990). Frontal systems impairment following multiple lacunar infarcts. *Archives of Neurology*, **47**, 129–32.

Zubieta JK, Bueller JA, Jackson LR, Scott DJ, Xu Y, Koeppe RA et al. (2005). Placebo effects mediated by endogenous opioid activity on μ-opioid receptors. *Journal of Neuroscience,* **25**, 7754–62.

Chapter 8

Defence mechanisms of the body in the course of evolution: from cellular to social responses

Summary and relevance to the clinician

1) This chapter is aimed at drawing some conclusions on the basis of all the mechanisms that have been described throughout this volume. Following the evolutionary and neuroscientific approach to the doctor–patient relationship, this special social interaction can be viewed as a defence mechanism which is capable of suppressing the patient's discomfort and influencing the course of illness.

2) The basic concept of defence mechanisms is that the body can protect itself from invaders, as the immune system does, and from damage, as the wound healing processes do. Likewise, simple reflexes, like the withdrawal reflex, or more complex behaviours, like the fight-or-flight response, are aimed at protecting the body against environmental dangers.

3) Complex cultural factors can also represent an important mechanism of defence. For example, cultural thermoregulation is a way to protect the body against extreme temperatures, which the normal thermoregulatory mechanisms are not able to tackle. With cultural thermoregulation, mankind was capable of making clothes and building heating machines to tackle extreme low temperatures.

4) Social and cultural factors are also important to promote health and well-being. Living in a social group is advantageous to health. For example, the social interaction with members of the same ethnic group may be beneficial to one's own health.

5) Within the context of body defence mechanisms and social interactions, the doctor–patient relationship represents a special case of beneficial social interaction which can be conceptualized as a true defence mechanism. This evolved to guarantee suppression of discomfort by a mere social event, that is, meeting the healer. For example, a person whose brain is capable of

shutting down pain when the presence of medical help is detected may have an advantage over someone whose brain lacks this capacity.

6) The central point is that the system 'patient–therapist' is at work regardless of whether the therapy is effective or ineffective. Even if the therapy is totally ineffective, i.e. it has no specific effects, expectation of benefit (the placebo response) may be sufficient to inhibit discomfort and eventually to influence the course of illness. Therefore, the whole system is capable of suppressing discomfort through the mere social interaction between patient and therapist.

7) Health professionals represent environmental variables that act on the patient's brain by inducing expectancies of benefit and hope. Health professionals are the crucial point in this process, for they promise good treatments and induce expectations and hope for the patient's future well-being. The patient's personal expectations play a key role here. If he wants to consult a healer, be he a shaman or a modern doctor, this is because of his personal beliefs about the healer's therapeutic capabilities. Therefore, the healer is the environmental variable that triggers those endogenous mechanisms of self-cure, e.g. the release of endogenous opioid painkillers.

8.1 A variety of defence mechanisms are present in living organisms

8.1.1 Cells respond to invaders and to damage

Different defence mechanisms are shared by different animal species, some of which are very old along the phylogenetic scale, from invertebrates to vertebrates. These mechanisms can be found at the cellular level in snails, insects, fish, reptiles, amphibians, birds, and mammals, thus they represent a very primitive set of elements with a variety of functions. Although these defence mechanisms are somehow quite different from each other, it goes without saying that the meaning is only one, that is, defence from damage, injury, external attacks, or, in a single word, survival. With some notable and sometimes obvious differences among species, the defence mechanisms are yet very similar, even between invertebrates, lower vertebrates and mammals, including human beings.

One of the classical mechanisms of defence in living organisms is represented by the immune system. The main objective of the immune system is to defend the organism from invaders, such as viruses and bacteria. The organization of this system is quite complex and there are many variations across species. For example, even simple unicellular organisms such as bacteria possess an immune system, however this is basically represented by enzyme systems that protect against viral infections. By contrast, vertebrates such as humans have a more sophisticated defence mechanism that consists of many types of proteins, cells, organs, and tissues, which interact in an elaborate and dynamic network (Fig 8.1A). As part of this more complex immune response, the human immune system adapts over time to recognize specific pathogens more efficiently. This adaptation process is referred to as adaptive immunity and creates immunological memory. Even plants possess a form of innate immunity but lack adaptive immunity (Beck and Gail 1996; Litman et al. 2005).

There is however a common conceptualization that can be applied to different organisms and different species. All living organisms have developed a highly complex cellular system that can recognize a foreigner and, accordingly, can neutralize it. In addition, once a foreigner has been identified, a mechanism of immune memory is capable of remembering which foreigner had invaded the organism in the past. This powerful memory system can induce a larger cellular reaction to the invader when the latter is identified. There is no need to go into the details of immune mechanisms for the purpose of this volume. What matters is the highly specialized character of this cellular system which warrants identification, elimination, and memory of the invader.

Other cellular systems respond to injury and damage rather than to external invaders. For example, the mechanical damage to a tissue is followed by an intricate cascade of biochemical and cellular events that guarantee wound recovery and healing. In this case also, these mechanisms are present in different species. In mammals as well as in other vertebrates, wound healing derives from a cascade of biochemical and mechanical events (Fig 8.1B). After an early inflammatory phase, a proliferative phase takes place, whereby angiogenesis, collagen deposition, and epithelialization represent the main events aimed at restoring the anatomy and physiology of the damaged tissue (Stadelmann et al. 1998; Midwood et al. 2004). A variety of growth factors take part in this process, like the epidermal growth factor, the vascular endothelial growth factor, the platelet-derived growth factor, and the fibroblast growth factors (Mitchell et al. 2007). Even more dramatic changes can be found in simple animals, such as regeneration. An organism is said to regenerate a lost or damaged part if the part re-grows so that the original function is restored. Regenerative capacity is inversely related to complexity: the more complex an animal is the less regeneration it is capable of (Bryant et al. 2002; Odelberg 2004).

Another mechanism of defence, which probably is also less understood, is neuronal regeneration. Axons and dendrites that are damaged can regenerate and sprout in order to re-occupy the synapses that have been left empty. In this case also, there are many variations across species (Kandel et al. 2000). For example, axons in the invertebrate central nervous system grow better after

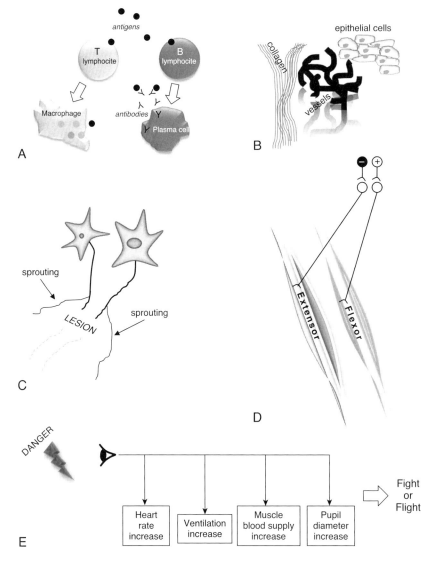

Fig 8.1 Examples of endogenous defence systems. (A) Some immune responses are mediated by T lymphocytes, which turn into macrophages, and B lymphocytes, which turn into plasma cells. Whereas macrophages destroy antigens through phagocytosis, plasma cells produce antibodies which bind to antigens and destroy them. (B) Three main events occurring during the proliferative phase of wound healing: collagen deposition, formation of new blood vessels (angiogenesis), and of new epithelial cells (epithelialization). (C) A lesion to axons or dendrites induces a sprouting of new terminals from the axonal or dendritic stumps. (D) The synaptic organization underlying the withdrawal reflex allows the contraction of flexor muscles while inhibiting extensor muscles (see also section 1.1.2 and fig. 1.2). (E) In the fight-or-flight response, the sight of a danger triggers a cascade of physiological events, like the increase of heart activity, respiration, and muscle blood supply, which aim to better fight or escape from the danger.

damage compared to those in vertebrates. In the latter, particularly in mammals, a real and efficacious axonal regeneration does not occur in the central nervous system and re-growing axons are often halted by the scar. What seems to be more important in mammals is not so much a real axonal regeneration but rather what is called sprouting, whereby small terminal fibres sprout for very short distances within the brain (Fig 8.1C). However, in this case also, a common conceptualization is present across different species, i.e. nervous fibres of living organisms have the potentiality of regenerating, albeit with different modalities, in order to restore the lost functions.

8.1.2 Living organisms protect themselves from a variety of dangers

Living organisms are also endowed with complex neuronal circuits responding to foreign attacks that are somehow different from viruses, bacteria, or mechanical damage. For example, the withdrawal reflex (see also section 1.1.2) is activated when a potential damage is present on the cutaneous surface, such as a painful stimulus. Of course, the purpose of such a reflex response is the very same as that of the immune response to viruses, i.e. the defence of the organism from a danger. The synaptic organization of the neurons subserving the withdrawal reflex allows an optimal response, with the contraction of the flexor muscles and the inhibition of the extensor muscles (Fig 8.1D). In this way, the limb can be withdrawn from the noxious stimulus.

A more complex and highly organized response to environmental dangers is represented by the fight-or-flight response, also known as stress response (Cannon 1929). In this case, when the organism faces a danger, for instance a prey facing a predator, it activates a series of behavioural and autonomic responses that are aimed at better surviving the dangerous situation. Regardless of whether the prey starts fighting with or escaping from the predator, its physiological functions tackle the new situation by increasing the physical performance for a better fight or flight. For example, in order to increase the efficiency of the muscles during the intense muscular effort for surviving, the heart increases its activity to provide more blood to the muscles, and ventilation increases to supply more oxygen to the muscles. At the same time, a vasodilation occurs in muscle vessels in order to favour a better supply of blood and oxygen (Fig 8.1E). In other words, the fight-or-flight response is a set of sympathetic-mediated physiological changes that prepare the organism to a better physical performance, thus increasing the probability of survival (Gleitman et al. 2004).

It is quite interesting to note that the fight-or-flight response can go in the opposite direction as well. Many animals freeze or play dead when in front of a predator in the hope that it will lose interest. Others have more exotic self-protection methods, for example some species of fish change colour swiftly in order to camouflage themselves. Therefore, it is important to realize that the conceptualization of the fight-or-flight response is broad and applies to many situations and behavioural repertoires. For example, somehow differently from prehistoric times, when the fight-or-flight responses emerged and evolved, in current times the fight response may be manifested in angry, argumentative behaviour, and the flight response may be manifested through social withdrawal and substance abuse (Friedman and Silver 2007).

8.2 Defence mechanisms can also involve cultural and social aspects

8.2.1 Thermoregulation as an example of physiological and cultural mechanism

In order to protect themselves against hypothermia and hyperthermia, living organisms have developed a set of adaptive mechanisms to both low and high temperatures. There are a number of ways by which organisms regulate their body temperature, from the lack of a real thermoregulatory centre in reptiles, which need to expose themselves to the sun in order to warm up, to dogs which pant to decrease body temperature. Thus thermoregulation is a powerful defence mechanism against dangerous variations in temperature.

For the sake of this volume, it is not necessary to go into the details of the physiology of thermoregulation. Instead, what is interesting is that humans may adopt several regulatory mechanisms, from unconscious physiological changes to conscious behavioural repertoires (Fig 8.2). Typically, human thermoregulation is accomplished through a set of physiological adjustments (Guyton and Hall 2006). For example, in order to adapt to cold environments, constriction of arterioles allows to avoid excessive heat loss, and repetitive muscle contractions and decontractions, i.e. shivering, allow heat production. Likewise, increased metabolic activity is warranted by increased activity of adrenal and thyroid glands. By contrast, adaptation to hot environments involves vasodilation of arterioles, sweating and reduced activity of adrenal and thyroid glands (Fig 8.2). Needless to say, all these physiological adjustments occur without any conscious activity. They are completely unconscious and are mediated by the hypothalamus.

However, sometimes physiological thermoregulation alone is not sufficient during exposition to excessively cold or hot environments. During evolution, mankind developed a sort of cultural thermoregulation, a powerful adaptive behaviour which typically involves the neocortex and a complex conscious

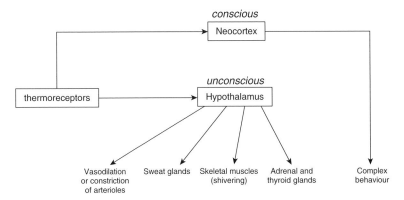

Fig 8.2 A simplified schema of thermoregulatory mechanisms in humans. Unconscious mechanisms in cold environments, such as arterioles vasoconstriction, no sweating, shivering, increased metabolism, and in hot environments, like arterioles vasodilation, sweating, no shivering, decreased metabolism, are mediated by the hypothalamus. However, conscious mechanisms may produce, via the neocortex, complex behavioural repertoires, such as wearing warm clothes or the construction of heating machines, also known as cultural thermoregulation.

behavioural repertoire (Fig 8.2). For example, human beings can produce and wear clothes when the temperature decreases. Likewise, the construction of heating systems and machines allows big environments to be heated even in extreme cold conditions. Similar systems and machines have been produced to adapt to hot temperatures as well (e.g. air conditioning).

Cultural thermoregulation is a good example of how human beings are capable of protecting themselves from extreme temperatures by adopting complex behaviours. Consequently, in our society, particularly in western society, low and high temperatures no longer represent a critical factor for survival.

8.2.2 Social groups can be advantageous to health in a number of ways

As described in sections 1.3 and 1.4, social cooperation is advantageous to the members of the social group. The advantages range from grooming and being groomed in nonhuman primates to the various forms of altruistic behaviour in humans (see section 1.3). In particular, social cooperation is advantageous to health and survival. For example, the daily provision of food in order to survive in harsh conditions was not guaranteed in early hominids, because of the high variability of hunting success. The first altruistic exchanges of food were likely to occur among relatives, but in the course of evolution further food exchanges occurred with non-kin that were less lucky on that particular hunting day. These non-kin recipients eventually returned this favour (see section 1.4.1). In a social group it is very important to help and support the weak, the sick, and the elderly. Individuals who cannot hunt and feed themselves are not abandoned, but rather they are looked after and fed. In section 1.4.1, we have seen some of the earliest examples of altruistic behaviour and social cooperation, for instance in the hominids found in the site of Dmanisi in the Eurasian Republic of Georgia, or in the Neanderthal's individuals at La Chapelle-aux-Saints and Shanidar caves.

The reasons why social cooperation and, in general, the social environment affects the health status of the single individual are many. First, according to Cassel (1976), the social environment alters host susceptibility by affecting neuroendocrine function, and the most feasible and promising interventions to reduce disease are to improve and strengthen the social supports rather than reduce the exposure to stressors. Second, political and economic processes in different societies are also involved in the health status of the population, and this may lead to social inequalities in health (Krieger 2001). Third, the so-called 'neighbourhood effect' has emerged as a potentially relevant group or context effect, whereby neighbourhoods possess both physical and social attributes which could plausibly affect the health of individuals (Diez-Roux 2007). For example, studies examining the effects of neighbourhood characteristics have reported what has been called a 'group density' effect on health, such that members of low status minority communities living in an area with a higher proportion of their own racial or ethnic group tend to have better health than those who live in areas with a lower proportion. In addition, members of ethnic minorities who live in areas where there are few like themselves are likely to be materially better off than those who live in areas with a higher concentration. However, they may be made more aware of belonging to a low status minority group by the majority community, and the psychosocial effects of stigma may offset any advantage. Therefore, the psychological effects of stigma are sometimes powerful enough to override material advantage (Pickett and Wilkinson 2008).

Neighbourhood effects are good examples of how the social group may affect the health of the individual who belongs to the group. These effects, of course, are not always positive and many factors may lead to a negative impact on health. Neighbourhood effects are also good examples of how living in an area with a higher proportion of the same ethnic group may represent a social defence mechanism which prevents, at least in part, the occurrence of illness. Whereas these effects are mediated by the social interactions with all the members of a group, in the next section the social interaction occurs with a single 'specialized' member of the group: the doctor or, more in general, the healer.

8.3 The doctor–patient interaction is a social mechanism of defence

8.3.1 The system works regardless of effective therapies

In this section, a summary of what has been described throughout the volume is presented, whereby the system 'patient+therapist' is considered as a whole, and some conclusions are drawn. Indeed, the social interaction between the patient and the therapist can be considered as a powerful mechanism of defence which is aimed at suppressing discomfort and at influencing the course of illness merely by means of this social encounter. We have seen in section 1.4.1 that shamanism is likely to have evolved from the cooperation among the members of a social group. Whereas at the very beginning all the members of the group were likely to take care of the weak, the sick, and the elderly, at a given point in the course of evolution a single member of the group, the shaman, acquired the power, and indeed the prestige, of taking care of sick individuals. Trusting the shaman and believing in his magic powers was likely to strengthen the effects of social interaction on health. In other words, taking care of the sick (i.e. 'medical care' in modern words) evolved from mere social cooperation to a special attribute that belonged to a single endowed individual, thus boosting trust, beliefs, hope.

The system 'patient+therapist' is depicted in Fig 8.3. The only difference between shamans and modern doctors is likely to be the effectiveness of therapies. Whereas shamanic procedures are likely to lack specific effects completely, at least in most circumstances, modern doctors rely on effective procedures and medications with specific mechanisms of action. The system of Fig 8.3 is at work regardless of the availability and use of effective treatments, thus it works with both shamanic and mainstream medicine procedures. The patient's feeling of sickness triggers a motivated behaviour which is aimed at seeking relief and suppressing discomfort. Here motivation and reward mechanisms aim to find a means to reach this goal, that is, to meet a therapist. The complex interaction between the patient and therapist, which is based on trust and hope on the one hand and empathy and compassion on the other, leads to expect therapeutic benefit and clinical improvement. At this point, when the therapy is administered, all the key elements of this complex social encounter are activated in the patient's brain, thus he is now ready to activate expectation and placebo mechanisms. The central point here is that this system is at work regardless of whether the therapy is effective or ineffective. Even if the therapy is totally ineffective, i.e. it has no specific effects, expectation of benefit (the placebo response) may be enough to inhibit discomfort, thus suppressing the feeling of sickness.

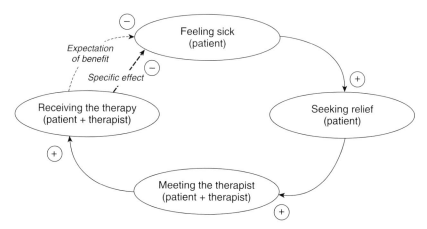

Fig 8.3 This figure summarizes what has been described throughout the volume and shows how the system 'patient+therapist' works. The feeling of sickness triggers (+ sign) a motivated behaviour (seeking relief) which is aimed at suppressing discomfort. This leads to meet a therapist who, in turn, is the means to suppress discomfort (− sign) through the administration of a therapy. The central point is that this system works regardless of whether the therapy is effective or ineffective. Even if the therapy is totally ineffective, i.e. it has no specific effects, expectation of benefit (the placebo response) may be sufficient to inhibit discomfort, thus suppressing the feeling of sickness. Therefore, the whole system represents a powerful defence mechanism which is capable of suppressing discomfort through the mere social interaction between patient and therapist.

Therefore, the whole system represents a powerful defence mechanism which is capable of suppressing discomfort through the mere social interaction between patient and therapist. Reasoning in this way, the only difference between shamans and doctors is represented by the fact that the latter were capable of developing effective procedures and treatments that have specific effects for the condition to be treated (see section 2.1). In this sense, the system 'patient+therapist' of Fig 8.3 can be compared to the thermoregulatory system of Fig 8.2. In the same way as there is a natural physiological thermoregulation, which is regulated by the hypothalamus, and a cultural thermoregulation, which involves the neocortex and a complex behavioural repertoire (e.g. building heating machines), so there is both a natural and a cultural component in the doctor–patient relationship. The first is represented by the mechanisms that have been described throughout this book and that are depicted in Fig 8.3. The second cultural component is represented by the development of medications and procedures that have specific effects for the disease to be treated.

The analogy between the 'doctor–patient interaction' system and other regulatory systems, such as thermoregulation, is even more evident by considering extreme conditions. In some extreme circumstances, these natural regulatory systems are not sufficient to guarantee the appropriate outcomes. For example, in extreme cold conditions the hypothalamus cannot regulate adequately all the physiological responses that are needed to maintain the body temperature constant, and the construction and use of heating machines is the only means to survive (cultural thermoregulation). Likewise, in severe medical conditions such as tissue damage or severely altered physiological parameters, the mere social encounter with a therapist and subsequent activation of expectation mechanisms cannot be sufficient to restore the lost function or suppress the discomfort. The only means to recovery from illness is the development and use of medications and procedures with specific effects (modern cultural medicine).

The emergence of complex motivated behaviours during evolution, like cultural thermoregulation and modern cultural medicine, is therefore a powerful means to compensate for those natural mechanisms that, otherwise, would not be sufficient for survival. Therefore, the system 'patient+therapist' depicted in Fig 8.3 can be considered a social mechanism of defence in all respects. It is at work in any medical encounter, but it is not always sufficient to warrant the appropriate therapeutic outcomes. In this latter case, modern cultural medicine either complements or replaces the natural systems of expectations and beliefs.

8.3.2 Why does the system work this way?

The doctor–patient relationship can be considered as a social mechanism with beneficial effects on the patient's health. An important issue is to understand why this social interaction is necessary in order to activate the endogenous mechanisms that are responsible for expectation and placebo effects. The reason why a social mechanism of this kind emerged in the course of evolution seems to be quite obvious. There are many advantages in altruism, social cooperation, and shamanic beliefs (see sections 1.3 and 1.4). Suppression of physical and psychological discomfort by general social interactions (with the members of the group) and by specific interactions (with a single 'specialized' member, the shaman) warrants a powerful means to recover, at least in part, from illness. From a natural selection perspective, only those social groups in which shamans were present and trust/hope were the key elements of the members, warranted well-being and longer survival.

Following evolutionary theory, the system can be even more complex and can acquire the characteristics of a true endogenous healthcare system. According to Humphrey (2002), the capacity to activate expectation and placebo mechanisms following the doctor–patient encounter is an emergent property of a specially designed procedure for 'economic resource management', that is, one of the key features of the 'natural healthcare service' which has evolved in animals, included humans, to help us deal with repeated bouts of sickness, injury, and other threats to our well-being. Humphrey (2002) argues that people's bodies and minds have a considerable capacity for curing themselves, but that sometimes this capacity for self-cure is not expressed spontaneously, but can be triggered by the influence of a third party, i.e. the doctor. Therefore, the central point is to understand why the patient–doctor encounter is needed in order to activate the self-cure mechanisms. On the basis of an 'economic resource management' and related costs/benefits conceptualization, the questions posed by Humphrey (2002) are the following: 'Is it indeed sometimes the case that there are benefits to remaining sick and, correspondingly, costs to premature cure? Is it, as we might guess, more usually the case that there are benefits to getting better and, correspondingly, costs to delayed cure? In either case, are there really costs associated with the process of cure as such?'.

Following Humphrey's thoughts, indeed it is sometimes more useful to maintain illness and to consider its cure as premature. For example, one of the main functions of pain is to avoid further injury and to remind us that the painful part of our body should be put at rest. Likewise, fever is a way of fighting off the invading bacteria or viruses and phobias serve to limit exposure to potential dangers. In these and other conditions there are benefits to delay the cure. If it is true there are sometimes benefits to remain sick, there are costs as well. Pain, for example, causes physical/psychological stress and hopelessness, fever may have side effects such as convulsions, and phobias may inhibit normal social interactions. Similarly, there are costs of the process of cure itself. For example, mounting an immune response is energy-consuming.

An endogenous healthcare system, with its 'economic resource management', must take all these costs and benefits into consideration in order to produce the optimal responses. This is well evident in different situations, such as stress-induced analgesia. To use the same example mentioned by Humphrey (2002), if a sprained ankle does not allow running, is it better to reduce the pain or not? In other words, will the pain actually do more harm than good? The answer is not simple. It very much depends on the situation and on the correct appraisal of the costs and benefits. If one is chasing a gazelle and the pain has made him stop, then it is going to save the ankle (benefit) even if it means losing the gazelle (cost). But if one is being chased by a lion, then if he stops it will likely be the end of him (only cost, no benefit). Indeed, in stress-induced analgesia (i.e. being chased by a lion), the endogenous opioid systems are activated and pain is inhibited, so as to allow running and escaping from the lion (see section 3.2.4 for the top-down modulation of pain).

The conceptualization of an endogenous healthcare system by Humphrey (2002) is very useful to understand why the doctor–patient encounter is necessary in order to trigger expectation and placebo mechanisms in the patient's brain. Shamans, healers, doctors and, in general, health professionals, represent environmental variables that act on the patient's brain by inducing expectancies of benefit and hope. Health professionals are the crucial point in this process, for they promise good treatments and induce expectations and hope for the patient's future well-being. The patient's personal expectations play a key role here. If he wants to consult a healer, be he a shaman or a modern doctor, this is because of his personal beliefs about the healer's therapeutic capabilities. Therefore, the healer is the environmental variable that triggers those endogenous mechanisms of self-cure, e.g. the release of endogenous opioid painkillers. It is like in the above example of stress-induced analgesia: being chased by a lion is the environmental variable that triggers the endogenous painkilling systems. Within the context of Humphrey's conceptualization of costs and benefits (Humphrey 2002), there are thus benefits in the doctor–patient encounter, for it triggers plenty of beneficial mechanisms, such as positive expectancies, hope, and related neurochemical systems. In other words, these endogenous mechanisms of healing are based on, and actually triggered by the figure of the doctor.

8.3.3 The doctor himself belongs to the system

From both an evolutionary and neuroscientific perspective, it is clear that in the scheme depicted in Fig 8.3 the therapist belongs to the system and has a central role in triggering all those mechanisms that take place in the patient's brain, from seeking and hopeful behaviour to expectation and placebo responses. The figure of the shaman, the healer, the doctor represents a product of evolution which evolved in any prehistoric social group and in any modern society. Many cultural differences do exist across different societies (see sections 2.2.2, 3.2.3, and 4.2.2), yet all societies rely on the central figure of somebody whom the sick needs to trust and from whom the sick expects empathic and compassionate behaviour.

As discussed in Chapter 1, health management may have evolved in a social context among different groups of hominids. The act of caring and curing must have become a powerful social stimulus that induced beliefs, trust, hope, and expectations of recovery. If a member of the social group trusts even only a single member of the group, he can improve his quality of life and maybe can survive longer. Therefore, individuals who trust a member of a social group, be he a shaman or a doctor, are better placed than those who do not. To be activated, these expectation and placebo mechanisms need the social contact with the person one trusts (Benedetti 2008). Wall (1999) claimed that pain is a need state, thus it can be terminated by specific consummatory acts, like hunger and thirst. According to Wall (1999), the consummatory acts that terminate pain can be either withdrawing one's hand from a noxious stimulus or care and attention from others. It is this purely social event that represents the evolutionary novelty in mankind (Evans 2002). For example, a person whose brain is capable of shutting down pain when the presence of medical help is detected may have an advantage over someone whose brain lacks this capacity (Evans 2003).

This evolutionary and neuroscientific approach to the doctor–patient relationship will hopefully make health professionals better understand their central role, as persons, in the healing process. A better understanding of the physiological, biochemical, and cellular mechanisms of this intriguing social interaction represents a challenge for cognitive and social neuroscience, with subsequent implications for routine medical practice as well as for insights into human biology. Hopefully, this new biological knowledge will boost not only health professionals' technical skills, but their empathic, compassionate, and humane behaviour as well.

References

Beck G and Gail SH (1996). Immunity and the invertebrates. *Scientific American*, **11**, 60–6.

Benedetti F (2008). *Placebo effects: understanding the mechanisms in health and disease.* Oxford University Press, Oxford.

Bryant SV, Endo T and Gardiner DM (2002). Vertebrate limb regeneration and the origin of limb stem cells. *International Journal of Developmental Biology*, **46**, 887–96.

Cannon W (1929). *Bodily changes in pain, hunger, fear, and rage.* Appleton, New York, NY.

Cassel J (1976). The contribution of the social environment to host resistance. *American Journal of Epidemiology*, **104**, 107–23.

Diez-Roux AV (2007). Neighborhoods and health: where are we and where do we go from here? *Revue d'Epidemiologie et de Sante Publique*, **55**, 13–21.

Evans D (2002). Pain, evolution, and the placebo response. *Behavioral and Brain Sciences*, **25**, 459–60.

—— (2003). *Placebo: the belief effect.* Harper Collins, London.

Friedman HS and Silver RC, eds. (2007). *Foundations of health psychology.* Oxford University Press, New York, NY.

Gleitman H, Fridlund AJ and Reisberg D (2004). *Psychology.* 6 edition. Norton, New York, NY.

Guyton AC and Hall JE (2006). *Textbook of medical physiology.* 11th edition. Saunders, Philadelphia, PA.

Humphrey N (2002). *The mind made flesh.* Oxford University Press, Oxford.

Kandel ER, Schwartz JH and Jessell TM (2000). *Principles of neural science.* 4th edition. McGraw-Hill, New York, NY.

Krieger N (2001). Theories for social epidemiology in the 21st century: an ecosocial perspective. *International Journal of Epidemiology*, **30**, 668–77.

Litman G, Cannon J and Dishaw L (2005). Reconstructing immune phylogeny: new perspectives. *Nature Reviews Immunology*, **5**, 866–79.

Midwood KS, Williams LV and Schwarzbauer JE (2004). Tissue repair and the dynamics of extracellular matrix. *International Journal of Biochemistry and Cell Biology*, **36**, 1031–7.

Mitchell RS, Kumar V, Abbas AK and Fausto N (2007). *Robbins basic pathology*. 8th edition. Saunders, Philadelphia, PA.

Odelberg SJ (2004). Unraveling the molecular basis for regenerative cellular plasticity. *PloS Biology*, **8**, E232.

Pickett KE and Wilkinson RG (2008). People like us: ethnic group density effects on health. *Ethnicity & Health*, **13**, 321–34.

Stadelmann WK, Digenis AG and Tobin GR (1998). Physiology and healing dynamics of chronic cutaneous wounds. *American Journal of Surgery*, **176**, 26S–38S.

Wall PD (1999). *Pain: the science of suffering*. Weidenfeld & Nicholson, London.

Index

Note: page numbers in *italics* refer to Figures.